AF682303

THE SQUIBB INSTITUTE FOR MEDICAL RESEARCH
LIBRARY
APR 11 1980
PRINCETON, N. J.

INDUCED DISEASE
DRUG, IRRADIATION, OCCUPATION

Edited by

Leslie Preger, M.B., Ch. B., D.R.C.O.G., F.R.C.R., F.F.R. (R.C.S.I.), F.A.C.R.

Clinical Professor of Radiology
University of California School of Medicine
San Francisco, California

Associate Clinical Professor of Radiology
University of California
Davis, California

Director, Department of Radiology
French Hospital
San Francisco, California

Foreword by

R.E. Steiner, M.D., F.R.C.P., F.A.C.R. (Hon), F.R.A.C.R. (Hon), F.R.C.R., F.F.R. (R.C.S.I.) (Hon)

President of the Royal College of Radiologists
Director and Professor, Department of Radiodiagnosis
Royal Postgraduate Medical School
London, England

Grune & Stratton

A Subsidiary of Harcourt Brace Jovanovich, Publishers
New York London Toronto Sydney San Francisco

Library of Congress Cataloging in Publication Data
Main entry under title:

Induced disease, drug, irradiation, occupation.

Includes bibliographical references and index.
1. Occupational diseases. 2. Drugs—Side effects.
3. Radiation—Toxicology. I. Preger, Leslie.
RC 964. 153 616.9′8 79-23147
ISBN 0-8089-1225-9

©1980 by Grune & Stratton, Inc.
All rights reserved. No part of this publication may be reproduced or transmitted in any form or by any means, electronic or mechanical, including photocopy, recording, or any information storage and retrieval system, without permission in writing from the publisher.

Grune & Stratton, Inc.
111 Fifth Avenue
New York, New York 10003

Distributed in the United Kingdom by
Academic Press Inc. (London) Ltd.
24/28 Oval Road, London NW 1

Library of Congress Catalog Number 79-23147
International Standard Book Number 0-8089-1225-9

Printed in the United States of America

Contents

PART 2. IRRADIATION-INDUCED DISEASE 121

PART 3. OCCUPATIONALLY INDUCED DISEASE 189

Acknowledgments

The French Hospital Medical Research Foundation has provided some of the funds necessary for the preparation of this volume. Mrs. Sunne Thomas has been very effectively responsible in her secretarial duties.

Foreword

Over the years modern civilization has progressively produced a considerable number of health hazards, to which medicine has made its own contribution. These hazards are multiplying at an alarming rate, and their effects are often appreciated and understood only after significant and irreparable damage has been done. The complexities and effects of damage on the various organ systems produced by chemicals and irradiation are such that today's student of medicine must find understanding and evaluation difficult, particularly when one considers the enormous amount of new information there is to absorb in the formative years in medical school. The same can be said about the postgraduate physician; here too it may be difficult to keep abreast of the new developments in the field of specialization.

It is therefore not only timely but helpful to all of us that the editor of this book, Leslie Preger, has brought together a number of experts to write short essays about chemical- or drug-induced disorders which are of importance to the practicing physician. The scope of this volume is very wide ranging; it covers most of the drug- and chemical-induced disease affecting the alimentary, respiratory, and other organ systems; it deals extensively with injuries to the respiratory system produced by inhalation; and it also analyzes the important aspects of radiation hazards, particularly to the fetus and the pregnant mother.

The reader of this volume will be confronted with the stark reality of ever-increasing hazards to our health, and will be made aware of the need to be much more alert to the possible effects, dangers, and risks of the explosively expanding use of new pharmaceuticals and chemicals.

The question may well have to be asked, "Can these man-made hazards be avoided?" Certainly, the relationship of the benefits of modern technology to the risks entailed in its use are not easily interpreted. Should we fail to do so correctly, however, man-made diseases will become more important and frequent than those that we are familiar with and that we have learned to treat in the past. If this is to be one of the medical advances of our time, the past centuries with their plagues may well be looked upon by future generations as periods of relative health.

R. E. Steiner
London, 1979

Preface

This book is intended for practicing clinicians and radiologists. The contributors reflect a wide range of specialties and include internists, surgeons, radiotherapists, radiodiagnosticians, biochemists, and a veterinarian. It is hoped that this balanced team will provide a broadbased account of induced disease suitable to the needs of the general medical community, but with special reference to the use of imaging procedures in the diagnosis and management of some of the problems presented by the various forms of induced disease.

The choice of subjects is somewhat arbitrary. Many of the topics have been included to reflect a wide general interest; for example, a balanced account of the risk–benefit ratios of the irradiation of women of child-bearing age, those who are pregnant, and the neonate. Other topics reflect a more narrow concern; they may elucidate the steps by which a hazard has been identified and show how future risks may be minimized. The clinical presentation of vinyl chloride is one such topic.

The use of experimental models to elucidate drug and industrial hazards is a timely subject. Polybrominated bipheyl is a synthetic chemical fire retardant used in the manufacture of plastics. PBB was first introduced in 1971; in 1973 thousands of pounds of PBB was inadvertently mixed with livestock feed in Michigan, causing not only much death and disease in farm animals and wildlife but much ill health in those eating meat from animals who had ingested PBB.

Many drugs have undesirable side effects. Some of these are described in depth, with special attention to radiologic findings.

Newer methods of imaging or modifications of older methods have a place in the diagnosis and management of the rapidly increasing numbers of industrial back injuries and those affected by asbestos inhalation. The current increase in coal mining merits a concise description of coal workers' pneumoconiosis and silicosis. Occupational medicine is no longer an esoteric matter to be ignored by the general medical community. Most physicians need be aware of the hazards which may affect not only those directly or occupationally involved, but those indirectly exposed, such as the household contacts of asbestos workers.

The harmful effects of the theraputic irradiation of certain organs is described, with suggestions on diagnosis and management.

Cost constraints have precluded the inclusion of some of the aspects of induced disease that one might like to include. The final choice has, of course, been a personal one. My sincerest thanks go to the contributors to this work, who have had to put aside so many demands upon their time in order to produce the scholarly contributions that they have.

Leslie Preger
San Francisco, 1979

Contributors

Henry A. Anderson, M.D.
Assistant Professor of Medicine
Environmental Sciences Laboratory
Department of Community Medicine
Mount Sinai School of Medicine of the
City University of New York
New York, New York

Brian T. Butcher, Ph.D
Assistant Professor of Medicine
Tulane University Medical Center
New Orleans, Louisiana

J. H. E. Carmichael, M.D., F.R.C.R., D.M.R.D., D.R.
Consultant Radiologist
Broadgreen Hospital
Lecturer in Radiodiagnosis
University of Liverpool
Liverpool, England

John K. Davidson, M.D., F.R.C.P. (Edin. and Glasg.), F.R.C.R.
Consultant Radiologist in Administrative Charge
Western Infirmary and Gartnavel General Hospital
Glasgow, Scotland

Michael Davis, M.D.
The Liver Unit
King's College Hospital and Medical School
London, England

Gordon M. Gamsu, M.D.
Associate Professor of Radiology
University of California
San Francisco, California

Jeffrey A. Golden, M.D.
Assistant Clinical Professor of Medicine
University of California
San Francisco, California

Ronald G. Grainger, M.D., F.R.C.P., F.R.C.R., F.A.C.R. (Hon), F.R.A.C.R. (Hon)
Consultant Radiologist
Hallamshire Hospital
Honorary Clinical Lecturer
University of Sheffield
Sheffield, England

Charles B. Higgins, M.D.
Professor of Radiology and Chief of Cardiac Radiology
San Diego Veteran's Administration Hospital
University of California, San Diego
Consultant Radiologist
Cardiology Service
Naval Regional Medical Center
San Diego, California

Reynold M. Karr, M.D.
Assistant Professor of Medicine
Tulane University Medical Center
New Orleans, Louisiana

Louis Kreel, M.D., F.R.C.P., F.R.C.R.
Consultant Radiologist
Northwick Park Hospital and Clinical Research Center
Harrow, England

John W. Laws, M.D., F.R.C.P., F.F.R., R.C.S.I. (Hon), F.A.C.R. (Hon), F.R.C.R.
Director, Department of Radiology
King's College Hospital and Medical School
London, England

Anthony Leyshon, M.D., F.R.C.S.
Senior Orthopaedic Registrar
Royal National Orthopaedic Hospital
London, England

Martin J. Lipton, M.B., Ch.B., M.R.C.P., F.R.C.P. (C)
Associate Professor of Radiology
University of California and Cardiovascular
Research Institute
San Francisco, California
Clinical Associate Professor of Radiology
Stanford University
Stanford, California

W.K.C. Morgan, M.D., F.R.C.P. (Ed), F.R.C.P. (C), F.A.C.P.
Director, Chest Diseases Unit
University Hospital
Professor of Medicine
University of Western Ontario
London, Ontario

Albert A. Moss, M.D.
Associate Professor of Radiology
University of California
San Francisco, California

Jack D. Noyes, M.D.
Clinical Instructor in Radiology
University of California, San Francisco
Radiologist
French Hospital and Shriner's Hospital
San Francisco, California

Heather B. Nunnerley, M.B., Ch.B., D.C.H., D.R.C.O.G., D.M.R.D., F.R.C.R.
Consultant Radiologist
King's College Hospital and Medical School
London, England

Stephen C. Pardys, M.D.
Division of Gastroenterology
Presbyterian Hospital, Pacific Medical Center
French Hospital
San Francisco, California

Landrus Pfeffinger, M.D.
Resident in Orthopedic Surgery
University of California and French Hospital
San Francisco, California

Leslie Preger, M.B., Ch.B., D.R.C.O.G., F.R.C.R., F.F.R. (R.C.S.I.), F.A.C.R.
Director, Department of Radiology
French Hospital
San Francisco, California
Clinical Professor of Radiology
University of California
San Francisco, California
Associate Clinical Professor of Radiology
University of California
Davis, California

Barbara M. Rohlfing, M.D.
Department of Radiology
St. Mary's Hospital and Medical Center
San Francisco, California
Assistant Clinical Professor of Radiology
University of California
San Francisco, California

C. John Rosenquist, M.D.
Associate Professor of Radiology
University of California
Davis, California

E. Nicholas Sargent, M.D.
Professor of Radiology
Los Angeles County/University of Southern California
Medical Center
Los Angeles, California

Irving J. Selikoff, M.D.
Professor of Medicine
Environmental Sciences Laboratory
Department of Community Medicine
Mount Sinai School of Medicine
City University of New York
New York, New York

Sam Silverman, D.V.M.
Associate Clinical Professor
Department of Radiological Sciences
University of California, Davis
Davis, California

T. C. B. Stamp, M.D., F.R.C.P.
Consultant Physician
Institute of Orthopaedics
Royal National Orthopaedic Hospital
London, England

John L. Stauffer, M.D.
Head of Pulmonary Disease Section
Department of Medicine
Veteran's Administration Medical Center
Fresno, California
Assistant Clinical Professor of Medicine
University of California Medical Center
San Francisco, California

Dennis J. Stoker, F.R.C.P., F.R.C.R.
Consultant Radiologist
Royal National Orthopaedic Hospital
London, England
Director of Radiological Studies
Institute of Orthopaedics
London, England

Anne E. Walker, M.D., F.R.C.P.
Consultant Dermatologist
The Royal Hospital Chesterfield
Derbyshire, England

William W. Wara, M.D.
Associate Professor of Radiation Oncology
University of California
San Francisco, California

J. A. Milford Ward, M.A., M.B., M.R.C. Path.
Director, Protein Reference Unit
Hallamshire Hospital Medical School
Sheffield, England

C. K. Warrick, C.B.E., F.R.C.P., F.R.C.S. (E), F.R.C.R.
Head, Academic Department of Radiology
University of Newcastle upon Tyne
Consultant Radiologist
Newcastle upon Tyne Area Health Authority
(Teaching)
Newcastle upon Tyne, England

Roger Williams, M.D.
The Liver Unit
King's College Hospital and Medical School
London, England

Roger Winkle, M.D.
Assistant Professor of Cardiology
Stanford University
Stanford, California

PART I

Drug-Induced Disease

Heather Nunnerley, John W. Laws
Michael Davis, Roger Williams

1

Chemical- and Drug-Induced Liver Tumors

While hepatic neoplasms can be induced in experimental animals by a variety of compounds, the relevance of many of these to the human situation remains to be established. In certain instances, however, strong associations have been documented in man between exposure to specific drugs and chemicals and the development of liver tumors; these associations, which have provided persuasive, if not absolute, evidence of a cause and effect relationship (Table 1-1), will be the subject of this review.

AFLATOXINS AND HEPATOCELLULAR CARCINOMA

Primary hepatocellular carcinoma is a rare condition in Europe and America but its incidence is higher in other parts of the world, and it is particularly common among the colored populations of South and West Africa. In Mozambique, hepatoma accounts for 65 percent of all cases of carcinoma among Bantus[1]—an incidence one hundredfold greater than that found in European South Africans[2], who seem no more prone to develop this condition than do Caucasians elsewhere in the world. This marked geographical and cultural distribution of primary hepatoma has led to the suggestion that a toxic environmental factor may be involved in its pathogenesis. Recently, much attention has been focused on the possible etiological role of aflatoxins in contaminating foodstuffs.

The aflatoxins are a group of compounds produced by the mold Aspergillus Flavus, which grows on nuts and grain when stored under warm, humid conditions. The staple diet of rural Africans is groundnuts

Table 1-1
Hepatic Neoplasms Associated With Chemicals and Drugs

Benign	
Adenoma	Anabolic steroids
	Oral contraceptives
Focal nodular hyperplasia	Oral contraceptives
MALIGNANT	
Hepatocellular carcinoma	Aflatoxins
	Anabolic steroids
	Oral contraceptives
Angiosarcoma	Vinyl Chloride
	Inorganic Arsenicals
	Copper Sulphate
	Thorotrast

(peanuts) and in some areas maize. The way in which these foodstuffs are traditionally stored, inadequately protected from rain, provides conditions ideal for colonization by Aspergillus Flavus.

Aflatoxins were first isolated in 1961[2] and have been shown to be potently hepatoxic and carcinogenic for a variety of animal species.[3] Furthermore, in a clinical study, histological evidence of toxic liver damage similar to that found in rats given aflatoxin, but different from the damage typical of viral hepatitis, was found in several native Africans having liver biopsies performed during an epidemic of hepatitis in 1963.[4] Three patients showing these liver lesions subsequently developed a hepatoma.

Surveys in Africa and Thailand, where primary hepatoma is also common, have shown that up to 65 percent of groundnuts sampled in the former country, and 30 percent of rice sampled in the latter was contaminated with aflatoxin.[5,6] Three separate surveys have demonstrated that the greater the quantity of aflatoxin consumed, the greater is the observed incidence of primary hepatoma.[7,8,9] Van Rensberg et al.[1] were able to show that aflatoxin consumption by natives living in the Inhamborne district of Mozambique was as uniquely high as the incidence of hepatoma in that area.

ROLE OF HEPATITIS B VIRUS INFECTION

Similar geographic parallels have been established between hepatoma incidence and the prevalence of hepatitis B virus infection or carriage. Among the early reports of this association was that of Vogel et al.[10] who, using relatively insensitive techniques, noted that 40 percent of their hepatoma patients had HBsAg in the serum. The figure was highest in the younger patients without underlying cirrhosis (70 percent of those under 30 years of age), whereas it was less frequent (17 percent) in patients over 50 years. In Britain, a study was conducted in the same year of 17 patients with HBsAg-positive chronic liver disease of at least six months' duration.[11] Five of these patients developed hepatoma; all were of Mediterranean stock. Later that year, a study performed in Greece found a 31 percent incidence of HBsAg-positivity in patients with hepatoma.[12]

If more sensitive techniques, such as radioimmunoassay and hemagglutination are employed, much higher rates are found, as in series reported from Taiwan,[13] South Africa (blacks),[14] Greece,[15] Thailand,[16] Senegal,[17] Uganda,[10] and South Vietnam,[18]—areas where HBsAg carriage in the normal population is at least as high as seven percent. HBsAg has been found less frequently with hepatoma in France and the United States, where HBsAg frequency in the normal population is very much lower.[19,20]

Screening for hepatitis B virus infection, however, may yield false negatives if only HBsAg, which represents the surface coat of the virus, is assayed. The determination of circulating antibody levels at the core of the virus (Hb_cAb) has been shown to yield a high positivity rate. Thus, Maupas et al. described anti-HBc antibody in 95 percent of African and Asian patients seen with hepatoma and suggested that, while there may be continuous production of core antigen, production of surface antigen may cease in some hepatoma patients.[21]

Kubo et al. reported that, while only 52.3 percent of a series of over 200 hepatoma sera were HBsAg-positive, anti-HBc was found in 81.3 percent.[22] Furthermore, in a recent survey of British patients with primary hepatocellular carcinoma, anti-HB_c was found in over two thirds of cases, less than half of whom were positive for HB_sAg.[23]

Since aflatoxin contamination of foodstuffs and carriage of hepatitis B virus often coexist in areas where hepatocellular carcinoma is common, it has been suggested that these two environmental factors may act synergistically as carcinogens; this requires further investigation. If a search for dietary aflatoxin contamination proved negative in a country such as Egypt where, despite a high rate of hepatitis B infection, hepatoma is uncommon, this hypothesis would be supported. An alternative suggestion is that the presence of HBs antigenemia indicates a defective immune response which is due to insult by the same toxin that is responsible for hepatocarcinogenesis. Aflatoxins have been shown to have immunosuppressive properties.[24,25]

ANGIOSARCOMA OF THE LIVER

Numerous case reports leave little doubt that workers who are chronically exposed to vinyl chloride monomer in the manufacture of PVC may develop angiosarcoma of the liver.[26-29] Similar tumors have been described in vineyard sprayers using "Bordeaux mixture", a fungicidal preparation consisting of copper sulphate and lime,[30] as well as in cases of long-term exposure to inorganic arsenicals found in pesticides[31] and in Fowler's solution[32], which is used for the treatment of psoriasis.

Angiosarcoma of the liver also occurs after exposure to the erstwhile radiological contrast agent thorotrast.[33-34] This colloidal suspension of 232-thorium dioxide localizes and persists in the liver and spleen, where it can be seen for many years on plain films of the abdomen. After a latent period of 20 years or more a high incidence of angiosarcoma of the liver occurs, as well as a significant increase in leukemia and blood dyscrasias. Although thorotrast is no longer employed, the long latent period between its administration and the development of neoplasia means that tumors produced by its previous use are still presenting.

HEPATIC TUMORS ASSOCIATED WITH ANABOLIC STEROIDS

Since the first report in 1965,[35] approximately 25 cases of liver tumors in long-term users of anabolic and androgenic steroids have been recorded.[36] In general, the doses taken have been high for the treatment of bone marrow aplasia, the correction of impotence, or the maintenance of male secondary sexual characteristics in female–to–male trans-sexuals.[37] In all reported cases a 17 α-alkylated steroid has been used. The oncogenic potential of the lower doses of androgenic steroids used in the treatment of menopausal symptoms is unknown.

While cases of benign hepatic adenoma have been reported,[37,38] the majority of androgen-related tumors have been histologically indistinguishable from primary hepato-cellular carcinoma. A feature of the neoplasms, however, is that they are frequently highly vascular;[36] the surrounding liver parenchyma may be infiltrated with dilated, blood-filled cysts characteristic of peliosis hepatitis, which may rupture into either the liver parenchyma or the peritoneal cavity. Cases of peliosis hepatis without liver tumor have also been reported in users of anabolic steroids,[39] who present with either hemoperitoneum or, when involvement is massive, liver failure.

There is some suggestion that the clinical course of these tumors may be different from other forms of hepato-cellular carcinoma in that they tend not to metastasize, and may even regress following the withdrawal of androgens.[40,41]

CASE HISTORY

A.W., a 29 year old mechanic, presented in December 1976 in a shocked state with acute central and right upper abdominal pain. At emergency laparotomy, a rupture in the right lobe of the liver was found with five liters of blood in the peritoneum. Following suture of the hepatic rupture, he was transferred to King's College Hospital for further assessment. Previous history revealed that, at age 21, he had been investigated for hypogonadism and had taken 50 mg. of methyl testosterone daily for five years.

Investigations included negative HB_sAg and α-fetoprotein. ^{99}Technetium liver scan revealed a large liver containing multiple filling defects, and arteriography (Fig. 1-1A) revealed multiple areas of tumor circulation that corresponded with these. Because of the unresectability of the tumor, cytotoxic therapy was considered, but the patient refused. After the withdrawal of androgens, the patient was observed.

During the period of follow up (21 months), serial scintiscans and ultrasound have shown a definite regression in the liver masses, and repeat hepatic arteriography four months after presentation has shown a diminution in tumor circulation (Fig. 1-1B).

HEPATIC TUMOR ASSOCIATED WITH ORAL CONTRACEPTIVES

Chemically related to the 17 α-alkylated anabolic steroids are the progestagen components of oral contraceptives. Since 1973[42] over 200 cases of liver tumors have been reported in women using the pill.[43] The majority, in contrast to tumors associated with anabolic steroids, have been benign, showing characteristics of either adenoma or focal nodular hyperplasia. However, while these two conditions are readily distinguishable histologically in typical cases (Table 1-2), in many tumors associated with oral contraceptives there has been overlap, and classification has often been difficult. At least 20 reported cases have had primary hepatocellular carcinoma,[43] and it is possible that benign lesions have the capacity to become malignant. In keeping with this are the cases[43,44] reporting areas of hepatocellular carcinoma found within benign adenomas, and areas of focal nodular hyperplasia.

A characteristic feature of these tumors is their extreme vascularity. Histologically, they show collections of dilated, thin-walled blood vessels resembling peliosis hepatis, and are similar to the lesions found in associa-

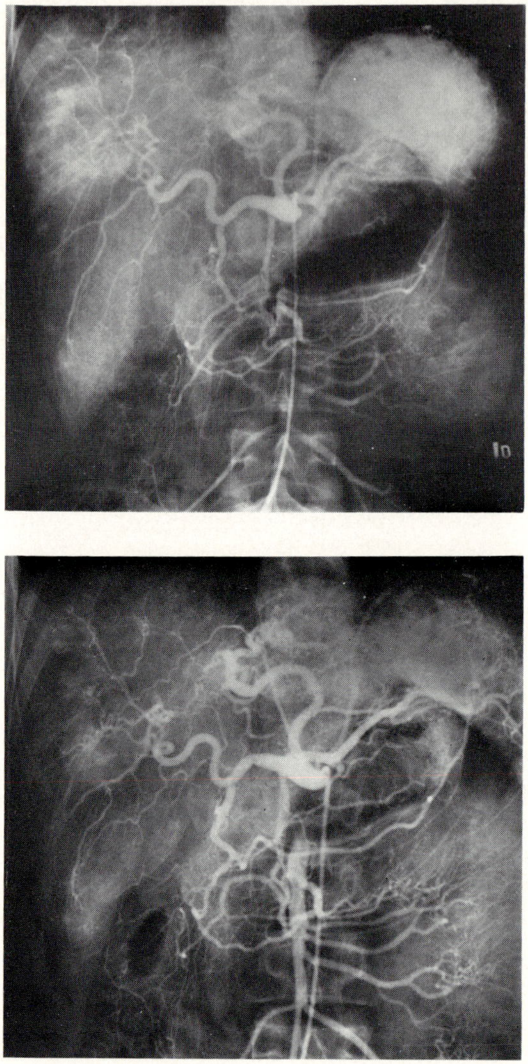

A

B

Fig. 1-1. A.W., male, 29 years: Hepatocellular carcinoma associated with anabolic steroids. A) Coeliac axis angiogram showing enlarged liver with many areas of vascular malignant circulation involving both lobes of the liver. B) Repeat angiogram after 4 months showing reduced size and vascularity of tumor masses.

A

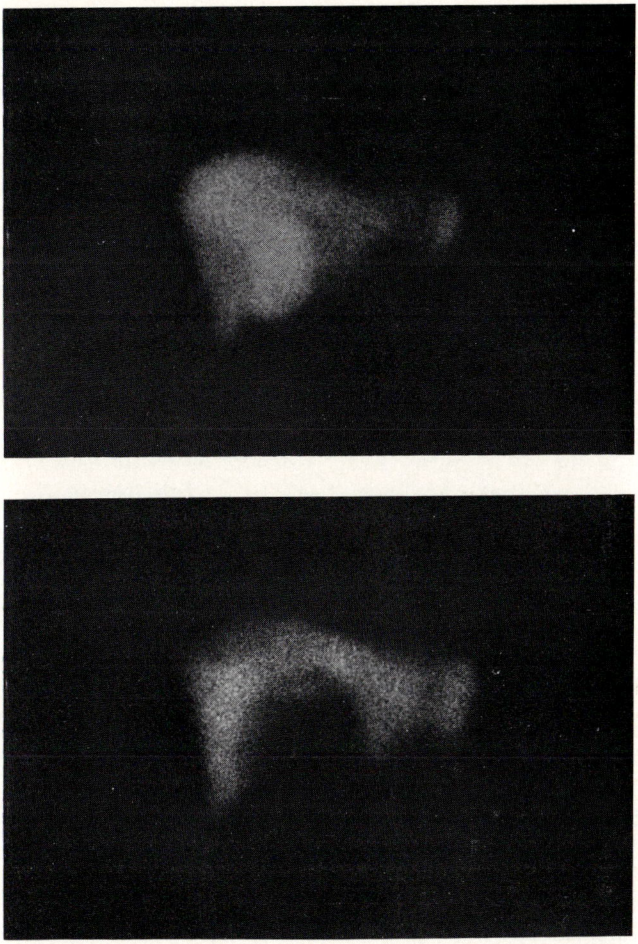

B

Fig. 1-2. S.H., female, 26 years: Benign "pill tumor." A) Technetium scintiscan of liver showing large central filling defect. B) Selenomethionine scintiscan showing take up of isotope in site of previous defect.

tion with anabolic steroids. As a result of this extreme vascularity, hemorrhage into the tumor, or rupture with hemoperitoneum are the most common modes of presentation, accounting in a recent review of the world literature for 55 percent of cases.[43] This complication appears to be associated with hepatic adenomas more frequently than with tumors classified as focal nodular hyperplasia.

In general, these tumors are associated with the long-term use of oral contraceptives; in two large series, 63 percent and 67 percent of cases had taken the pill continuously for four years or more,[45,46] and in another

Table 1-2
Some Histological Features Differentiating Hepatic Adenoma From Focal Nodular Hyperplasia

	ADENOMA	FOCAL NODULAR HYPERPLASIA
Capsule	Present	Absent
Central scar + fibrous septa	Absent	Present
Bile ducts	Absent	Present

series the mean duration of contraceptive use in tumor patients was 73.4 months—nearly double that of a group of age—matched controls.[47] Edmondson and colleagues have calculated that women who use the pill continuously for five to seven years run five times the risk of developing this complication, and the figure rises to 25 fold for those taking oral contraceptives for nine years or more.[47] These tumors are not, however, restricted to longterm users of the pill; in one survey exposure had been as brief as six to 12 months in ten percent of cases.[43]

DIAGNOSIS

Apart from the androgen and oral contraceptive associated liver tumours, which frequently present as acute abdominal crises, the most common mode of presentation for hepatic neoplasms is with right upper quadrant discomfort and general deterioration in health. Some cases, however, may present with an asymptomatic upper abdominal mass. With highly vascular hepatocellular carcinomas and angiosarcomas, a bruit may be heard over the liver.

Biochemical liver function tests are not helpful in diagnosis. The most common abnormality is an elevated serum alkaline phosphatase, especially if the tumor has infiltrated widely into the liver. In hepatic tumors due to oral contraceptives, abnormalities in liver function tests have been shown to be the exception rather than the rule.[43]

Estimations of levels of serum α-fetoprotein are useful in diagnosing hepatocellular carcinoma, but not angiosarcoma, and the test has proved uniformly negative in oral-contraceptive-associated tumors.[43] Using radioimmunoassay, elevated levels of α-fetoprotein can be demonstrated in 70–80 percent of cases of hepatocellular carcinoma in Great Britain.[48] Using such sensitive methods, some elevation in α-fetoprotein level may also be detected in acute hepatitis and cirrhosis without tumor, and occasionally, even in other gastrointestinal, testicular, and embryonal tumors. However, levels are rarely found to exceed 500 μg/ml in benign liver disease, and values greater than 1,000 μg/ml are virtually diagnostic of hepatocellular carcinoma. Serial estimation of serum α-fetoprotein in high risk patients can be of value in providing early warning of malignant transformation.

In addition to hepatic scintiscanning with ^{99}Technetium, which detects tumors as multiple or solitary space-occupying lesions, the use of selenomethione to show uptake of isotope by areas not taking up technetium is useful in the diagnosis of hepatocellular carcinoma (Figs. 1-2A and B). Although such selective uptake of selenomethione does not occur with all cases of hepatocellular carcinoma, it has been reported in a benign pill-associated tumour.[43] The main disadvantage of hepatic scintiscanning, which limits its use as an aid to screening for drug- and chemical-induced liver tumors, is that it will not detect smaller neoplasms (4 cm. diameter).

Assessment of hepatic histology is important for two reasons: first, to distinguish a benign from a malignant neoplasm, and second, to determine whether the tumor has formed on a normal or cirrhotic liver. If cirrhosis is present, surgical resection and hepatic devascularization procedures (see below) are contraindicated.

Grey scale ultrasound is another important diagnostic tool useful in detecting and evaluating liver tumors. It is a non-invasive technique of relatively low cost. Besides showing the extent of the tumour, it is possible in some cases to distinguish between a normal and a cirrhotic liver. This examination is of particular value in following the progress of patients with known disease. One of the disadvantages is that the gas pattern in the upper abdomen in a significant number of patients makes it impossible to obtain a technically satisfactory scan. The echogenic pattern of the tumor gives no indication of its vascularity or pathology.

Conventional radiographic techniques provide accurate information about the general state of the liver as well as the size and extent of vascularity of the tumor.

While plain radiographs of the abdomen give an estimate of the sizes of the liver and spleen, they also demonstrate any calcification within the tumor (Fig. 1-3A). Pulmonary metastases may be demonstrated by radiography of the chest, including whole lung tomography.

Arteriography is essential if extremely detailed information about the tumor is sought: its size, whether or not it is multi-focal, and the extent of vascularity. The branches of the hepatic artery feeding the tumor can be identified. The state of the rest of the liver, as well as the patency of the portal vein, can be assessed. This information is all essential for planning the treatment of the patient.

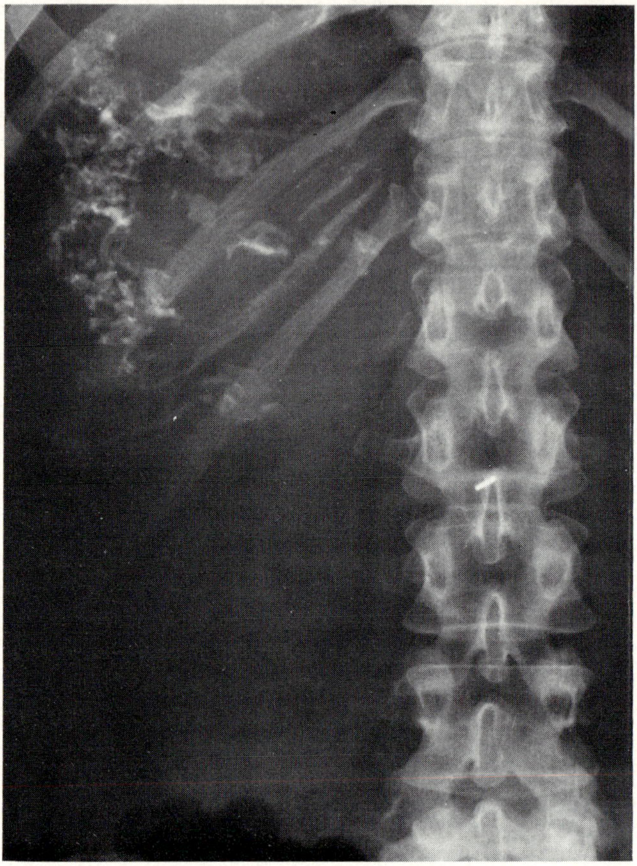

Fig. 1-3A. C.E., female, 25 years: Benign "pill tumor." Plain film showing dense calcification within tumor in liver.

The examination is generally performed using local anesthesia with heavy sedation. Although it is possible to start with selective angiography, we generally start with a free flush aortogram in order to demonstrate the arterial supply to the liver, which is variable, and to help exclude extra hepatic disease. This free flush aortogram has the disadvantages of increasing overall density of the abdominal organs, including the liver, and reducing the total amount of contrast that can be used on subsequent selective arterial injections.

An attempt should be made to correct any bleeding tendency or coagulation defect before undertaking angiography. If the prothrombin time (PT) is more than six seconds—prolonged in comparison with a control, vitamin K should be given for five days and the test repeated. If the PT is still prolonged, an infusion of fresh frozen plasma should be given immediately before, and during the procedure. Disseminated intravascular coagulation may occur in some patients with liver tumor, and the platelets may be deficient in number and quality. If the platelet level is below 50,000/cc., a platelet infusion should be given before angiography.

The hepatic artery should be catheterized selectively if possible. Separate injections should be made into the right and left branches if this is helpful. As contrast material has become less toxic and less painful on injection, the volume used has tended to increase. For selective injections we now employ 50 to 80 ml. Urographin 370 at a rate of 8 to 15 ml. per second, depending upon the size of the artery and the rate of flow through it. If it is not possible to enter the hepatic artery, injection of the coeliac axis artery provides useful but less exact information, while at the same time demonstrating the portal vein. A sequence of films is taken to cover both the early arterial and the late hepatogram phases. The precise sequence of films and number of different views will vary with each patient and depend upon the size and type of tumor as well as the possible mode of management. For example, if there appears to be a possibility of a partial hepatectomy, oblique films with the right side raised may be necessary in order to demonstrate that the tumor is confined to one lobe of the liver and that the other is completely free of tumors.

If arterial embolization is being considered as a method of treatment, it is necessary to demonstrate that the portal vein is patent and detailed information of the exact blood supply to the liver is required. This is usually shown in the late films after contrast has been injected into the splenic artery, coeliac axis artery or superior mesenteric arteries or a combination of these vessels simultaneously. Alternatively, a splenic venogram may be necessary to do this. It is essential that the portal vein be patent in order to supply nourishment to the liver if the hepatic artery is to be occluded.

If surgery—either partial resection or transplantation—is being considered, an attempt must be made to exclude extrahepatic spread of the tumour. Inferior vena cavography with both anterior–posterior and lateral projections is necessary. Lymphangiography has not proved helpful in excluding spread to abdominal lymph nodes.

Percutaneous cholangiography may be helpful if the patient presents with obstructive jaundice; it proved to be of use in one of our patients who was shown to have dilated ducts within the liver, a distended gall bladder and a tumor causing obstruction high up in the common bile duct. Endoscopic retrograde cannulation of the common bile duct confirmed the lower end of the common bile duct to be normal.

The place of computerized tomography in the diagnosis of hepatic tumors remains to be defined. Its main value will be in demonstrating accurately the limits of the tumor, and the presence or absence of distant

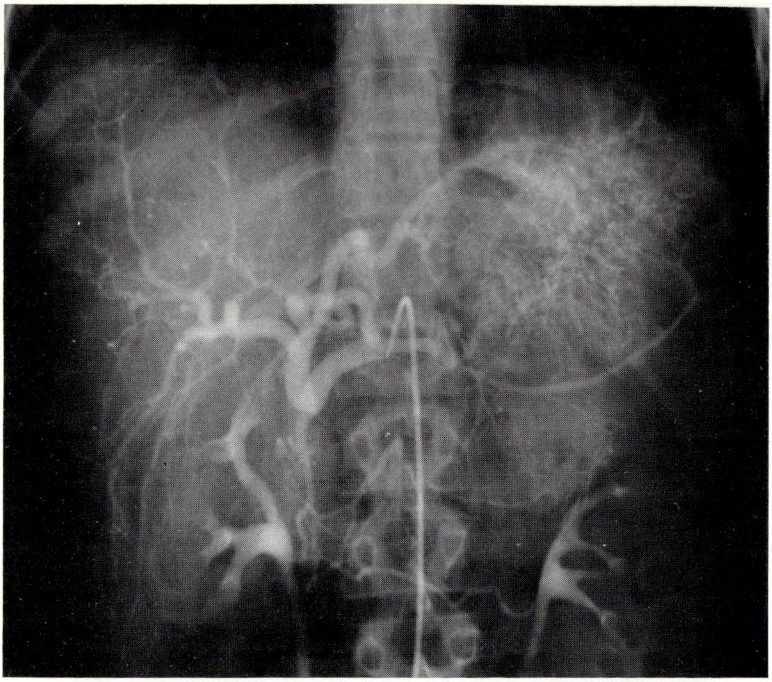

Fig. 1-5. G.H., female, 22 years: Benign "pill tumor." Hepatic angiogram showing vascular tumor in the left lobe of the liver with larger arteries curved around the tumor mass and many small vessels arising from them. Small areas of abnormal vascularity are seen in the right lobe.

ASPECTS OF MANAGEMENT

Benign Tumors Associated with Oral Contraceptives

The majority of these tumors have been solitary, and for this reason, surgical resection has been feasible. A few, however, have been multifocal; management of such cases has been a problem because little is known of the natural history of these neoplasms. Several cases have now been reported in which regression has been documented following cessation or oral contraceptives,[51–53] but a number of cases have presented clinically months and years after stopping the pill, so regression is not the rule in all cases.[54–57]

Where resection is not possible, some form of arterial occlusion should probably be carried out. This is the only means of securing hemostasis in some patients who present with hemorrhage. Further, in at least one instance, necrosis of the tumor was reported to follow.

As an alternative to a direct surgical attack on the hepatic artery, embolization of the major arterial supply to the tumor should be considered. The patency of the portal vein should be demonstrated, usually by aortoportography, prior to embolization of a major hepatic artery because

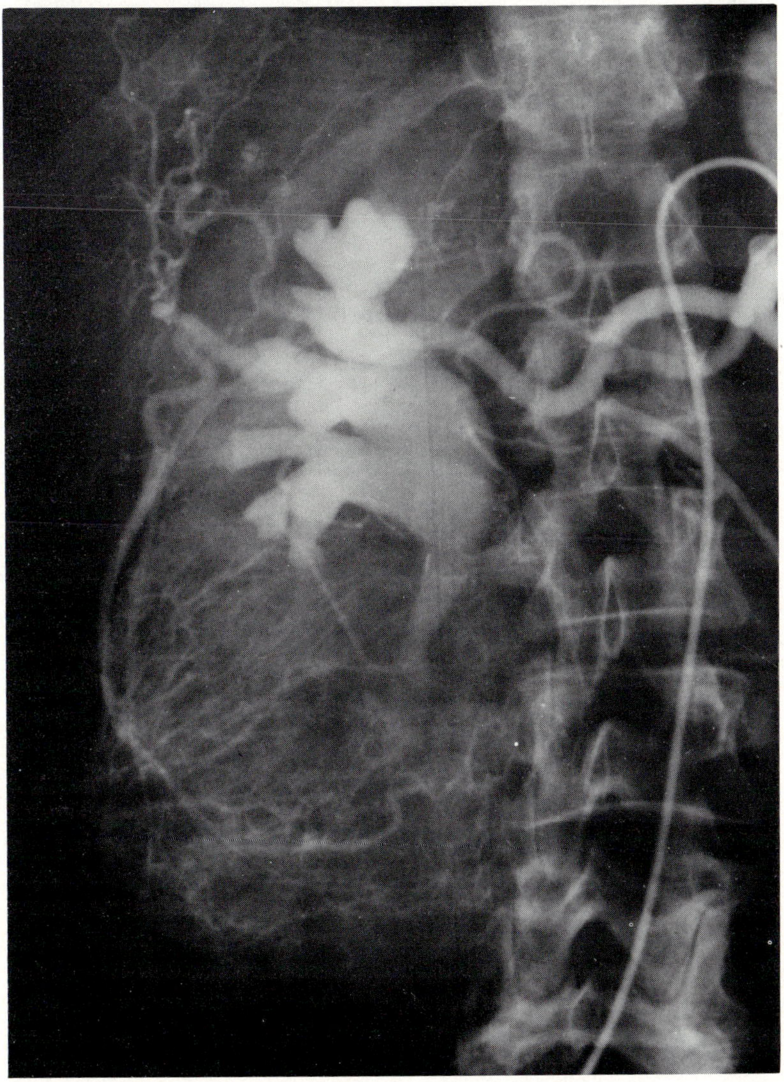

Fig. 1-6A. A.S., female, 40 years: Malignant "pill tumor." Hepatic angiogram showing circumscribed vascular tumor in right lobe of the liver.

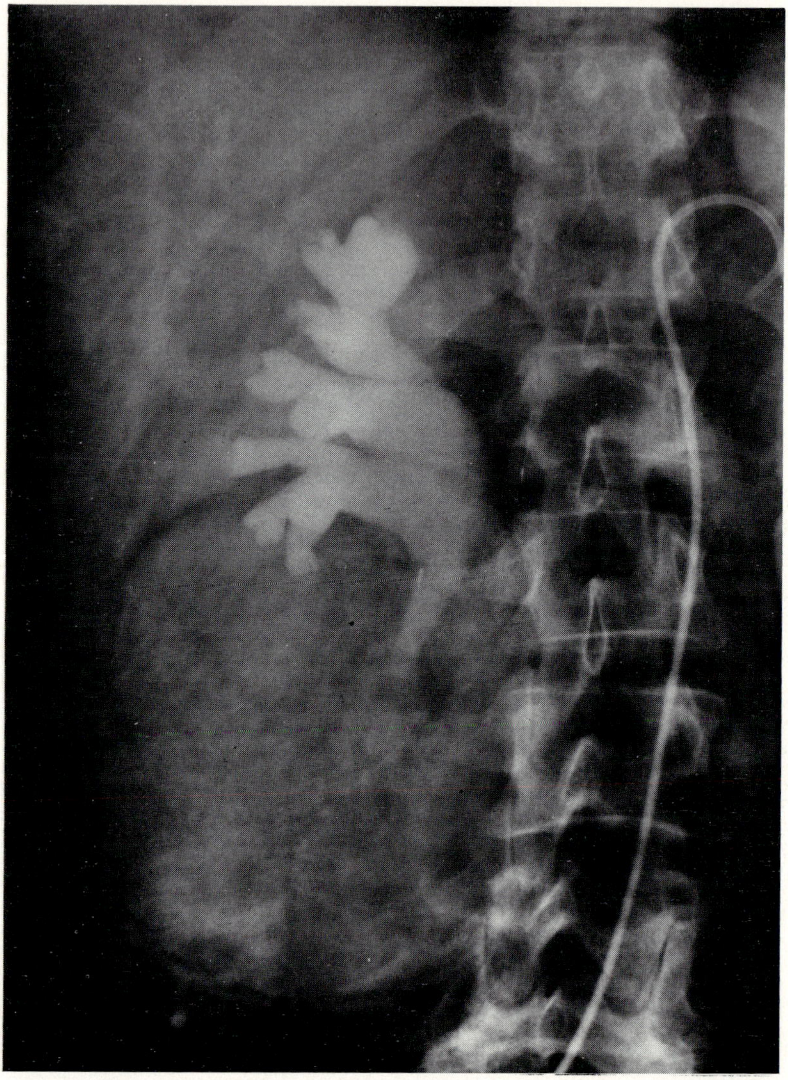

Fig. 1-6B. Hepatogram phase of A.S. showing patent vein and well circumscribed tumor which was histologically malignant.

of the risk of precipitating hepatic necrosis (by arterial occlusion) in the presence of a blocked portal vein.

To perform embolization it must be possible to place the catheter tip in an optimal position to occlude the artery or arteries supplying the tumor. Preferably this should be beyond the origins of the gastroduodenal artery and the cystic artery.

It is better to carry out the procedure under general anesthesia. The patient should be covered by antibiotics, for example, penicillin and flagyl; afterwards, adequate analgesia should be made available. Most patients experience pain, nausea, rigors, fever, and perhaps vomiting.

A variety of materials may be used in embolization. We favor Gelfoam, which is safe, but possibly not permanent. It is chopped into small 4 × 2 × 2 mm. fragments which are placed in a tuberculin syringe. Contrast is added before injection down the catheter. The course of the Gelfoam fragments can be observed and the gradual cessation of arterial flow noted. Small particles of human dura mater, 3 × 2 × 2 mm. soaked in contrast, can be added to the Gelfoam to give a more permanent result. As the flow in the artery will gradually halt, it is important to stop injecting particles before a reflux into other branches supplying the normal liver or other organs occurs. An inflatable balloon catheter may be of use in this process.

Following embolization the tumor usually becomes smaller, as demonstrated by serial isotope scans, ultrasound, or repeat angiography. Liquefaction of the tumor may occur with the formation of a sterile abscess. On one occasion this required surgical drainage. It appeared as though the entire tumor had sloughed, leaving a thin-walled cavity within the liver. After drainage, the patient made an uninterrupted recovery.

CASE REPORT

S.E., a 30 year old British housewife, presented in July 1977 with a painless epigastric mass. Laparotomy revealed a large bosselated tumor overlaid by large tortuous vessels arising from the surrounding liver, which appeared normal. Liver biopsy was non-diagnostic and she was transferred to King's College Hospital for assessment. The patient had been taking different oral contraceptive preparations for ten years: breakthrough bleeding in the early years had necessitated a high dose preparation.

Hepatic arteriography (Figs. 1-7A and B) revealed a highly vascular tumor in the right lobe of the liver that was supplied by many large arterial branches, each of which gave rise to numerous smaller vessels. The hepatogram showed an intense "blush" of contrast in the tumor, as well as several small areas of increased vascularity elsewhere in the right lobe. The general vascularity of the rest of the liver was poor because of the "steal" by the tumor.

In November 1977, she underwent hepatic artery embolization under a local anesthetic, using gelfoam and human dura. The catheter was placed just beyond the origin of the gastroduodenal artery. The emboli were seen to pass preferentially to the very vascular tumour. The patient had considerable post-embolization pain, rigor, and fever. This settled, but within a month an ultrasound examination of the liver revealed a cavitatory lesion in the area previously occupied by the tumor. A plain film showed a fluid and air-filled cavity (Fig. 1-7C). Hepatic arteriography at this stage demonstrated virtual disappearance of the tumour circulation (Fig. 1-7D).

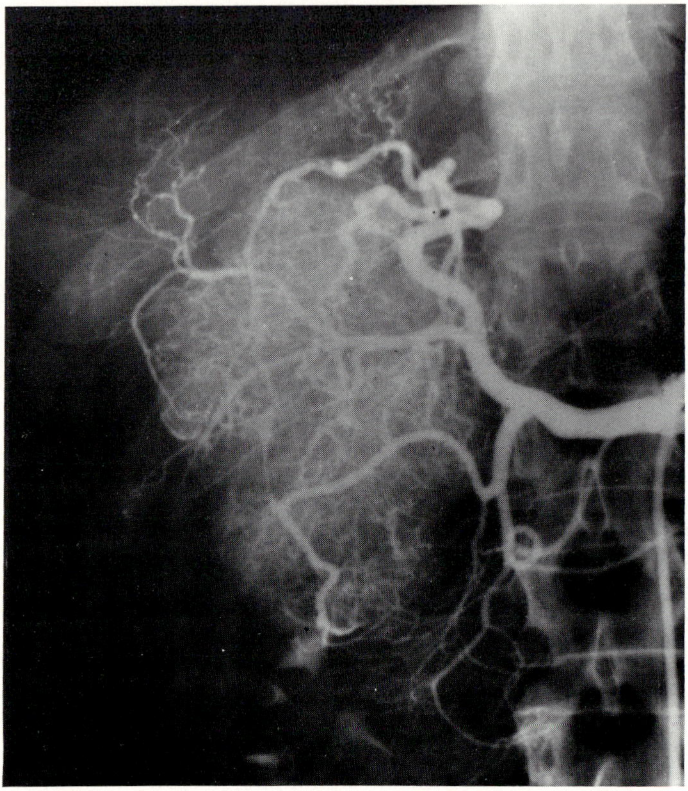

Fig. 1-7A. S.E., female, 30 years: Benign "pill tumor." Early phase of hepatic arteriogram showing large vessels supplying tumor mass in right lobe.

Malignant Tumours

Management depends on the extent of the tumour. In patients without cirrhosis, up to seven eighths of the liver may be removed in an extended right hepatic lobectomy, characterized by removal of the right lobe and the median segment. Regeneration of the remaining liver occurs within ten to 14 days of operation, but tumor may recur even after intervals of three to four years. The number of cases suitable for this form of radical surgery is very small.

Symptomatic relief (particularly from pain) and shrinkage of the tumor mass can be derived from hepatic artery ligation, since the tumor derives its blood supply almost exclusively from this vessel; the remaining liver (under normal circumstances) receives adequate blood supply from the portal vein. As a less invasive approach, hepatic artery embolization should be attempted first (see above). We have treated two patients with

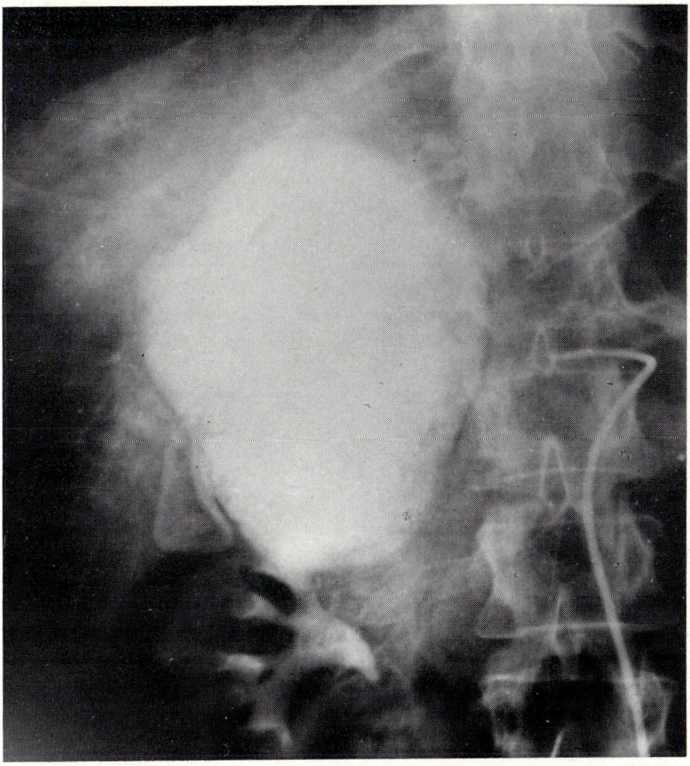

Fig. 1-7B. Hepatogram phase of S.E. showing intense vascularity of main tumor with small areas of hypervascularity elsewhere in the right lobe.

histologically-proven hepatocellular carcinoma, employing gelatin foam.[58] In both, α-fetoprotein levels fell precipitously. Subsequent cytotoxic therapy with adriamycin was initiated when the levels plateaued at a very low level. Both remain well and symptom-free four to six months later.

Neither partial hepatectomy nor hepatic artery ligation can be carried out in patients with underlying cirrhosis for two reasons. First, the functional reserve is so limited that surgery would lead to hepatic decompensation; second, the liver is heavily dependent on the hepatic artery for its blood supply, and when cirrhosis is present, portal vein blood is already diverted away from the cirrhotic liver into collateral channels.

Patients whose tumors have extended throughout the liver, but who are without demonstrable metastases, may be suitable for liver transplantation. Over 65 such operations have now been carried out by Cambridge-King's College Hospital teams,[59] and, since a better technique for establishing the biliary tract anastamosis was developed, results have improved considerably. Although recurrence of tumor will occur in 70

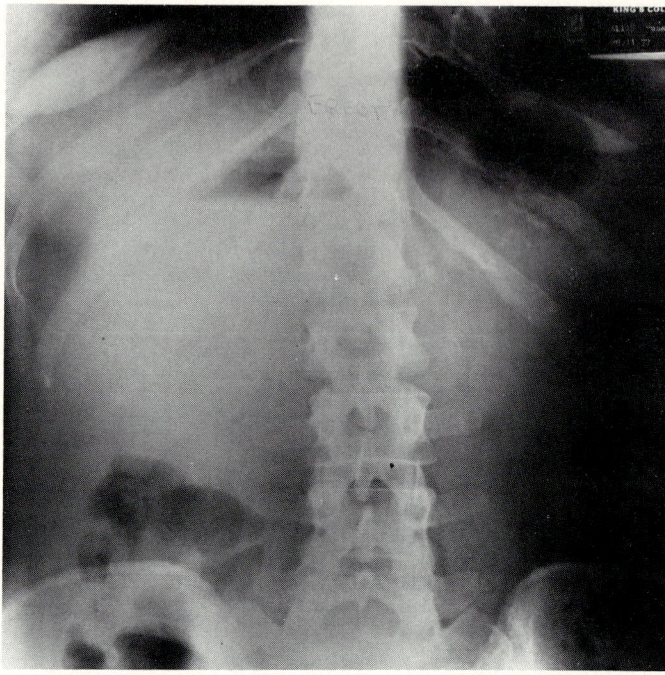

Fig. 1-7C. Plain film of S.E. showing a gas/fluid level in position of previously demonstrated tumor.

percent of patients, useful palliation for up to two years has been obtained in five patients, while six are presently alive and well with no evidence of recurrence, one of these at four years.

In many cases the tumor will have spread outside the liver, or the patient will be too ill for any surgical procedure. In such cases chemotherapy is the only available approach, although, until recently, it was questionable whether the minimal palliation obtained was worth the side effect of these drugs. Noteworthy results have been obtained from the use of adriamycin (Doxorubicin), an anthracycline derivative.[60] To date we have used this drug in 61 patients with primary hepatocellular carcinoma who were unsuitable for surgery or transplantation because of extensive tumor growth or poor clinical condition. In 19 of these a clinical remission has been obtained, and in five the remission has been complete, as judged by the disappearance of tumor circulation on arteriography or the disappearance of tumor mass on ultrasound examination. This is the first time that objective evidence of tumor regression has been obtained in a significant number of patients following any form of chemotherapy for hepatocellular carcinoma. In addition, two patients have had prolonged survival (12 and 15 months) despite evidence of incomplete regression.

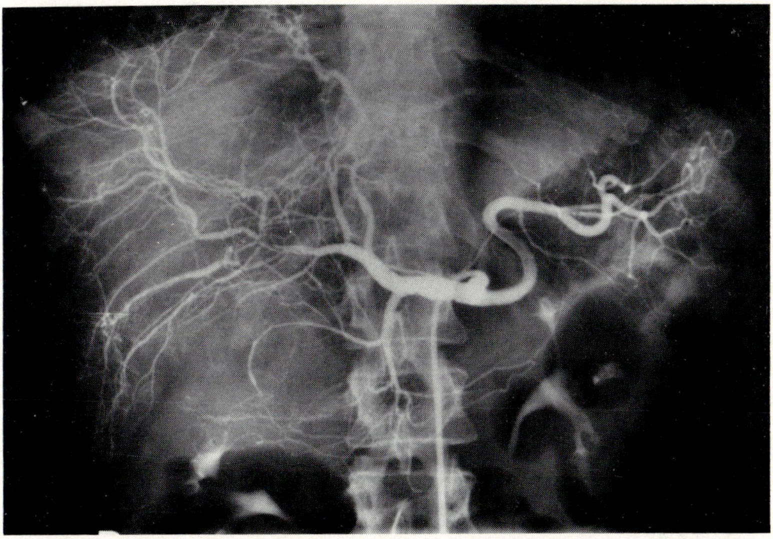

Fig. 1-7D. Hepatic angiogram of S.E. after embolization of tumor showing tumor mass now almost avascular and many normal branches of the hepatic artery not demonstrated on previous angiogram.

In the patients who showed a complete remission and in whom serum values of α-fetoprotein were initially elevated, there was a sharp drop in α-fetoprotein levels, to less than 20 percent of pretreatment values, within five weeks of the first injection of adriamycin. In contrast, levels continued to rise in patients who showed no response, while in those showing incomplete clinical remission an intermediate pattern of response was observed. Recurrence of tumor following initially successful chemotherapy was associated with a rise in α-fetoprotein levels. Using this technique, it is possible both to determine at an early stage which patients will respond to chemotherapy, and to make an early diagnosis of tumor recurrence, which can then be delineated by radiological examination.

REFERENCES

1. van Rensberg SJ, van der Watt JJ, Purchase IFH et al: Primary liver cancer rate and aflatoxin intake in a high cancer area. S African Med J 48:2508A–2508D, 1974
2. Sargeant K, Sheridan A, O'Kelly J, Carnaghan RBA: Toxicity associated with certain samples of groundnuts. Nature (London) 192:1096–1097, 1962
3. Newberne PM, Butler WH: Acute and chronic effects of aflatoxins on the liver of domestic and laboratory animals—a review. Cancer Research 29:236–241, 1969

4. Torres FO, Purchase IFH, van der Watt JJ: The aetiology of primary liver cancer in the Bantu. J Pathol 102:163–166, 1970
5. Shank RC, Wogan GN, Gibson JB: Dietary aflatoxins and human liver cancer. Food and Cosmetic Toxicology 10:51–70, 1972
6. Alpert ME, Wogan G, Davidson CS: Aflatoxin and hepatoma in Uganda. Gastroenterology 149:54–58, 1968
7. Shank RC, Gordon JE, Wogan GN, Nondasuta A, Subhaurand B: Dietary aflatoxins and human liver cancer III: Field survey of rural Thai families for ingested aflatoxins. Food Cosmet Toxicol 10:71–80, 1972
8. Shank RG, Bhamarapravati N, Gordon JE, et al: Dietary aflatoxins and primary liver cancer in two municipal populations of Thailand. Food Cosmet Toxicol 10:171–9, 1972
9. Peers FG, Linsell CA: Dietary aflatoxins and liver cancer—a population based study in Uganda. Brit J Cancer 27:473–484, 1973
10. Vogel CL, Anthony PP, Mody N, et al: Hepatitis associated antigen in Ugandan patients with hepatocellular carcinoma. Lancet 2:621–624, 1970
11. Sherlock S, Fox RA, Niazi SP, et al: Chronic liver disease and primary liver cell cancer with hepatitis-associated (Australia) antigen in serum. Lancet 1:1243–1247, 1970
12. Hadziyannis SJ, Merikas GE, Afroudakis AP: Hepatitis associated antigen in chronic liver disease. Lancet 1:100, 1970
13. Tong NY, Sun SC, Schaeffer BT, et al: Hepatitis-associated antigen and hepatocellular carcinoma in Taiwan. Ann Intern Med 75:687–691, 1971
14. Kew MC, Geddes EW, MacNab GM, et al: Hepatitis B antigen and cirrhosis in Bantu patients with primary liver cancer. Cancer 34:538–541, 1974
15. Theodoropoulos G, Archimandritis A, Angelopoulos B: Australia antigen and malignant hepatoma. Ann Intern Med 82:809–810, 1975
16. Chainuvatti T, Viranuvatti V, Pongpipat D: Relationship of hepatitis B antigen in cirrhosis and hepatoma in Thailand. Gastroenterology 68:1261–1264, 1975
17. Prince AM, Szmuness W, Michon J, et al: A case/control study of the association between primary liver cancer and hepatitis B infection in Senegal. Int J Cancer 16:376–383, 1975
18. Welsh JD, Bram JD, Arnold K, et al: Hepatitis B_s antigen, malaria titers and primary liver cancer in South Vietnam. Gastroenterology 70:392–396, 1976
19. Prince AM, LeBlanc L, Krohn K, et al: SH antigen and chronic liver disease. Lancet 2:717–718, 1970
20. Alpert E, Isrelbacher KJ: Hepatitis-associated antigen and hepatoma in the U.S. Lancet 2:1087, 1971
21. Maupas P, Werner B, Larouze B, et al: Antibody to hepatitis B core antigen in patients with primary hepatic carcinoma. Lancet 2:9–11, 1975
22. Kubo Y, Okuda K, Musha H, Nakashima T: Detection of hepatocellular carcinoma during a clinical follow up of chronic liver disease: observations on 31 patients. Gastroenterology 74:578, 1978
23. Bassendine MF, Chadwick RG, Lyssiotis T, et al: Hepatitis B virus and primary liver cancer. Britain Digestion (in press)
24. Auksandrowicz J, Urasinski I, Lisiewicz J, et al: Cytotoksyczny wply afatoksyny B l na lymphocyty w hodowi z titohemaglutyna. Przegl lek 28:689–692, 1971
25. Savel H, Forsyth B, Schaeffer W, et al: Effect of aflatoxin B, on phytohaemogglutinin-transformed human lymphocytes. Proc Soc Exp Biol Med 134:1112–1115, 1970
26. Creech JL, Johnson MN: Angiosarcoma of liver in the manufacture of polyvinyl chloride J Occup Med 16:150–157, 1974
27. Block JB: Angiosarcoma of the liver following vinyl chloride exposure. JAMA 229:53–54, 1974

28. Lee FI, Harry DS: Angiosarcoma of the liver in a vinyl chloride worker. Lancet 1:1316–1318, 1974
29. Thomas LB, Popper H, Berk PD, et al. Vinyl chloride-induced liver disease. From idiopathic portal hypertension (Bantu's syndrome) to angiosarcomas. N Engl J Med 292:17–22, 1975
30. Pimentel JC, Menezes AP: Liver disease in vineyard sprayers. Gastrotenterology 72:275–283, 1977
31. Roth F: Arsen-leber-tumoren (Hamangioendotheliom). Z Krebsforsch 61:468–503, 1957
32. Regelson W, Kim U, Ospira J, et al: Hemangioendothelial sarcoma of liver from chronic arsenic intoxication by Fowler's solution. Cancer 21:514–522, 1968
33. MacMahon HE, Murphy AS, Bates M: Endothelial cell sarcoma of liver following thorotrast injections. Am J Pathol 23:585–595, 1947
34. Horta JS: Late effects of Thorotrast on the liver and the spleen and their efferent lymph nodes. Ann NY Acad Sci 145, 676–699, 1967
35. Recant L, Lacy P: Fanconi's anemia and hepatic cirrhosis. Am J Med 39:464–475, 1965
36. Paradinas FJ, Bull TB, Westaby D, et al: Hyperplasia and prolapse of hepatocytes into hepatic veins during longterm methyltestosterone therapy: Possible relationship of these changes to the development of peliosis hepatis and liver tumours. Histopathology 1:225–246, 1977
37. Westaby D, Ogle SJ, Paradinas FJ, et al: Liver damage from longterm methyltestosterone. Lancet 2:261–263, 1977
38. Bruguera M: Androgen-induced hepatoma. Lancet 1:1295, 1975
39. Bagheri SA, Boyer JL: Peliosis hepatitis associated with androgenic-anabolic steroid therapy: a severe form of hepatic injury. Ann Intern Med 81:610–618, 1974
40. Farrell GG, Joshua DE, Uren RF, et al: Androgen-induced hepatoma Lancet 1:430–2, 1975
41. Johnson FL, Feagler JR, Lerner KG, et al: Association of androgenic-anabolic steroid therapy with development of hepatocellular carcinoma. Lancet 2:1273–1276, 1972
42. Baum JK, Holtz F, Bookstein JJ, et al: Possible association between benign hepatomas and oral contraceptives. Lancet 2:926–929, 1973
43. Klatskin G: Hepatic tumours: possible relationship to oral contraceptives. Gastroenterology 73: 386–394, 1977
44. Davis M, Portmann B, Searle M, et al. Histological evidence of carcinoma in a hepatic tumour associated with oral contraceptives. Br Med J 4:496–498, 1975
45. Nissen ED, Kent DR, Nissen SE, et al. The association of liver tumours with oral contraceptives. Obstet Gynecol 48:49–55, 1976
46. Christopherson WM, Mays ET Liver tumours and contraceptive steroids: experience with the first one hundred registry patients. J Natl Cancer Inst 58:167–171, 1977
47. Edmondson HA, Henderson B, Benton B: Liver cell adenomas associated with oral contraceptives. New Engl J Med 294:470–472, 1976
48. Johnson P, Williams R: Serial AFP estimation and measurement of doubling time in patients with hepatocellular carcinoma: Influence of therapy and value in early detection. Gut (in press)
49. Baum JK, Holtz E, Bookstein JJ, et al: Possible association between benign hepatomas and oral contraceptives. Lancet 2:926–929, 1973
50. Reuter SR, Redman HC: Tumours, in E.J. Ratchen (ed): Gastrointestinal Angiography. London, W.B. Saunders, 1977, pp 132–139
51. Kay S, Shatzki PF: Ultrastructure of a benign liver cell adenoma. Cancer 28:755–762, 1961
52. Ross D, Pina J, Mirpa M et al. Regression of focal nodular hyperplasia after discontinuation of oral contraceptives. Ann Intern Med 85:203–204, 1976

53. Edmondson HA, Reynolds TB, Henderson B, et al: Regression of liver cell adenomas associated with oral contraceptives. Ann Intern Med 86:180–182, 1977
54. Davis JB, Schenken JR, Zimmerman O: Massive hemoperitoneum from rupture of benign hepatocellular adenoma. Surgery 73:181–184, 1973
55. Antoniades K, Brooks CE: Hemoperitoneum from liver cell adenoma in a patient on oral contraceptives. Surgery 77:137–139, 1975
56. Model DG, Fox JA, Jones RW: Multiple hepatic adenomas associated with an oral contraceptive. Lancet 1:865, 1975
57. Mays ET, Christopherson WM, Barrows GH: Focal nodular hyperplasia of the liver: possible relationship to oral contraceptives. Am J Clin Pathol 61:735–746, 1974
58. Wheeler PG, Melia W, Dubbins P, Jones B, Johnson PJ, Nunnerley H, Williams R: Non-operative arterial embolisation in the management of primary liver tumour. Brit Med J 2:242–244, 1979
59. Calne RY, Williams R: Orthotopic liver transplantation: the first 60 patients. Brit Med J 1:471–6, 1977
60. Johnson PH, Williams R, Thomas H, et al: Induction of remission in hepatocellular carcinoma with adriamycin. Lancet 1:1006–1009, 1978

T. C. B. Stamp

2
Drug- and Chemical-Induced Rickets (and Osteomalacia)

Certain drugs and chemicals may interfere with vitamin D metabolism or function and lead occasionally to clinical rickets or osteomalacia. Mechanisms for this vary widely from the nephrotoxic effect of heavy metals such as cadmium to the hepatic-enzyme-inducing effect of anticonvulsant drugs such as phenytoin. Other agents such as diphosphonates may produce similar disease by direct action on bone. Significant problems in industrial toxiology are set by cadmium and to a lesser extent fluoride, but all other forms of the disease arise as unwanted side-effects from administered drugs. By far the greatest amount of recent work has concerned the effects of anticonvulsant drugs in epilepsy and, while we have tried to list all forms of drug-produced rickets, this problem is the most comprehensively discussed.

APPLIED VITAMIN D METABOLISM

Classification of the heterogeneous collection of drugs which we need to consider can be simplified by brief reference to the functional metabolism of vitamin D, shown in Fig. 2-1.[1] Vitamin D reaches the body either by the action on skin of solar or artificial ultraviolet light, which converts the physiological precursor 7-dehydrocholesterol (stored in the deeper layers of the epidermis) to cholecalciferol (vitamin D_3), or by ingestion of the vitamin in the diet. While it is highly unlikely that ultra-violet barrier preparations such as Mexenone or Padimate (British Pharmacopoeia approved names) will be incriminated in human rickets they are worth a

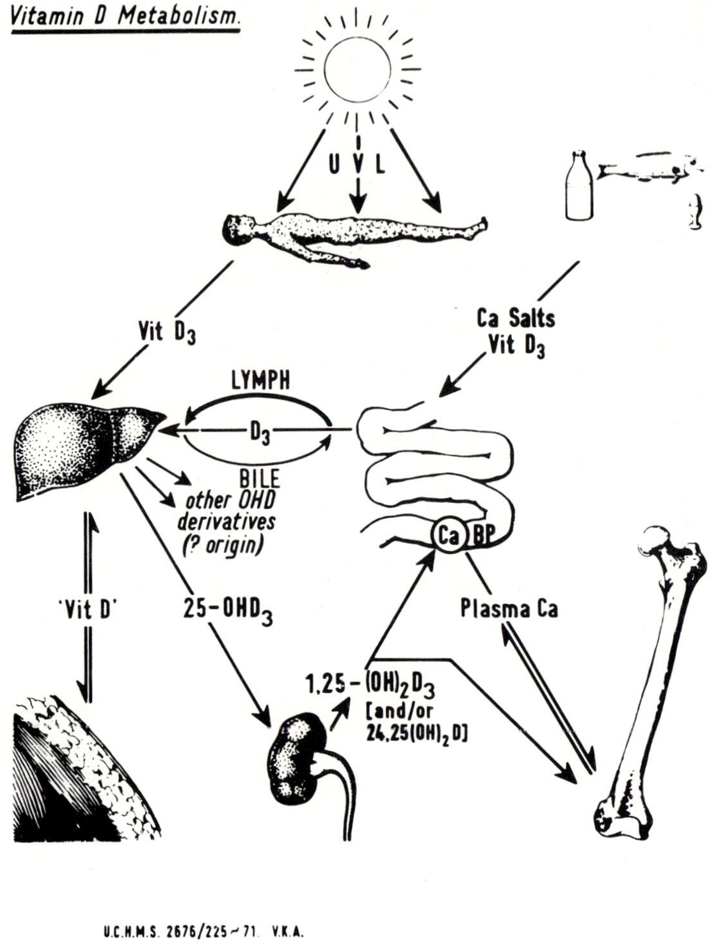

Fig. 2-1. Major pathways of vitamin D metabolism in man.[1] Pathways represented are through skin, liver, small intestine, kidney, bone and storage reservoir of muscle and adipose tissue. 25-HCC = 25-hydroxycholecalciferol, 1,25-DHCC = 1,25-dihydroxycholecalciferol, CaBP = calcium-binding protein.

mention from this physiological standpoint: solar ultraviolet light may provide adequate protection against rickets in the presence of vitamin D-deficient diets[2] and its rigid exclusion can produce gross human rickets as shown in Fig. 2-2. Dietary vitamin D, either cholecalciferol or the synthetic ergocalciferol (vitamin D_2), is absorbed throughout the small intestine and possible malabsorption by purgative abuse will be considered. Bile salts appear necessary for vitamin D absorption, via the lymphatics, and there is significant entero-hepatic recirculation of conjugated

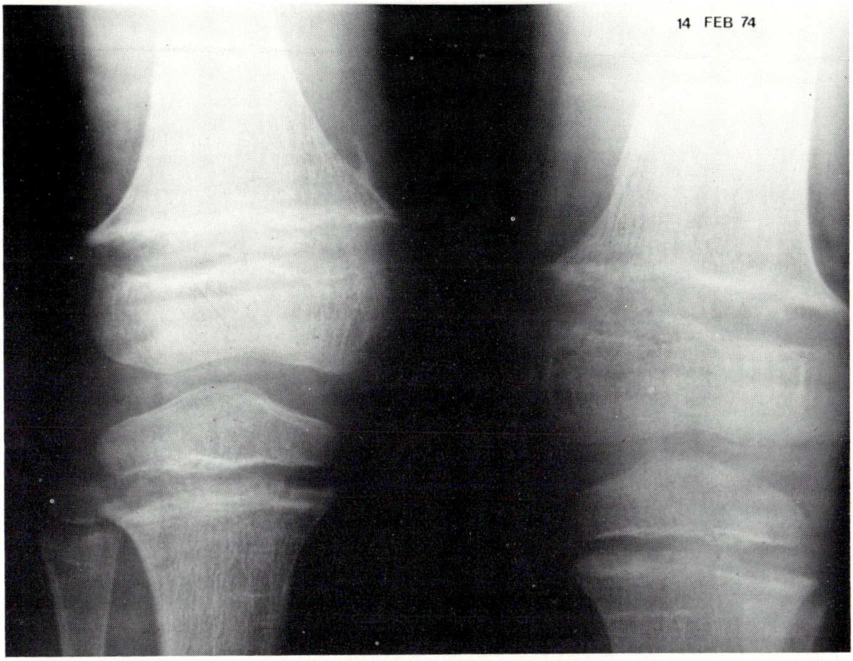

Fig. 2-2. Gross rickets in a seven year old with myositis ossificans progressiva, produced by exclusion both of dietary vitamin D and of sunshine (he wore a perspex "space-helmet" out of doors). Progress of the primary disease was not discouraging. (Earlier x-rays are shown in Fig. 2-5, patient of the late Professor C. E. Dent, London.)

vitamin D metabolites. We will consider below the action of cholestyramine in binding bile-acids. Vitamin D is hydroxylated in liver to its 25-hydroxyderivative and this compound (25-OH D) is the major circulating metabolite. 25-OH D is hydroxylated further in kidney tubules to a true hormone, 1,25-dihydroxyvitamin D (D_2 or D_3) which is the active principle in target organs, intestine, bone and possibly others. Synthesis of 1,25-dihydroxyvitamin D ($1,25(OH)_2D$) is meticulously regulated by mechanisms chief among which is stimulation by parathyroid hormone. Compounds which interfere with $1,25(OH)_2D$ production may therefore be potent causes of drug-induced rickets. $1,25(OH)_2D$ prevents its specific deficiency disease(s), rickets and osteomalacia, by its actions in promoting active intestinal transport of calcium and phosphorus and in resorbing bone in areas of provisional calcification.[1,3,4] Drugs may interfere with target organ actions of $1,25(OH)_2D$, or may themselves produce bone changes similar to rickets.

We can now fit into this scheme the wide variety of drugs and chemicals that interfere with one or more of these steps. They are classified in Table 2-1 according to the site at which they interfere with vitamin D metabolism.

Purgatives

Purgatives, even when abused over long periods, must be an extremely rare cause of osteomalacia. Hypocalcemia and tetany have been reported without correction for hypoalbuminaemia,[5-7] but these abnormalities are likely to be multifactorial and associated with alkalosis, hypokalemia, hypomagnesaemia and other deficiencies. Osteomalacia has been described on very few occasions[8,9] and has been associated with arthropathy.[10] Osteomalacia in this situation is also likely to be multifactorial and could be associated with dietary vitamin D deficiency, sunshine

Table 2-1
Drug- and Chemical-Induced Osteomalacia

Agents are listed according to their known (or presumed) sites of action. Possible or presumed actions are shown with a question mark. Agents active in experimental situations only are given in parentheses.

A. Acting in the small intestine.
   1. Purgatives; e.g. phenolphthalein, ricinoleic acid, and many other combinations.
   2. Cholestyramine.
   3. Phosphate-binders; aluminium hydroxide, magnesium hydroxide.

B. Acting in the liver (enzyme-inducing drugs).
   4. Anticonvulsants;* phenobarbitone
      phenytoin
      primidone
      pheneturide
      carbamazepine
   5. ? Hypnotics; glutethimide.

C. Acting in kidney.
   6. Metals; cadmium
      (strontium)
      (? beryllium)
   7. ? Acetazolamide.

D. Acting in bone.
   8. Diphosphonates*
   9. Fluoride.

* See text for discussion of additional possible sites of action of anticonvulsants in intestine and bone, and of diphosphonates in kidney.

lack, and even chronic renal failure, which is sometimes observed in these patients.

Cholestyramine

Cholestyramine binds bile-acids in the intestine and is frequently given to control itching in primary biliary cirrhosis and in other forms of long-standing obstructive jaundice. It may reduce vitamin D absoprtion in experimental animals.[11] Clinical osteomalacia after ileal resection has been attributed to cholestyramine.[12] Stronger evidence that cholestyramine may diminish absorption of vitamin D (actually 25-hydroxyvitamin D) and hasten osteomalacia has been reported recently by Compston and Thompson.[13]

Phosphate-Binders

Although sufficient phosphate restriction produces rickets in experimental animals even without vitamin D deficiency, the high phosphorus content of all human diets makes dietary phosphorus deficiency virtually impossible in man. However, it has long been known that non-absorbable antacids containing aluminium hydroxide can bind phosphate in the gut and limit its intestinal absorption.[14] Excessive consumption of aluminium and magnesium hydroxide gels, taken as self-medication for dyspepsia, has been reported as a cause of human osteomalacia.[15,16,17A,17B] Aluminum hydroxide is also regularly prescribed in patients with chronic renal failure and phosphate retention in order to reduce the two dangers of ectopic calcification and hyperparathyroid bone disease (osteitis fibrosa). Overvigorous therapy may more readily produce osteomalacia in this situation.[17]

Anticonvulsant Drugs

Since the first reports of an osteopathy occurring among epileptic patients receiving these drugs[18,19] and its confirmation as osteomalacia[20] a vast amount of experimental, clinical and epidemiological data has been accumulated. Although florid, clinical rickets and osteomalacia are rare, case reports have carefully excluded other etiologies and emphasized the metabolic (i.e., vitamin D-resistant) nature of the disorder (Fig. 2-3).[20–25]

The first biochemical survey of epileptic patients was conducted by Richens and Rowe[26], who recorded hypocalcemia in 22 percent and raised alkaline phosphatase levels in 28 percent: both bone and liver phos-

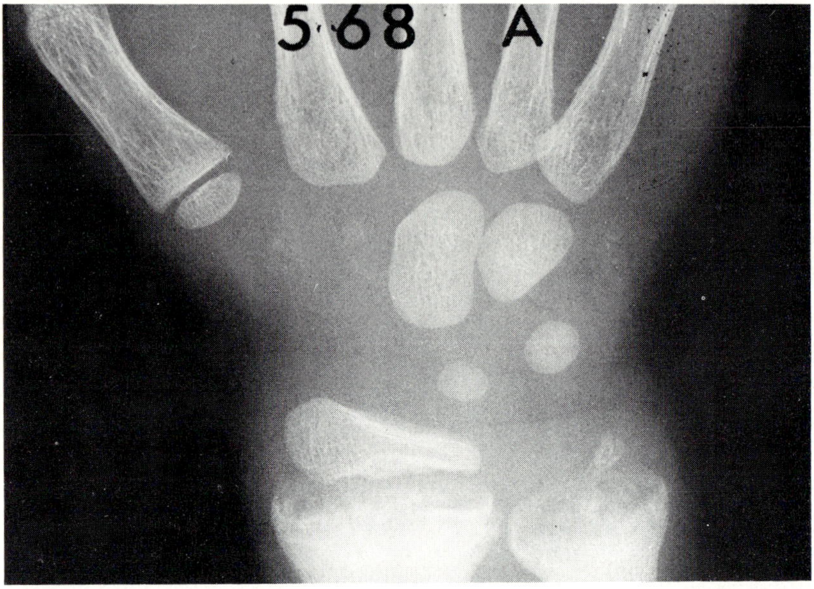

Fig. 2-3A. Anticonvulsant rickets treated 4 mo. with vitamin D 1000 i.u./day.

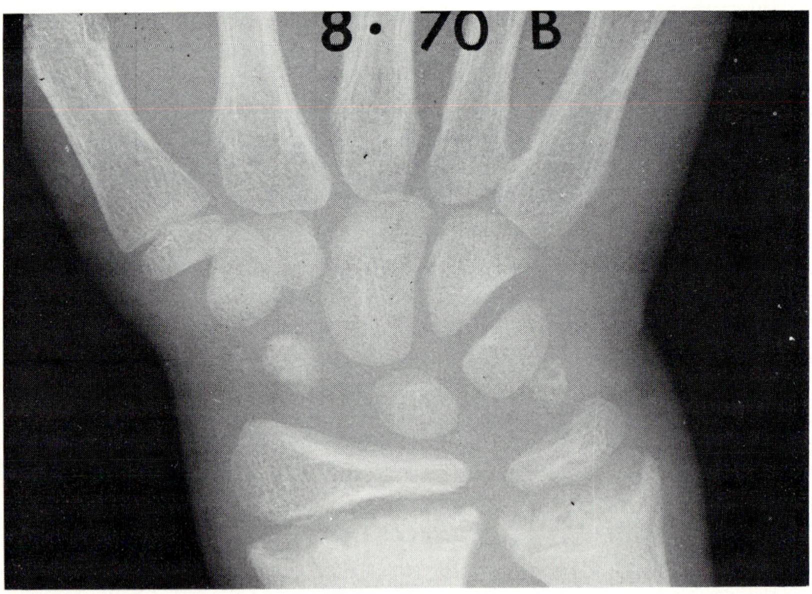

Fig. 2-3B. Anticonvulsant rickets treated further 27 mo. with increasing doses of vitamin D (1600 i.u./day plus two parenteral injections).

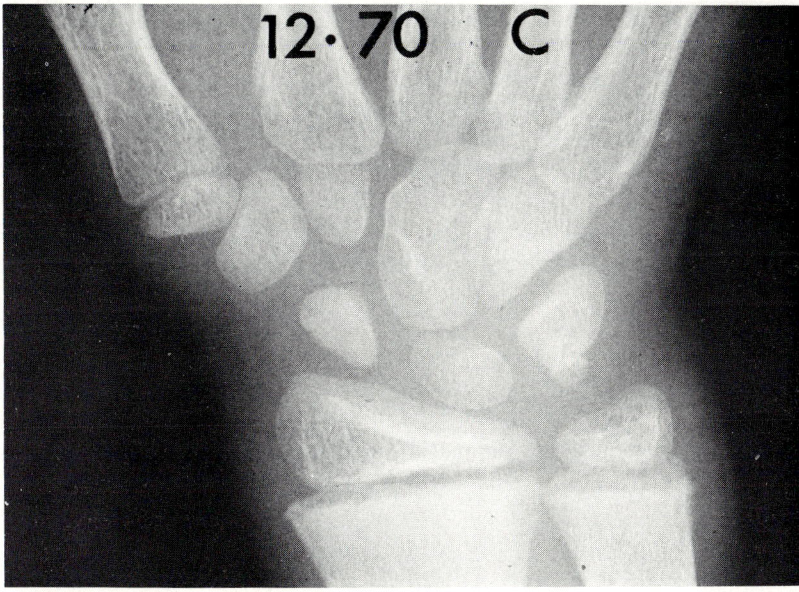

Fig. 2-3C. Anticonvulsant rickets treated 4 mo. with still higher doses of vitamin D (5000 i.u./day).

phatase iso-enzymes were significantly raised. Since then a number of surveys on both sides of the Atlantic have amply confirmed the scale of these disturbances, hypocalcemia sometimes occurring less frequently (seven percent was the lowest incidence) and raised alkaline phosphatase being sometimes seen in over 40 percent.[27-33] Not all workers have accepted these figures uncritically, some believing that changes are virtually confined to the mentally retarded.[34] Nevertheless, most workers now accept the evidence as overwhelming. Several early case reports carried confirmatory histological proof of osteomalacia, and more recent histological surveys based on iliac crest bone biopsies have reported abnormalities consistent with osteomalacia in as many as over 50 percent of patients.[35,36]

All the anticonvulsant drugs incriminated in osteomalacia have the ability to induce hepatic microsomal enzyme synthesis.[37,38] Such enzymes are mixed function oxidases involving the cytochrome P450 system and, through mechanisms of hydroxylation, conjugation, and transfer reactions, they play an important role in the catabolism and excretion of numerous drugs and endogenous metabolites including steroid hormones. The first survey of Richens and Rowe related the degree of hypocalcemia to drug dosage.[26] This was followed by another study relating the degree of hypocalcemia to indices of enzyme induction.[27] The first contention that osteomalacia was produced by enzyme induction that enhanced vitamin D catabolism through pathways other than (physiological) 25-hydroxylation was speculative and based on circumstantial evidence only.[20] It was soon followed, however, by firmer evidence: low 25-OH D levels were found among epileptics in general[21] as well as in relation to dietary vitamin D intake.[28] Furthermore, experimental studies appeared to confirm a catabolic effect of anticonvulsants on vitamin D metabolism in vitro.[39] All patients with frank clinical osteomalacia have had appropriately deficient 25-OH D levels whenever these have been measured, and unequivocal proof of a causative role of the appropriate drugs in experimental rickets has recently been forthcoming.[40] One report has partially incriminated the enzyme-inducing hypnotic agent glutethimide as a further cause of osteomalacia.[41]

Nevertheless, a growing body of evidence suggests that enzyme induction is not the sole mechanism by which these drugs disturb mineral metabolism. First, phenytoin inhibits parathyroid hormone-induced bone resorption in tissue culture—a form of functional hypoparathyroidism. Phenobarbitone does not have this property although it is, experimentally, the strongest enzyme-inducing drug. Second, phenytoin inhibits $1,25(OH)_2D$-stimulated calcium transport in intestinal organ culture, hardly a result of enzyme induction.[43] Phenytoin which, experimentally, is not as strong an enzyme-inducing drug as phenobarbitone, is in the writer's experience of 12 florid cases of osteomalacia the only consistently associated drug.[20,21,25] Third, in a group of patients with biochemical abnormalities suggestive of osteomalacia (other status unknown), circulating $1,25(OH)_2D$ levels may be normal.[44] Finally, treatment with 25-OH D_3 may not restore low ionised plasma calcium to normal, and treatment with vitamin D, although it abolishes the correlation between plasma calcium and plasma 25-OH D in these patients, may not alter the strong correlation between plasma total calcium and other indices of enzyme induction.[45] Fig. 2-4 shows the effect of enzyme-inducing drugs on indices of calcium metabolism and enzyme induction in a population of 47 adolescent males resident in a hospital school and, therefore, reasonably controlled for diet and sunshine exposure. Those on drugs were taking a wide range including phenytoin, primidone, carbamazepine, ethosuximide, methsuximide, diazepam, sulthiame and sodium valproate of which only the first three are known enzyme inducers; through that hospital's practice none were taking phenobarbitone. Because of the enormous problem of classifying drug intake and dosage, the simplest scheme was adopted. Patients were grouped according to whether they were taking no enzyme-inducing drugs (Group 1), one such drug (Group 2), or more than one of the first three in the above list (Group 3). All other

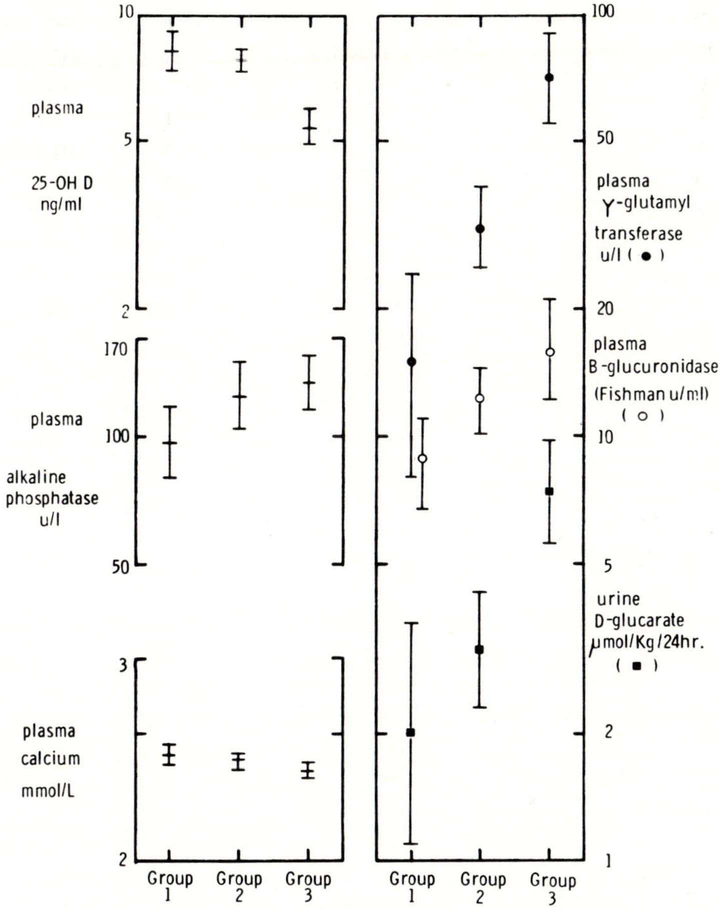

Fig. 2-4. Mean plasma levels of calcium, alkaline phosphatase, 25-OH D, γ-glutamyl transpeptidase, β-glucuromidase and urinary D-glucarate excretion in 49 boys grouped according to drug treatment (see text.) Bars indicate mean and limits of 2 × SEM after log transformation and reconversion (from Ref. 45, with permission of the publishers).

influences were therefore broadly controlled. The effects of these drugs were well illustrated.

The relationships between indices of calcium metabolism and of enzyme induction, and the effects of vitamin D treatment (vitamin D_3 0.25 mg. orally for eight weeks, followed three months later by follow-up) in this same population are shown in Table 2-2.[45] These data strongly suggest that plasma calcium relationships in epilepsy are not primarily mediated

Table 2-2
Baseline, Treatment, and Follow-up Correlation Coefficients (r) Among Total Population

		log plasma y-GT	log urine D-glucarate excret'n: conc'n:	Plasma calcium
log Plasma 25-OHD:	Baseline	−0.46**	−0.39**	0.31*
	Vit. D-treatment	−0.20 (NS)	—	0.02 (NS)
	Follow-up	−0.29 (NS)	—	0.28 (NS)
Plasma calcium:	Baseline	−0.52**	−0.25 (NS) −0.35**	
	Vit. D-treatment	−0.48**	—	
	Follow-up	−0.56**	—	
Urine D-glucarate:	Baseline	0.56**	(excretion)	

* $p < 0.05$; ** $p < 0.01$; NS = not significant

by the state of vitamin D nutrition, which was restored to a high level in all these patients.

It seems likely that, in addition to problems of diminished dietary vitamin D intake and restricted sunshine exposure in epileptic patients, drug-mediated abnormalities in calcium and bone metabolism may be multifactorial. The relative importance of any of the factors discussed is likely to prove extremely difficult to establish. Complicating the issue still further is the observation by Dent and Watson[46] that grand mal epilepsy was a feature in seven of their 80 younger patients with pure *osteoporosis* studed in a metabolic ward. Most of these patients led normal lives while on small doses of phenobarbitone only, and the possible involvement of this drug in the etiology of osteoporosis must be questionable. A problem of osteoporosis in epilepsy may, however, further confuse interpretation of x-rays or of bone mineral densitometry.

Metals—Particularly Cadmium

Heavy metals such as cadmium, mercury, gold and lead have long been known for their nephrotoxic effects in man.[47] Long-term cadmium exposure is a particular industrial hazard in the cadmium pigment industry[48] and among alkaline battery workers.[49] In all these cases a Fanconi syndrome may result, with renal tubular proteinuria, glycosuria, phosphaturia, amino-aciduria, acidosis and osteomalacia. More recently, disease endemic to the Jintzu and Itchi river basins in Toyama Prefecture (Japan), known since the 1940s as itai-itai (literally "ouch-ouch") disease has been confirmed as being caused by cadmium poisoning from industrial effluent.[50]

Cadmium binds to a specific protein, a metallothionein in the kidney. Whether toxic effects are exerted only by the ionic cadmium remaining after saturation of the binding protein with the metal is not known, nor is the mechanism of cadmium intoxication fully understood. There is evidence that free cadmium ion may inhibit the renal tublar ATP-Na-K-ATPase transport system.[51] Recent work suggests that altered membrane permeability may be a cause of transport defects in the experimental toxic Fanconi syndrome produced by sodium maleate.[52] Possible interference by cadmium and other heavy metals in renal tubular or intestinal vitamin D metabolism is uncertain, but cadmium is particularly effective in displacing calcium from the vitamin D-dependent calcium-binding protein system.[53]

Other forms of rickets produced by metals are of theoretical interest only. Industrial beryllium poisoning (berylliosis) is not associated with the rickets that experimental poisoning can produce. The mechanism of such rickets is unknown: earliest work showed interference with alkaline phosphatase, but complex beryllium compounds have peculiar effects in bone characterised by marked endosteal bone proliferation and frequent progression to osteogenic sarcoma.[54] Work has not been done to establish whether beryllium has similar effects on vitamin D metabolism to strontium. Strontium, when replacing calcium in the diet, is known to induce severe vitamin D resistant rickets. Corradino and Wasserman[55] showed that intestinal calcium resorption was depressed in this condition, and De Luca and co-workers proved that strontium acted by severely inhibiting renal $1{,}25(OH)_2D$ production.[56]

Acetazolamide

The diuretic acetazolamide, a carbonic anhydrase inhibitor, has not been proved to cause osteomalacia. However, two cases of severe anticonvulsant osteomalacia have been reported in which acetazolamide, given concurrently with standard agents for control of atypical seizures, may have accelerated development of the disease.[57] In these patients discontinuation of acetazolamide produced a marked fall in urinary calcium excretion and a rise in renal tubular phosphate reabsorption (without change in serum levels of either). It is clearly possible that the renal effects of acetazolamide, suggested by these observations, contributed to the bone mineral abnormality.

Diphosphonates

These compounds are analogues of pyrophosphate and contain a P-C-P bond in place of the P-O-P bond of pyrophosphate. They are resistant to the ubiquitous pyrophosphatases in vivo and inhibit both accretion and dissolution of hydroxyapatite crystals in vitro. They have marked effects on mineral metabolism in vivo and the prototype ethane hydroxy-1-diphosphonate (EHDP, Sodium etidronate) is marketed in the United States for the treatment of Pagets disease of bone. Long term studies have shown both symptomatic relief of bone pain in this disease and improvement in the biochemical indices with falling levels of plasma alkaline phosphatase and urinary total hydroxyproline excretion.[58-60] However, experimentally and in humans, higher doses (15–20 mg. per kg. body weight) have been clearly shown to produce histological osteomalacia[60,61] and pathological fractures have been noted in treated patients on these dosages.[62] This property of EHDP in inhibiting mineralization of osteoids has been employed in the treatment of myositis (fibrodysplasia) ossificans progressiva. Figure 2-5 shows the development and progress of a pathological fracture (result of tripping on a living room carpet) in a five year old boy with the disease who had been receiving

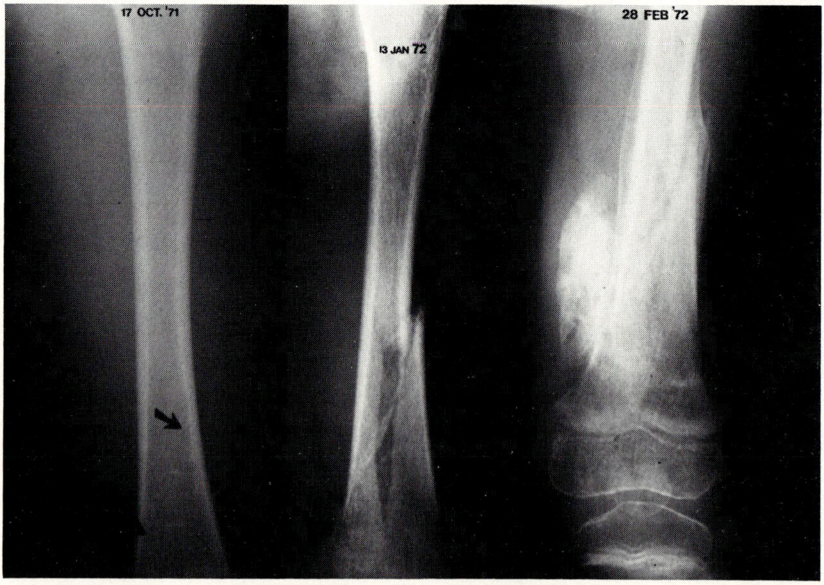

Fig. 2-5. Inhibition of mineralization in a pathological fracture produced by diphosphonate therapy in a 5 year old with myositis ossificans progressiva, with permission of the publishers (Ref. 63.) See text for discussion.

EHDP treatment (20 mg/kg) for one month before his minor accident. Three months later there was no radiological evidence of calcification in callus (Fig. 2-5b) although the fracture appeared clinically united. EHDP was discontinued because of the unacceptable x-ray appearance, and one month later, abundant calcification had occurred (Fig. 2-5c). The calcifications became permanent, indicating that muscle tissue had ossified. (This patient is the same as that illustrated in Fig. 2-2, two years earlier and before vitamin D restriction had begun.)

In addition to the direct action of EHDP on bone, the compound also profoundly affects vitamin D metabolism in the renal tubule. In high concentration it severely inhibits $1,25(OH)_2D$ production.[56] While this property would be expected to contribute to the rickets experimentally, in clinical practice the dosage levels prescribed are far below those at which this renal effect is seen. EHDP does have a second renal effect, however, which may be observed regularly in patients under treatment—namely, an increase in renal tubular phosphate reabsorption, which produces a mild rise in plasma phosphorus levels.

Fluoride

Excessive ingestion of fluoride over many years produces the classical appearances of fluorosis, with the extreme increase in bone density that is so striking radiographically. Associated with this is extra-skeletal ossification usually visible as bone spicules radiating out from the ribs, pelvis and other bones into aponeuroses, ligaments and tendon insertions. Degrees of marrow cavity obliteration are also seen. Despite its density fluorotic bone is weaker than normal and pathological fracture can occur.

Fluorosis is an industrial hazard in aluminium workers and also occurs endemically where water supplies (usually well water) contain high concentrations of fluoride (at least 20 parts per million, compared with the one part per million recommended for prophyllaxis of dental caries). It is seen in pockets throughout the world, particularly in parts of the Persian Gulf, Nigeria and northern India.

Histological appearances show excessive osteoblastic activity with poor mineralization of abundant osteoid and some evidence of increased osteoclastic resorption—an osteomalacic picture.[64,65] Evidence of secondary hyperparathyroidism is forthcoming from other sources.[66,67]

If fluoride is administered with heavy calcium supplements to women with post-menopause osteoporosis, with or without extra vitamin D, histological and microradiographical appearances improve. Such regimes have received long-term trials and enthusiastic support from their adherents.[68-70] Whether simultaneous calcium supplements will prevent ultimate fluorosis in treated osteoporotic patients, and whether improved histology will ultimately mean no more vertebral crush fractures or height loss in these patients remain to be seen.

CONCLUSION

Any complex metabolic pathway requiring and involving the participation of different organs and systems may be disrupted, at some point, by a wide variety of drugs and chemicals. The vitamin D endocrine system surveyed here illustrates this point well. Other drugs yet to be developed will doubtless be seen to exert unwanted side effects somewhere in this pathway.

REFERENCES

1. Stamp TCB: Vitamin D Metabolism. Recent Advances Arch Dis Childh 48:2–7, 1973
2. Stamp TCB, Round JM: Nature (London) 247:563–565, 1974
3. De Luca HF: Recent advances in our understanding of the vitamin D endocrine system. J Lab Clin Med 87(1):7–26, 1976
4. Haussler MR, McCain TA: Basic and clinical concepts related to vitamin D metabolism and action. New Eng J Med 297:974–983, 1041–1050, 1977
5. Coghill NF, McAllen PM, Edwards F: Electrolyte losses associated with the taking of purges investigated with the aid of sodium and potassium radioistopes. Br Med J 1:14–19, 1959
6. Rawson MD: Cathartic colon. Lancet 1:1121–1124, 1966
7. Staffurth JS, Allott EN: Paralysis and tetany due to simultaneous hypokalaemia and hypocalcaemia, with other metabolic changes. Amer J Med 33:800–806, 1962
8. Meulengracht E: Osteomalacia of spine following abuse of laxatives. Lancet 2:774–776, 1938
9. Frame B, Guiang HL, Frost HM, et al: Osteomalacia induced by laxative (phenolphthalein) ingestion. Arch Intern Med 128:794
10. Frier BM, Scott RDM: Osteomalacia and arthropathy associated with prolonged abuse of purgatives. Br J Clin Pract 31(1–3):17–19, 1977
11. Thompson WG, Thompson GR: Effect of cholestyramine on the absorption of vitamin D_3 and calcium. Gut 10:717–722, 1969
12. Heaton KW, Lever JW, Barnard D: Osteomalacia associated with cholestyramine therapy for postiliectomy diarrhoea. Gastroenterology 62:642–646, 1972
13. Compston JE, Thompson RPH: Intestinal absorption of 25-hydroxyvitamin D and osteomalacia in primary biliary cirrhosis. Lancet i:721–724, 1977
14. Fawley GB, Ivy AC, Terry I, et al: Attempt to prevent postoperative jejunal ulcer by aluminium hydroxide therapy. Amer J Digest Dis 5:792–796, 1939
15. Lotz, M, Ney R, Bartter FC: Osteomalacia and debility resulting from phosphorus depletion. Trans Assoc Am Phys 77:281–295, 1964
16. Dent CE, Winter C: Osteomalacia due to phosphate depletion from excess aluminum hydroxide ingestion. Br Med J 1:551–552, 1974
17. Baker L, Ackrill P, Cattell WR, et al: Iatrogenic osteomalacia and myopathy due to phosphate depletion. Br Med J 3:150–152, 1974

17A. Cooke N, Teitelbaum S, Avioli LV: Antacid induced osteomalacia and nephrolithiasis. Arch Int Med 138:1007–1009, 1978
17B. Bloom WL, Flinchum D: Osteomalacia with pseudofracture caused by the ingestion of aluminum hydroxide. JAMA 174:1327–1330, 1960
18. Schmid F: Osteopathien bei antiepileptischer Dauerbehandlung. Fortschr Med 85:381–385, 1967
19. Kruse R: Osteopathien bei antiepileptischer langzeittherapie (vorlaufige Mitteilung). Monatsschr Kinderheilk 116:378–381, 1968
20. Dent CE, Richens A, Rowe DJF, et al: Osteomalacia with anticonvulsant therapy in epilepsy. Br Med J 4:69–72, 1970
21. Stamp TCB, Round JM, Rowe DJF, et al: Plasma levels and therapeutic effect of 25-hydroxycholecalciferol in epileptic patients taking anticonvulsant drugs. Br Med J 4:9–12, 1972
22. Borgstedt AD, Dryson MF, Young LW, et al: Long term administration of antiepileptic drugs and the development of rickets. J Paediat 81:9–13
23. Genuth SM, Klein L, Rabinovitch S, et al: Osteomalacia accompanying chronic anticonvulsant therapy. J Endocrinol Metab 35:378–380, 1972
24. Sotaniemi EA, Hakkarainen HK, Puranen JA, et al: Radiologic bone changes and hypocalcaemia with anticonvulsant therapy in epilepsy. Ann Intern Med 77:389–394, 1972
25. Stamp TCB: Effects of long-term anticonvulsant therapy on calcium and vitamin D metabolism. Proc Roy Soc Med 64:69–72, 1974
26. Richens A, Rowe DJF: Disturbance of calcium metabolism by anticonvulsant drugs. Br Med J 4:73–76, 1970
27. Hunter J, Maxwell JC, Stewart DA, et al: Altered calcium metabolism in epileptic children on anticonvulsants. Br Med J 4:202–204, 1971
28. Hahn TJ, Hendin BA, Scharp CR, et al: Effect of chronic anticonvulsant therapy on serum 25-hydroxycalciferol levels in adults. New Eng J Med 287:900–904, 1972
29. Lifschitz F, Maclaren NK: Vitamin D-dependent rickets in institutionalized, mentally retarded children receiving long-term anticonvulsant therapy. 1. A survey of 288 patients. J Paediatr 83:612–620, 1973
30. Tolman KG, Jubiz W, Sannella JJ, et al: Osteomalacia associated with anticonvulsant drug therapy in mentally retarded children. Paediatrics 56:45–51, 1975
31. Hahn TJ, Hendin BA, Scharp CR, et al: Serum 25-hydroxycalciferol levels and bone mass in children on chronic anticonvulsant therapy. New Eng J Med 292:550–554, 1975
32. Crosley CJ, Chee C, Berman PH: Rickets associated with long-term anticonvulsant therapy in a pediatric outpatient population. Pediatrics 56:52–57, 1975
33. Winnacker JA, Yeager H, Saunders JA, et al: Rickets in children receiving anticonvulsant drugs. Am J Dis Child 131:286–290, 1977
34. Livingston S, Berman W, Pauli LL: Anticonvulsant drugs and vitamin D metabolism. J Amer Med Ass 224:1634–1635, 1973
35. Mosekilde L, Melsen F: Anticonvulsant osteomalacia determined by quantitative analysis of bone changes. Acta Med Scand 199:349–355, 1976
36. Mosekilde L, Christensen MS, Lund B, et al: The interrelationships between serum 25-hydroxycholecalciferol, serum parathyroid hormone and bone changes in anticonvulsant osteomalacia. Acta Endocrinol 84:559–565, 1977
37. Conney AH: Pharmacological implications of microsomal enzyme induction. Pharmacol Rev 19:317–366, 1967
38. Kuntzman R: Drugs and enzyme induction. Ann Rev Pharmacol 9:21–26, 1969
39. Hahn TJ, Birge SJ, Scharp CR, et al: Phenobarbital-induced alterations in vitamin D metabolism. J Clin Invest 51:741–748, 1972

40. Harris M, Rowe DJF, Darby AJ: Anticonvulsant osteomalacia induced in the rat by diphenylhydantoin. Calc Tiss Res 25:13–18, 1978
41. Greenwood RH, Prunty FTG, Silver J: Osteomalacia after prolonged glutethimide administration. Br Med J 1:643–645, 1973
42. Jenkins MV, Harris M, Wills MR: The effect of phenytoin on parathyroid extract and 25-hydroxycholecalciferol-induced bone resorption: adenosine 3′,5′ cyclic monophosphate production. Calc Tiss Res 16:163–167, 1974
43. Corradino RA: Diphenylhydantoin: direct inhibition of the vitamin D_3-mediated calcium absorptive mechanism in organ-cultured duodenum. Biochem Pharmacol 25:863–864, 1976
44. Jubiz W, Haussler MR, McCain TA, et al: Plasma 1,25-dihydroxyvitamin D levels in patients receiving anticonvulsant drugs. J Clin Endocrinol Metab 44:617–621, 1977
45. Stamp TCB, Flanagan RJ, Richens A, et al: Anticonvulsant osteomalacia, in, Copp DH, Talmage RV (eds): Endocrinology of Calcium Metabolism. Amsterdam, Excerpta Medica, 16–22, 1978
46. Dent CE, Watson L: Osteoporosis. Postgrad Med J suppl. October, 1966
47. Nicaud P, Lafitte A, Gros A: Les troubles de l'intoxication chronique par le cadmium. Arch Mal Prof 4:192–202, 1947
48. Kazantzis G, Flynn FV, Spowage JS, et al: Renal tubular malfunction and pulmonary emphysema in cadmium pigment workers. Quart J Med 32:165–192, 1963
49. Adams RG, Harrison JF, Scott P: The development of cadmium-induced proteinuria, impaired renal function and osteomalacia in alkaline battery workers. Quart J Med 38:425–443, 1969
50. Nogawa K, Ishikazi A, Fukushima M, et al: Studies on the women with acquired Fanconi syndrome observed in the Itchi river basin polluted by cadmium. Environmental Res 10:280–307, 1975
51. Gonick H, Indraprasit S, Neustein H, et al: Cadmium-induced experimental Fanconi syndrome. Curr Probl Clin Biochem 4:111–118, 1976
52. Bergeron M, Dubord L, Hausser C, et al: Membrane permeability as a cause of transport defects in experimental Fanconi syndrome. J Clin Invest 57:1181–1189, 1976
53. Wasserman RH, Taylor AN, Fullmer CS: Vitamin D-induced calcium-binding protein and the intestinal absorption of calcium, in Fraser DR (ed): The Metabolism and Function of Vitamin D. Biochem Soc Spec Publ (London) 3:55–74, 1974
54. Schneider M, Resnick MI, Wellmann K: Increased bone formation in rabbits following intravenous and intra-osseous injection of zinc beryllium selicate. Clin Orthop 92:251–259, 1973
55. Corradino RA, Wasserman RH: Strontium inhibition of vitamin D_3-induced calcium-binding protein (Ca BP) and calcium absorption in chick intestine. Proc Soc Exp Biol Med 133:960–963, 1970
56. De Luca HF: Regulation of functional vitamin D metabolism: a new endocrine system involved in calcium homeostasis, in Fraser DR (ed): The Metabolism and Function of Vitamin D. Biochem Soc Spec Publ (London) 3:5–26, 1964
57. Mallette LE: Acetazolamide-accelerated anticonvulsant osteomalacia. Arch Intern Med 137:1013–1017, 1977
58. Russell RGG, Smith R, Preston C, et al: Diphosphonates in Pagets disease. Lancet 1:894–898, 1974
59. Hosking DJ, Bijvoet OLM, Aken JV, et al: Pagets bone disease treated with diphosphonate and calcitonin. Lancet 1:615–617, 1976
60. Khairi MRA, Altman RD, De Rosa GP, et al: Sodium etidronate in the treatment of Pagets disease of bone. A study of long-term results. Ann Intern Med 87:646–663, 1977

61. Russell RGG, Fleisch H: Pyrophosphate and diphosphonates in skeletal metabolism. Clin Orthop 108:241–263, 1975
62. Kantrowitz FG, Byrne MH, Schiller A, et al: Clinical and biochemical effects of diphosphonates in Pagets disease of bone. Arth Rheum 18:407, 1975
63. Dent CE: Metabolic forms of rickets (and osteomalacia), in, Bickel H, Stern J (ed): Inborn Errors of Calcium and Bone Metabolism, Lancaster, MTP Press, p 141, 1974
64. Burkhart JM, Jowsey J: Effect of variations in calcium intake on the skeleton of fluoride-fed kittens. J Lab Clin Med 72:943–950, 1968
65. Jowsey J, Schenk RK, Reutter FW: Some results of the effect of fluoride on bone tissue in osteoporosis. J Clin Endocrinol Metab 28:869–874, 1968
66. Faccini JM, Care AD: Effect of sodium fluoride on the ultra-structure of the parathyroid glands of the sheep. Nature 207:1399–1401, 1965
67. Teotia SPS, Teotia M: Secondary hyperparathyroidism in patients with endemic skeletal fluorosis. Br Med J 1:637–640, 1973
68. Jowsey J, Kelly PJ, Hoffman DL: Effect of combined therapy with sodium fluoride, vitamin D and calcium in osteoporosis. Amer J Med 53:43–49, 1972
69. Riggs BL, Jowsey J, Kelly PJ, Hoffman DL, Arnaud CD: Studies on pathogenesis and treatment in post-menopausal and senile osteoporosis, in, Clinics in Endocrinology and Metabolism, Vol. 2. Philadelphia, WB Saunders Co, 1973, pp 317–332
70. Jowsey J: Metabolic Diseases of Bone. Philadelphia, WB Saunders, 1977, pp 296–304

Barbara M. Rohlfing
John L. Stauffer

3 Drug-Induced Pulmonary Disease

Pulmonary complications account for but five percent of all drug-induced disease; however, since five percent of all hospitalizations are for treatment of drug-induced disease, and 18 percent of all hospitalized patients develop adverse drug reactions, the number of cases of drug-induced pulmonary disease is relatively large and increasing with the current rapid expansion of the pharmacopoeia.[1] The mechanisms by which drug therapy may result in adverse reactions are multiple (Table 3-1). Although the number of drugs capable of causing pulmonary disease is also great, the ability of the lung to respond to these is limited (Table 3-2). The majority of the various pulmonary manifestations of drug-induced diseases may be divided into the four groups to be discussed in this chapter: Pulmonary fibrosis, pulmonary infiltrates, systemic lupus erythematosus syndromes, and hilar and mediastinal diseases. Each of the drugs will be discussed with reference to: 1)incidence, 2)pathology induced, 3)clinical signs and symptoms of toxicity, 4)laboratory findings, 5)roentgenographic findings, and 6)therapy.

PULMONARY FIBROSIS

Drug therapy may cause pulmonary disease by producing either parenchymal fibrosis or pleural fibrosis, or both (Table 3-3). The drugs in question will be discussed in their approximate order of clinical significance.

gen exposure, and cortisone administration, in which, though the reactions are similar, there is desquamation of *intact* cells without loss of lamellated bodies. The classical bizarre type II pneumocytes may be identified in sputum and bronchial washings, although one must take care not to confuse them with neoplastic cells, to which they bear some resemblances.[14]

The main clinical difference among manifestations of busulfan, cyclophosphamide, and bleomycin toxicity is the time of onset of abnormality.[14] Clinically, the patient presents with insidious onset of cough, fever without leukocytosis, and dyspnea. Dry, end-inspiratory rales are heard. Pulmonary function testing in busulfan toxicity shows a marked decrease in diffusing capacity.[15] Although a decreased diffusing capacity may occur with bleomycin toxicity, the only consistent abnormality of pulmonary function testing is a marked decrease in forced vital capacity (FVC). A sudden drop in FVC may herald the development of bleomycin fibrosis before clinical symptoms appear,[9] making it a helpful means of early detection.

Gallium 67 citrate has been found to accumulate in pulmonary lesions of bleomycin toxicity, thereby indicating abnormality at the onset of early symptoms, when the radiograph is only minimally abnormal.[16] As this agent also localizes in a wide variety of neoplastic and inflammatory tissue, however, such localization is non-specific.

Radiographs demonstrate a nonsegmental linear interstitial pattern in all three drug toxicities which is most obvious at the bases (Figs. 3-1 A and B).

Steroids have been used in treating the fibrotic reaction of bleomycin[9] with partial or complete success in clearing clinical and radiographic findings. One percent of all bleomycin patients who are treated with steroids die of the pulmonary toxicity, while the morbidity rate is ten percent for patients receiving more than 500 mg. total dose. In those who do respond to steroid therapy, the radiographic appearance and the clinical symptoms may improve markedly over several months. Although steroids have also been used in the treatment of busulfan fibrosis, they appear to be ineffective in this case; death usually ensues within six months of the onset of clinical symptoms. Several cases of cyclophosphamide-induced infiltrates have been treated successfully with steroid therapy.[6]

PARENCHYMAL FIBROSIS DUE TO OTHER CANCER CHEMOTHERAPEUTIC AGENTS

Pulmonary fibrosis has also been reported with cancer chemotherapeutic agents other than busulfan, cyclophosphamide, and bleomycin, but the occurrence of pulmonary toxicity from these agents is much lower; the clinical experience is, therefore, more limited. BCNU [1,3-bis(2-chloroethyl)-1-nitrosourea] has been found to cause hyperplasia of type II alveolar pneumocytes with obliteration of air spaces and thickening of alveolar walls into dense fibrous tissue, and edema.[17,18,19] The reaction has been reported to occur from 22 to 36 months after the beginning of therapy consisting of between 2 and 3.3 g total dose. The clinical presentation is similar to that of busulfan: cough, fever, and dyspnea, without effusion or eosinophilia. Steroids do not appear to be helpful.

Four reports of pulmonary fibrosis following long-term, anti-leukemic chlorambucil therapy have been reported,[20,21] with pulmonary symptoms beginning one to two years after the initiation of therapy. In at least two of these cases, it seems likely that the drug was causative, producing a histological picture somewhat similar to that produced by busulfan. Steroid therapy has been attempted to no avail.

Single reports of pulmonary fibrosis have been reported to have resulted from the anti-neoplastic agent melphalan[22] and the immunosuppressive agent azathioprine.[23] The relationship between the use of the drug and the pulmonary reaction in these patients is not certain; if a relationship does indeed exist, it must be rare.

PULMONARY FIBROSIS DUE TO NITROFURANTOIN

The chronic form of nitrofurantoin pulmonary toxicity is distinctly different from and less common than the acute form (see PULMONARY INFILTRATES); the exact incidence is not certain. The histological picture is most commonly that of nonspecific (''usual'') interstitial pneumonitis with fibrosis[24], although desquamative interstitial pneumonitis may occur.[25] There is no substantial evidence to indicate an immunological basis for the reaction, although the presence of lymphoid aggregates, plasma cells, and eosinophilia in biopsy specimens has raised the suspicion of an underlying immune process.[25] Pulmonary symptoms begin insidiously from six months to six years after the beginning of therapy. Cough and dyspnea appear, but without fever and (unlike the acute reaction) without effusions or eosinophilia. Radiographically, diffuse, non-specific interstitial infiltrates are seen (Fig. 3-1C). The response to steroids and withdrawal of the drug may be favorable, with a return to normal pulmonary well-being following after a few months[25]; this response to therapy is unfortunately the exception rather than the rule.

PULMONARY FIBROSIS DUE TO OXYGEN THERAPY

Oxygen therapy may result in pulmonary infiltrates which, if the oxygen therapy is continued, progress to pulmonary fibrosis.[26,27] The incidence and extent of damage to the alveolar–capillary membrane is

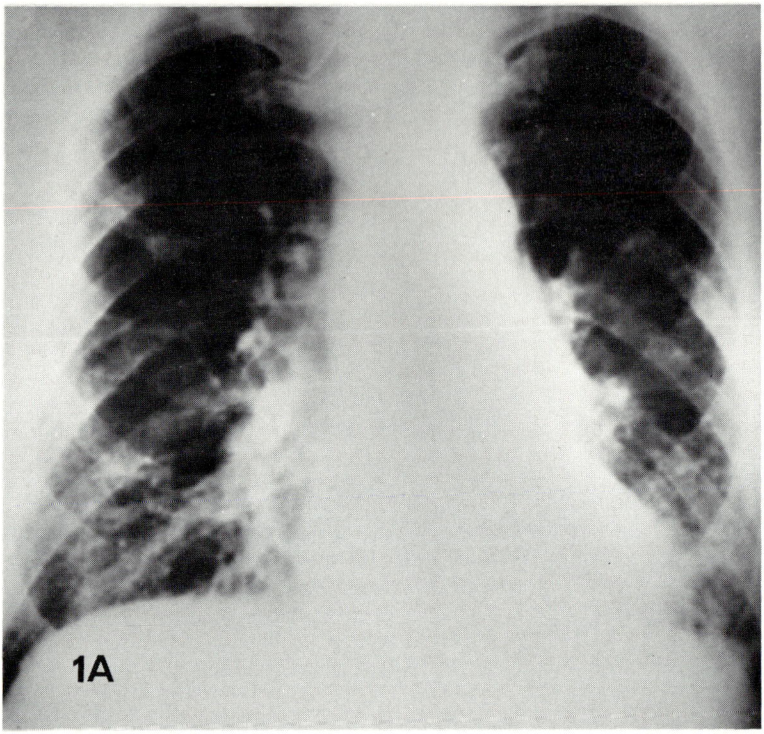

Fig. 3-1A. Pulmonary fibrosis (busulfan interstitial fibrosis.) This patient had been receiving busulfan for several years; his chest radiograph had been normal six months prior. At the time of presentation he complained of chronic dyspnea, cough, and fever. Note the bilateral basilar interstitial fibrosis.

dose-related; with an inspired oxygen content of 100 percent damage may occur within 24 to 48 hours. With inspired oxygen concentrations in the range of 60 to 70 percent, a longer period is needed for the condition to develop.Two phases of the disease exist: an acute exudative stage, and a subacute or chronic proliferative stage. During the early phase, there is edema, vacuolization, and fragmentation of the capillary endothelial cells with leakage of fluid into the interstitium[11], as well as intraalveolar hemorrhage and fibrinous exudates. During the acute phase a nonproductive cough, substernal discomfort, low-grade fever, throat irritation, and increased secretions develop. Ronchi and rales may be heard. As oxygen therapy continues, there is disappearance of type I (membranous) pneumocytes, with subsequent proliferation of type II granular pneumocytes. Desquamation of intact type II pneumocytes results, followed by pulmonary fibrosis. Therapy is directed towards providing for adequate oxygenation with lower levels of inspired oxygen, as may be achieved with positive end expiratory pressure ventilation (PEEP).

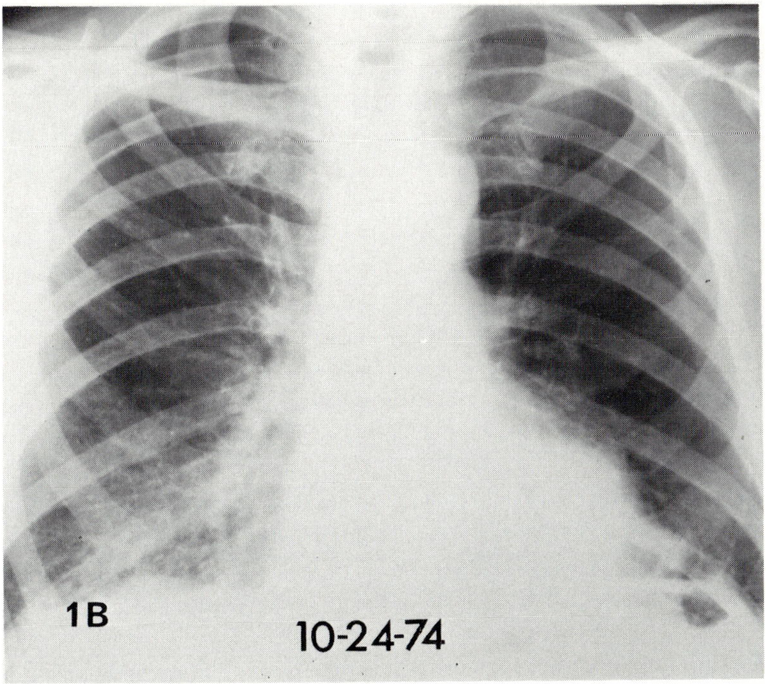

Fig. 3-1B. Pulmonary fibrosis (bleomycin interstitial fibrosis.) This patient had received a total dose of 300 mg. bleomycin when he presented with acute onset of severe dyspnea. The chest radiograph was normal three months prior. There are bibasilar interstitial densities.

Oxygen toxicity also occurs in newborn infants requiring high inspired oxygen for long periods of time. Northway[28] has described four stages of abnormality: Stage 1 occurs several days after the onset of respiratory distress and is manifested radiographically by the "ground glass" appearance of hyaline membrane disease. Stage 2 begins four to ten days after onset of distress and is characterized pathologically by necrosis and repair of alveolar epithelium, with focal thickening of capillary basement membrane and proliferation of pericapillary reticulin, bronchiolar necrosis, squamous metaplasia, and intraluminal exudate. Radiographically, the lungs are opacified, usually with evident air bronchograms. Stage 3 occurs ten to twenty days after the onset of symptoms, with alternating areas of atelectasis and emphysema seen pathologically. This stage assumes a spongy radiographic appearance. Stage 4 develops in those surviving beyond age one month who will require oxygen therapy. In these infants, large emphysematous areas develop, with hypertrophy of the peribronchial smooth muscle; these emphysematous areas are visible radiographically.

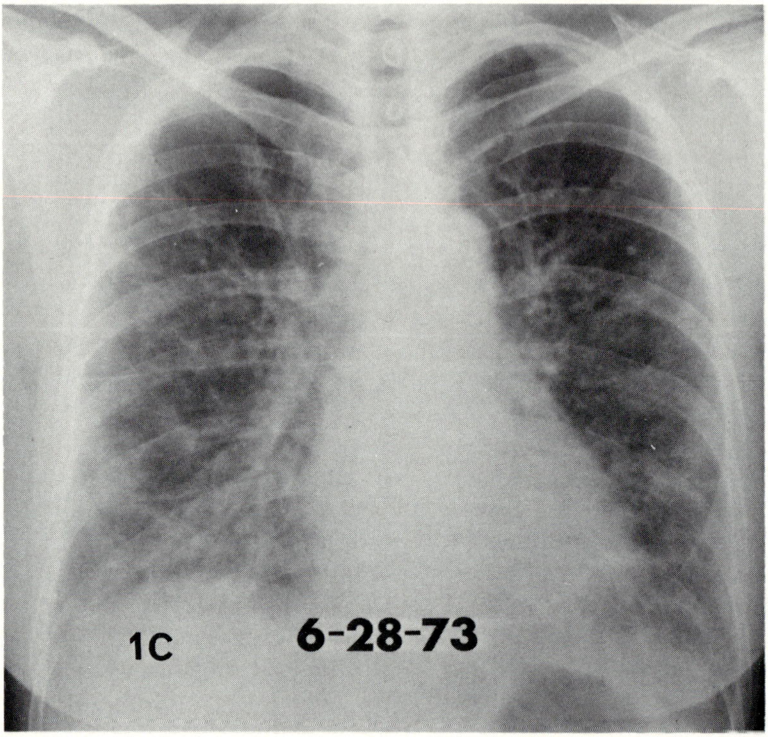

Fig. 3-1C. Pulmonary fibrosis (chronic nitrofurantoin fibrosis.) This patient had been on nitrofurantoin for three years when she presented with a three-month history of cough and dyspnea, but no fever. Her diffusing capacity was markedly decreased and eosinophilia was absent. The diffuse bilateral infiltrates became much less prominent within one month of withdrawal of the drug.

PARENCHYMAL FIBROSIS DUE TO GOLD THERAPY

Gold sodium thiomalate, used in the therapy of arthritis, has resulted in a reversible form of diffuse interstitial pulmonary fibrosis.[29] The reaction has been seen after a total dose of 300 to 400 mg. Biopsy reveals thickened alveolar septae with proliferation of loose fibrous connective tissue, plasma cells, and lymphocytes. Hyperplasia of type II pneumocytes is present, but intra-alveolar desquamation of pneumocytes and alveolar macrophages is absent. The patient presents with chronic cough and dyspnea without fever. The white blood cell count is normal to minimally elevated, with mild eosinophilia (four to five percent). Radiographically, nonspecific interstitial fibrosis is seen at the lung bases; effusions are absent. Resolution of clinical and radiographic findings occurs several weeks or months after sufficient steroid therapy and cessation of intake of the drug.

PARENCHYMAL FIBROSIS DUE TO PARAQUAT

Ingested paraquat, an herbicide, has long been recognized as a potent agent, capable of causing severe, irreversible pulmonary fibrosis.[30] Paraquat is highly toxic in doses as small as 4 mg./kg.[31] Paraquat preferentially accumulates in the lungs; its concentration in the lungs is 50 times its concentration in the plasma, and its half-life in the lungs is weeks, though in the blood it is only hours. The potential for toxicity, therefore, is greatest in the lungs. Early histologic changes, as revealed through electron microscopy, comprise damage to the alveolar epithelium without damage to capillary endothelium. Within days intra-alveolar and interstitial fibrinous edema with hemorrhage, hyaline membrane formation, and epithelial proliferation develop. Selenium deficiency enhances this effect.[32] The mechanism of pulmonary damage is the production of oxygen-free radicals in the lung.[1] Because of this production of lethal oxygen-free radicals oxygen therapy actually enhances the severity of lung damage. With ingestion of large amounts of paraquat, mouth and gastrointestinal ulcers, diarrhea, and renal failure develop one to three days after ingestion. If the patient survives this initial phase, there is a clinically asymptomatic "silent" period of several days before the development of respiratory failure. No more than a week after ingestion, the patient develops severe respiratory failure with diffuse infiltrates, hypoxia with cyanosis, and decreased lung volumes with low compliance and a decreased diffusing capacity. Radiographically, nonspecific interstitial and alveolar edema are seen. Prior modes of therapy (glutathione, D-propanolol, steroids, forced diuresis, potassium iodide expectorants, and gastro-intestinal adsorbants) have been of little or no value; current research is directed at lessening the effects of oxygen-free radicals.* The parenteral use of superoxide dismutase converts the oxygen-free radical, superoxide anion, to hydrogen peroxide; it is hoped that this conversion will lessen the cytotoxic effect of free radicals. Therapy with superoxide dismutase must be continuous to be effective; intermittent use does not improve survival.[33] It may be that other reducing agents, such as Vitamin E, are also helpful in treating this condition. Because of recent allegedly widespread contamination of marijuana by paraquat, it was feared pulmonary fibrosis due to inhaled paraquat might become a major health problem. However, even in clinics where large numbers of heavy marijuana users are seen (those who had smoked allegedly contaminated marijuana),[34] no definite cases of paraquat-induced pulmonary insuf-

* Oxygen-free radicals are compounds with an unpaired electron; because of this property, these radicals appropriate an electron from any available source. In the water milieu within a cell this results in disruption of the water molecule, with cellular disorganization. In addition, as a result of the disruption of water molecules, additional free radicals are formed, resulting in a chain reaction of further molecular disruption.

ficiency or fibrosis have been seen. These patients have been followed for only a few months, however, and long-term effects cannot be excluded.

PULMONARY FIBROSIS DUE TO SULPHASALAZINE

Although sulphasalazine most often causes a hypersensitivity reaction with pulmonary infiltrates and eosinophilia, it has reportedly caused a single case of reversible[35] and a single case of irreversible[36] fibrosing alveolitis. Biopsy evaluation has not included electron microscopy; light microscopy reveals alveoli filled with mononuclear cells, edema fluid, and desquamated cells. The alveolar walls are thickened by fibroblasts and reticulin fibers. Honeycombing with fibrotic destruction of the alveolar pattern is also seen. The onset of symptoms is acute, with dyspnea and hypoxia, but no cough or fever. Eosinophilia (three percent) was present in both cases. Radiographically, bilateral diffuse interstitial densities appear. In one case, removal of the drug and subsequent steroid therapy resulted in clinical and radiographic resolution, as well as disappearance in the eosinophilia; reinstitution of the drug resulted in the recurrence of all findings. In the other case, use of steroids and removal of the drug proved to be to no avail, and the patient died in pulmonary failure.

PULMONARY FIBROSIS DUE TO DIPHENYLHYDANTOIN (PHENYTOIN)

Moore[37] has described the development of diffuse bilateral asymptomatic nodular fibrosis in patients taking hydantoin. The evidence presented, however, was not convincing radiographically, and histopathological proof was not submitted. In addition, in a large study of patients on long-term diphenylhydantoin therapy, Livingston[38] was unable to confirm the occurrence of pulmonary fibrosis. However, Hazlett[39] has found impairment of gas exchange in patients on long-term diphenylhydantoin. Forty patients with normal chest radiography who had taken diphenylhydantoin for more than two years were evaluated; 45 percent had a decreased steady state diffusing capacity (D_{LCO}) and abnormal blood gas tension during exercise. In addition, one half had an abnormally great difference between resting and exercise alveolar-arterial oxygen tensions and/or failed to appropriately increase their D_{LCO} with exercise. Those who had started diphenylhydantoin therapy prior to age eight had abnormalities of gas exchange twice as often as those who began therapy after age eight. As these patients were clinically asymptomatic, no tissue was obtained for pathologic evaluation. Diphenylhydantoin is known to stimulate the growth of normal fibroblasts in tissue culture. A fibrogenic action of the drug may be responsible for these observed abnormalities of gas exchange during its use, and it may be that the effect of this fibrogenic action is greatest on the growing lung. Diphenylhydantoin may also cause pulmonary infiltrates due to a hypersensitivity reaction (see PULMONARY INFILTRATES).

PULMONARY FIBROSIS DUE TO ANTI-HYPERTENSIVE AGENTS (HEXAMETHONIUM, PENTOLINIUM, AND MECAMYLAMINE)

Hexamethonium, pentolinium, and mecamylamine, used in the therapy of hypertension, have been found to cause pulmonary fibrosis[40], but are no longer in use clinically.

Pleural Fibrosis

PLEURAL FIBROSIS DUE TO METHYSERGIDE

Methysergide inhibits or blocks the effects of serotonin, and therefore is used in the treatment of vascular headaches. It is well recognized as a cause of retroperitoneal fibrosis. It may also result in pleural fibrosis, pulmonary fibrosis, localized mass-like pleuro-parenchymal fibrosis (usually in the posterior portion of the lower lobes) and aortic and mitral valve insufficiency.[41] The exact incidence of such pulmonary and cardiac reactions is uncertain, though they probably occur rarely. Cough and dyspnea without fever are the presenting symptoms, occurring insidiously six months to several years after the beginning of therapy. The most common pulmonary manifestation is pleural fibrosis. Eosinophilia is absent; pulmonary function tests reveal restrictive disease. Radiographically, a fine, ground-glass haze is seen overlying the lungs (Fig. 3-2). The pleural, pleuro-parenchymal, and pulmonary fibrosis and the valvular lesions regress when the drug is withdrawn.

PLEURAL FIBROSIS DUE TO PRACTOLOL

Pleural fibrosis has also been found to result from practolol therapy.[42,43] A beta-blocker, anti-hypertensive agent, practolol was withdrawn from the market in 1976 because it caused sclerosing peritonitis and keratitis superficialis; it was never marketed in the U.S. It has now been reported that delayed pleural and parenchymal fibrosis may result, with symptoms of dyspnea beginning in some patients many months after removal of the drug (although all patients, while on the drug, exhibited abnormal chest radiographs.) Pulmonary function tests show diffuse airway obstruction. Effusions may be seen, and gallium-67 citrate scans show pulmonary uptake. A systemic lupus erythematosus syndrome may develop. Steroids are of little use. Although the frequency of pulmonary reaction has been high in patients receiving practolol, the number of

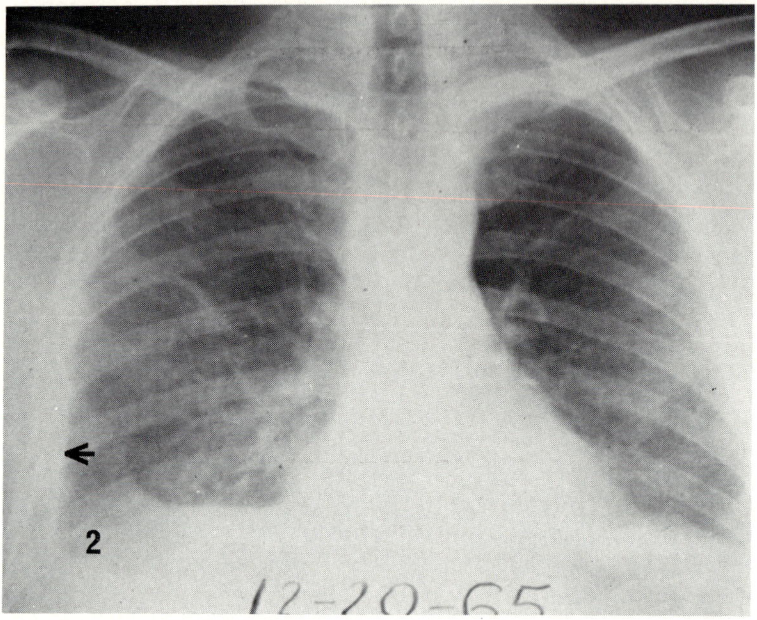

Fig. 3-2. Pleural fibrosis (methysergide pleuropulmonary fibrosis.) This patient had received methesergide for several years for migraine headaches. Note the ill-defined haze, especially on the right, a manifestation of diffuse pleural disease. In addition, pleural thickening can be seen laterally on the right (arrow). A pleural effusion was present on the right as well.

individuals affected is so small that the occurrence of practolol-induced fibrosis is uncommon.

PULMONARY INFILTRATES

Drug-induced pulmonary infiltrates may occur with or without eosinophilia. It is important to differentiate drug-induced disease from the PIE Syndrome (pulmonary infiltrates with eosinophilia), which is due to other etiologies[44] (Table 3-4). This may be possible only after a careful study of the patient's history has been made.

Pulmonary Infiltrates with Eosinophilia

The agents that most commonly cause pulmonary infiltrates with eosinophilia are para-aminosalicyclic acid (PAS), isoniazid, penicillin, nitrofurantoin, aspirin, and sulfonamides, although a large number of other drugs may be causative (Table 3-4). The reaction may be a hypersensitivity reaction in many of these situations. Because of the ubiquitous use of these agents, an exact incidence is uncertain. Pathological proof is uncommon, as the pulmonary disability is usually self-limited when the drug is removed. Characteristic in most patients are fever, dyspnea, and cough; although all of these drugs may cause eosinophilia, the eosinophilia may be absent in some patients with infiltrates. Radiographically, transient patchy infiltrates, occasionally with pleural effusion, are seen. The withdrawal of the drug results in gradual regression of the infiltrates, usually over a few days to two weeks. In some cases, the use of steroids has also been helpful.

Special mention should be made of the pulmonary reaction brought about by several cancer chemotherapeutic agents that cause pulmonary infiltrates: methotrexate, procarbazine, and bleomycin.

Methotrexate is a folic acid antagonist used in the therapy of acute lymphatic leukemia, psoriasis, choriocarcinoma, lymphosarcoma, Wegener's granulomatosis, and occasionally carcinoma. The development of drug-induced infiltrates may occur any time in the course of therapy[5,59,60] and is not strictly dose related, although it has not been reported in patients receiving less than 20 mg. per week. Multiple drug therapy seems to increase the incidence of methotrexate pneumonitis, and it seems that prior adrenalectomy may predispose to an especially severe and protracted course.[61]

Table 3-4
Causes of Pulmonary Infiltrates With Eosinophilia (PIE Syndrome)†

Loeffler's syndrome
Parasites
Drugs
Fungi
Viruses
Bacteria
Sarcoidosis
Exogenous antigens
Microfilaria
Allergic aspergillosis
Polyarteritis nodosa
Hypersensitivity angiitis
Allergic granulomatosis
Wegener's granulomatosis
Lymphoma

† Modified from Citro, et al[44]

Histologically, non-caseating granulomata, containing multinucleated giant cells and large mononuclear cells, are present, with perivascular cuffing of small vessels by lymphocytes. There is pronounced desquamation of cells lining the alveoli and bronchioles.[62] The patients present with headache, malaise, non-productive cough, dyspnea, fever, crepitant rales, and often cyanosis. Fifty percent of patients will have peripheral eosinophilia as high as 16 percent. Radiographically, a diffuse, acute rapidly-progressive process involving both lungs is present. Early perihilar interstitial changes may be seen, progressing to a mixed acinar and interstitial pattern (Fig. 3-3). Hilar adenopathy may occur, and may be very prominent: differentiation from adenopathy due to the underlying disease may be difficult. The presence of clinical remission suggests that the adenopathy is not due to the primary disease. Effusions are absent. Although steroid therapy has been used with apparent dramatic success in some cases,[62,63,64] the radiographic and clinical abnormalities appear to be

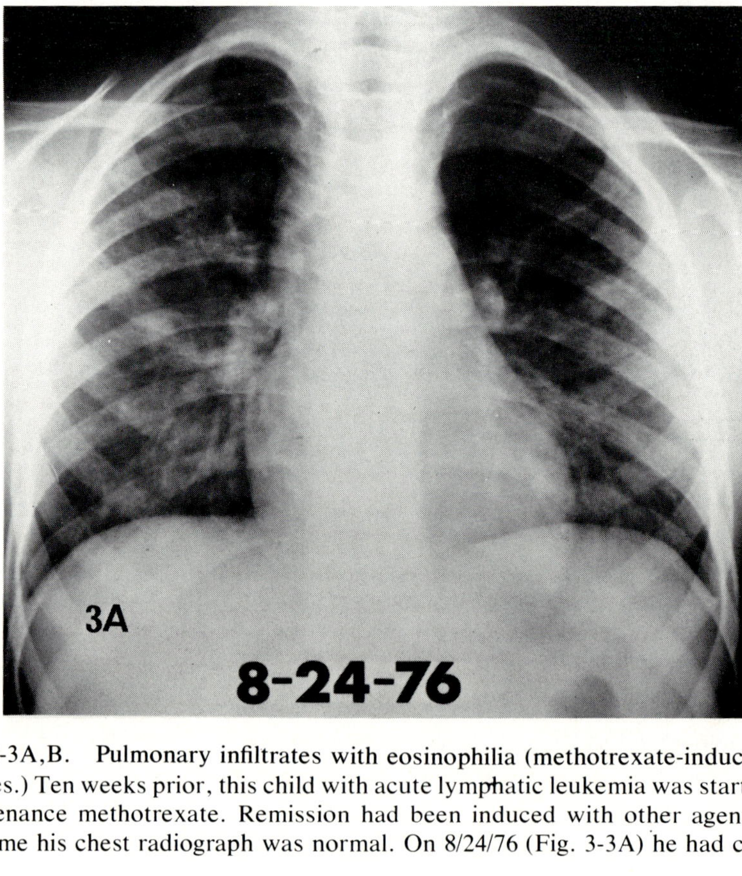

Fig. 3-3A,B. Pulmonary infiltrates with eosinophilia (methotrexate-induced infiltrates.) Ten weeks prior, this child with acute lymphatic leukemia was started on maintenance methotrexate. Remission had been induced with other agents. At that time his chest radiograph was normal. On 8/24/76 (Fig. 3-3A) he had cough,

self-limited. Early reports suggested that low-dose daunorubicin therapy might be helpful, but in view of the apparent self-limited nature of the illness, this therapy does not appear warranted and has not found widespread acceptance. In fact, the pneumonitis may resolve spontaneously, even if the methotrexate is not withdrawn and no steroids are administered. The pneumonitis may not recur even if methotrexate is reinstated. Resolution usually occurs in ten to fourteen days, although it may take up to 60 days. The diagnosis is one of exclusion and is made by lung biopsy, since *Pneumocystis carinii* pneumonia and radiation pneumonitis may be indistinguishable clinically and radiologically from methotrexate pneumonitis and may also occur during periods of remission. Hilar adenopathy, which forms in association with recurrent tumor, can also appear identical to methotrexate-related adenopathy. Leukemic pulmonary infiltrates, which may appear radiologically similar, are rarely visible

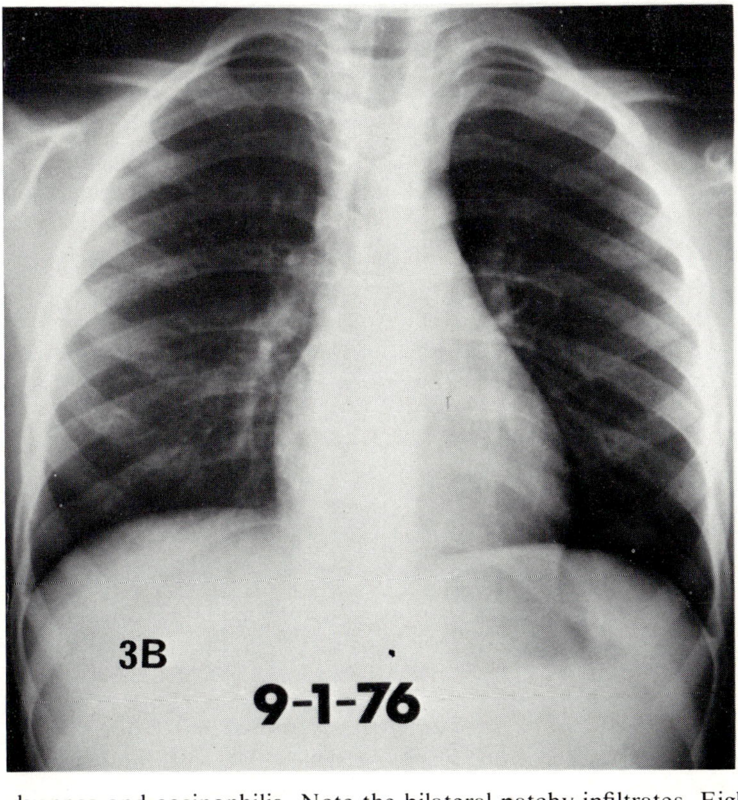

fever, dyspnea and eosinophilia. Note the bilateral patchy infiltrates. Eight days later (Fig. 3-3B, p. 58), after withdrawal of methotrexate, the infiltrates had cleared. (Courtesy Hideyo Minagi, M.D.)

radiographically, except pre-terminally, and would not occur during remission. It is unlikely that the occurrence of methotrexate pneumonitis is due to a hypersensitivity reaction because of: 1) spontaneous regression of the pneumonitis despite continuation of the drug, 2) failure of the pneumonitis to recur with re-institution of the drug, 3) onset of pneumonitis during periods of steriod therapy, and 4) the inherent immuno-suppressive and anti-inflammatory effects of methotrexate.

PULMONARY INFILTRATES DUE TO PROCARBAZINE

Procarbazine is a methylhydrazine derivative used in the therapy of lymphoma. A true hypersensitivity reaction to procarbazine has been reported[54] in which the sudden onset of chills, fever, cough, and eosinophilia is accompanied by bilateral interstitial and alveolar infiltrates and pleural effusion. The reaction begins shortly (9 to 14 days) after beginning therapy initially, or after resuming cyclic therapy. A skin rash may occur. The infiltrates, eosinophilia, and clinical signs and symptoms disappear a day or two after discontinuation of the drug.

PULMONARY INFILTRATES DUE TO BLEOMYCIN

Although the most common pulmonary reaction to bleomycin is pulmonary fibrosis, a much rarer hypersensitivity pneumonitis has been reported,[18] presenting as bilateral, patchy interstitial infiltrates (less pronounced than those with bleomycin fibrosis.) Histologically, there is eosinophilic infiltration of alveoli and focal hyperplasia of type II granular pneumocytes, without the bizarre appearance and extrusion of lamellated bodies seen in bleomycin-induced fibrosis. No intrinsic abnormality of the type I pneumocytes is seen, and there is no deposition of immune complexes in the epithelial or endothelial basement membranes. The absence of tissue IgG, IgA, and IgM mitigates against this being a Type II or Type III hypersensitivity reaction, and the absence of tissue granulomata indicates that it is unlikely to be a Type IV reaction; it may well represent a Type I (IgE-dependent) immunologic reaction.* Unlike bleomycin-induced fibrosis, there is an associated eosinophilia, varying in degree from 12 to 16 percent. Effusions are absent, as are the dry, end-inspiratory rales heard in pulmonary fibrosis. The patient may be

* The four types of allergic reactions responsible for hypersensitivity diseases of the lungs are: Type I (IgE dependent), Type II (cytotoxic; tissue-specific antibody), Type III (immune-complex disease), and Type IV (cell-mediated, delayed hypersensitivity). Type I reactions occur with asthma, eczema, and parasitic infestation. Type II reactions include thrombocytopenia, hemolytic anemia, and membranous glomerulonephritis and Goodpasture's syndrome. Type III reactions include extrinsic allergic alveolitis, serum sickness, and drug sensitivity. Type IV reactions are responsible for graft rejection, graft versus host reaction, reactions to tuberculous and fungal infections, and probably tumor immunity.

asymptomatic or tachypneic and complain of dyspnea; the forced vital capacity may be decreased. The pneumonitis clears after four to eight weeks of steroid therapy.

PULMONARY INFILTRATES DUE TO L-ASPARAGINASE

A hypersensitivity type reaction also occurs commonly with the use of L-asparaginase;[65] 20 percent of patients receiving the drug develop a pulmonary hypersensitivity reaction with shortness of breath.

PULMONARY INFILTRATES DUE TO 6-MERCAPTOPURINE

Four cases of pulmonary infiltrates due to 6-mercaptopurine therapy have been reported.[5] In each of these cases, diffuse, finely nodular infiltrates developed within a few days of beginning therapy. Histologically, round cell infiltration and exuberant epithelial proliferation were present, without fibrosis. In at least one patient, recovery was spontaneous after removal of the drug.

PULMONARY INFILTRATES DUE TO DIPHENYLHYDANTOIN (PHENYTOIN)

A hypersensitivity reaction to diphenylhydantoin has also been reported,[54] in which miliary, reticulo-nodular pulmonary infiltrates associated with eosinophilia developed. An immune-complex origin of tissue injury is postulated, since the serum complement was depressed and returned to normal after withdrawal of the drug. The reversible nature of this reaction and the presence of eosinophilia differentiate it from the fibrotic reaction induced by diphenylhydantoin, which was discussed earlier.

Pulmonary Infiltrates without Eosinophilia

As indicated previously, eosinophilia, though commonly present, may be absent in certain cases of infiltrates induced by the drugs in Table 3-4. In addition, any drug that causes pulmonary edema or hemorrhage due to capillary damage may result in the radiographic appearance of what seem to be pulmonary infiltrates without eosinophilia. Such agents causing edema include amitryptyline, codeine, dextran 40, epinephrine, heroin (Fig.3-4), hydrochlorothiazide, intra-bronchial aqueous radiographic contrast media, methadone, phenylbutazone, propoxyphene, ethylchlorvinyl, and salicylates.[26] The pulmonary infiltrates last 24 to 48 hours; therapy is supportive, occasionally requiring oxygen and diuretic therapy. Pulmonary edema resulting in the radiographic appearance of infiltrates

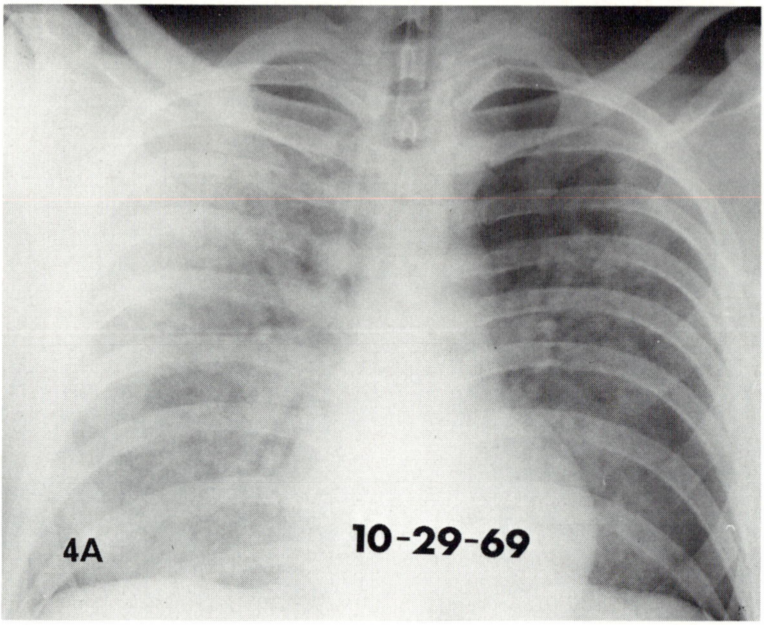
4A
10-29-69

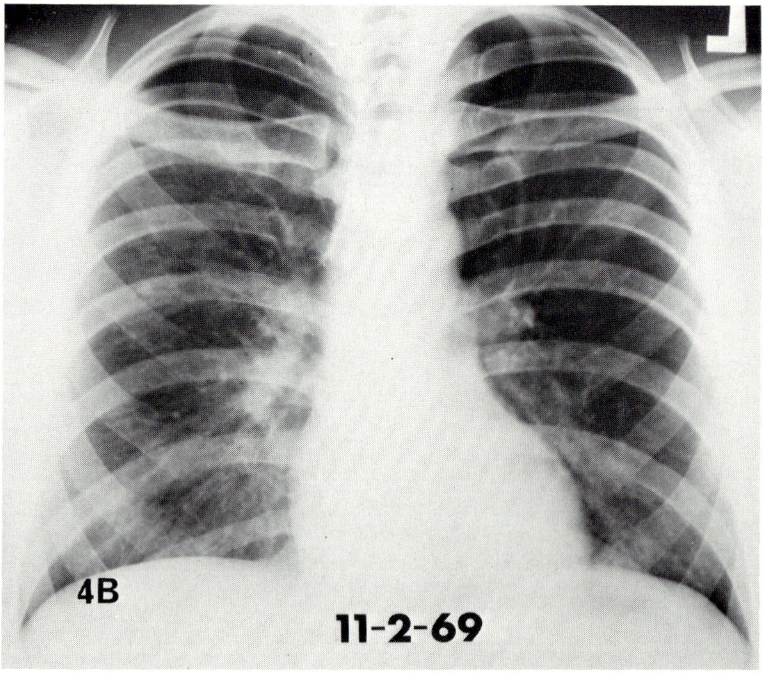
4B
11-2-69

may occur early in the course of oxygen toxicity (see PULMONARY FIBROSIS above). Pulmonary hemorrhage has been reported during anti-coagulant therapy[66] and following lymphangiography.[67] The diagnosis of pulmonary hemorrhage may be made by seeing hemosiderin-laden macrophages in lavage fluid. Therapy is supportive; in the former instance, anti-coagulation is reversed. The infiltrates resolve after five to ten days.[68]

SYSTEMIC LUPUS ERYTHEMATOSUS SYNDROME

Since the first report of hydralazine-induced systemic lupus erythematosus (SLE) in 1954, 38 drugs have been implicated as iatrogenic causes of SLE[69] (Table 3-5). Although the ANA (anti-nuclear antibody) test, the LE cell preparation, and tests for single-stranded DNA antibodies may be positive in drug-induced SLE, the presence of double-stranded (native) DNA antibody is almost diagnostic of idiopathic SLE.* (Rarely, antibodies to double-stranded DNA may be seen in hydralazine-induced lupus.)

Procainamide is the most common cause of drug-induced lupus. The reaction is dose-related; although a 1,400–3,600-gram total dose is usually required, a daily dose of as little as 500 mg. has been reported to be causative. Although the ANA test is positive in a high percentage of patients taking procainamide, only five percent of those taking the drug for more than six months will have symptoms of SLE. The female : male distribution in drug-induced SLE is 3:2, while in idiopathic SLE it is 9:1. The amine and hydrazine moieties are metabolized by acetylation via the hepatic N-acetyltransferase system. Persons who are phenotypically rapid acetylators metabolize procainamide more rapidly than do slow acetylators; the duration of therapy required for induction of procainamide-related SLE in phenotypically rapid acetylators is four times that required in slow acetylators.[72] The time from beginning of therapy to onset of symptoms varies from three months to two years, with

* Double-stranded DNA is naturally occurring (native) DNA; antibodies to double-stranded DNA are, for all practical purposes, indicative of idiopathic systemic lupus erythematosus syndrome. Antibodies to chemically denatured DNA (single-stranded DNA), as measured by the ANA test, are a non-specific finding, which may occur with collagen vascular diseases, as well as with many other clinical syndromes.

Fig. 3-4A,B. Pulmonary infiltrates without eosinophilia (heroin pulmonary edema.) This patient was admitted in coma, hypoxia due to heroin overdose. Note the extensive pulmonary edema with normal cardiac size (Fig. 3-4A). The pulmonary edema resolved in 48 hours with only supportive therapy (Fig. 3-4B, p. 62). (Courtesy Hideyo Minagi, M.D.)

Table 3-5
Drugs Which May Result in Systemic Lupus Erythematosus Syndrome†

Allopurinol	Methysergide
Alpha-methyldopa	Oral contraceptives
Acetylsalicylic acid	Oxyphenylbutazone
Carbamazepine	Penicillin
Chlorpromazine	Phenelzine[70]
Clofibrate	Phenylbutazone
Corticosteroids	Practolol
Corticosteroid withdrawal	Prazosin
Diphenylhydantoin*	Primidone
D-penicillamine	Procainamide
Ethosuximide	Propanolol
Gold compounds	Propylthiouracil
Guanoxan	Quinidine
Hydralazine	Reserpine
Isoniazid**	Streptomycin
Levodopa	Sulfonamides
Mephenytoin	Tetracycline
Mesantoin	Trimethadione
Methylthiouracil	Vitamins

* Steroids required to reverse, so does not fit strict criteria for drug-induced
** Accounts for 90% of cases
† Modified from Jones, et al[69]

an average of slightly more than six months. In rare cases it may occur as early as two weeks, or as late as four-and-a-half years after the beginning of therapy. Clinically, patients may present with arthralgias, pleuritic chest pain, cough, and/or dyspnea. Pleuritis occurs in 30 percent of patients sustaining procainamide-induced SLE; one half will have pulmonary infiltrates. Pericardial effusion may occur (Fig. 3-5). As with other types of drug-induced SLE, removal of the drug results in disappearance of the syndrome, usually after about two weeks. Although the clinical symptoms may improve, the serological findings may persist for months or years.

Hydralazine-induced SLE occurs in two to 21 percent of treated patients, and is also dose- and duration- dependent. Dosages greater than 400 mg./day are often associated with the syndrome, especially if the drug is taken for three months or more. The syndrome occurs on the average 17 months after the beginning of therapy, but may be seen between three weeks and ten to 20 years later. There seems to be an inverse relationship

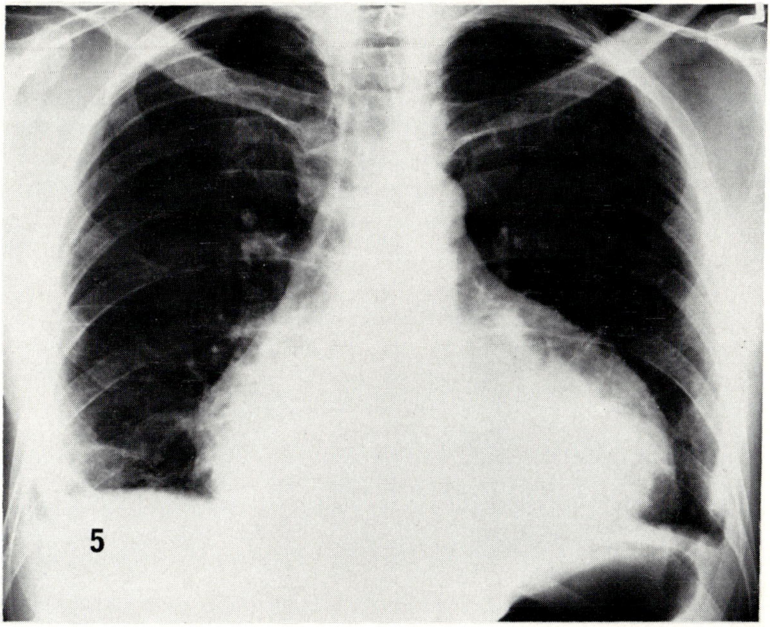

Fig. 3-5. Procanamide-induced SLE. This patient had been on procainamide for many months. The patient developed SLE clinically, as well as a pericardial effusion, all of which resolved after the withdrawal of the drug.

between SLE symptoms and blood pressure response to therapy. Pericarditis with tamponade may occur.

HILAR AND MEDIASTINAL DISEASE

It has long been recognized that diphenylhydantoin (phenytoin) may produce hilar and mediastinal adenopathy, or "pseudolymphoma." Pseudolymphoma is a benign chronic inflammatory process of unknown cause, involving the pulmonary parenchyma. It is manifested by small, irregularly marginated lesions, 3–6 cm. in diameter. These often contain non-homogeneous areas or air-bronchograms. In 25 percent of patients adenopathy is seen.[73] The radiographic and even histological differentiation from lymphoma in such cases can be difficult,[74] although the use of immunoperoxidase staining may be helpful.[73] The adenopathy and pulmonary parenchymal changes usually regress within one to two weeks of withdrawal of the drug. It is known that diphenylhydantoin can cause lymphoma in laboratory animals; it is now reported that the drug may also

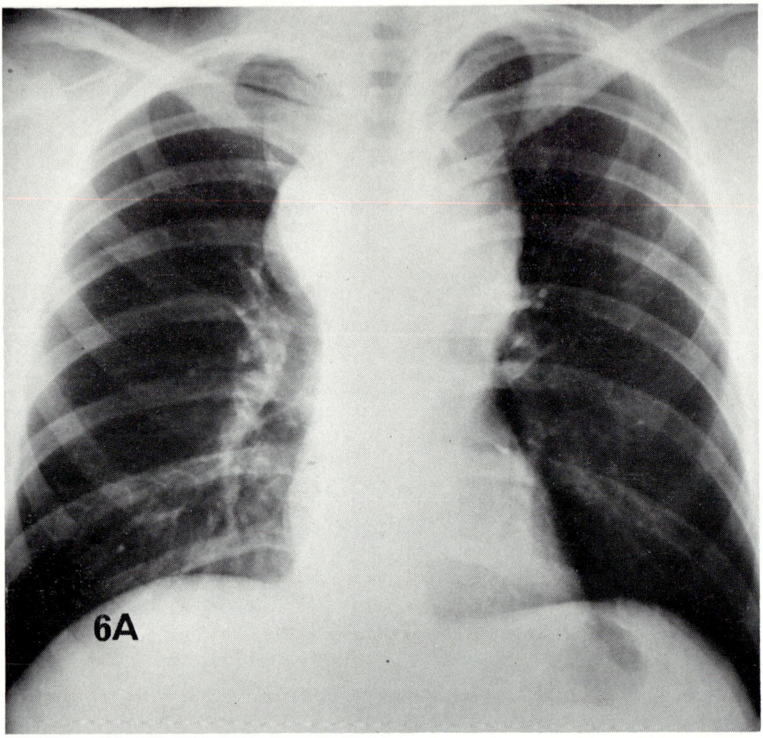

Fig. 3-6A. Mediastinal and hilar disease (possible hydantoin-induced lymphoma.) This patient had received diphenylhydantoin for five years when he developed diffuse, poorly differentiated lymphocytic lymphoma. Note the extensive superior and anterior mediastinal mass.

produce true lymphoma in humans.[75] The patient seen in Fig. 3-6A may represent such a case.

Methotrexate may cause hilar and mediastinal adenopathy, which regresses spontaneously within a few weeks, even if intake of the drug is continued. Oral potassium iodide therapy may result in hilar adenopathy, which may be associated with eosinophilia. The adenopathy regresses promptly when the drug is withdrawn.[76]

Steroid therapy may result in widening of the mediastinum due to depostion of fat in the mediastinum and pericardium (Figs. 3-6B and C).[77] Although several months of steroid therapy are usually required before such deposition is apparent, when large doses are used (as in brain tumor therapy), it may occur as early as six weeks after initial therapy. This mediastinal fat does not compress the trachea, and its upper border is

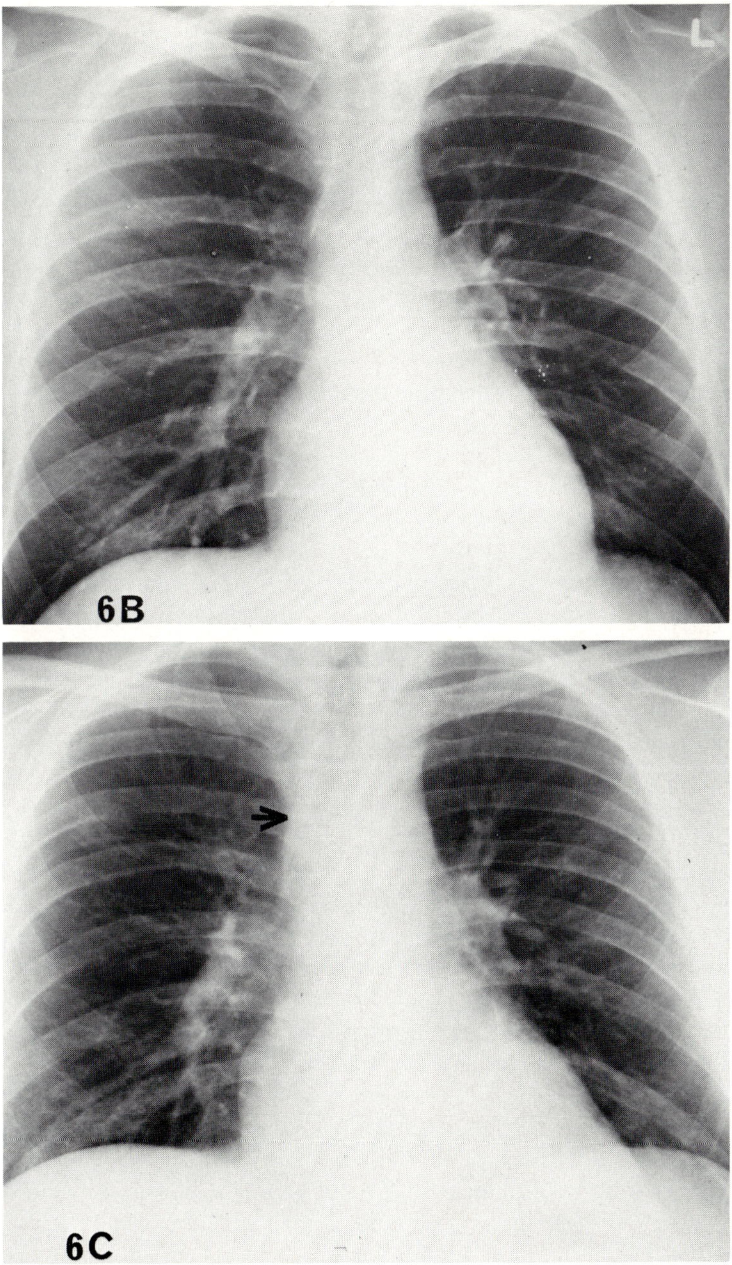

Fig. 3-6B,C. Mediastinal and hilar disease (mediastinal fat deposition.) At the time of renal transplantation (Fig. 3-6B), the superior mediastinum is normal. After eighteen months of steroid therapy to prevent transplant rejection, the superior mediastinum is widened due to fat deposition (Fig. 3-6C). Note the right paratracheal widening (arrow, Fig. 3-6C); the margins of the mediastinum fade indistinctly superiorly.

indistinct, fading out at the level of the clavicles. It is often less dense than other mediastinal masses. This fat disappears when steroids are withdrawn.

EVALUATION OF THE PATIENT WITH SUSPECTED DRUG-INDUCED LUNG DISEASE

Drug-induced lung disease is rarely diagnosed with certainty by the clinician, radiologist, or pathologist. This is because the features of adverse pulmonary drug reactions are rarely specific for a given drug and because the signs and symptoms of drug-induced lung disease are usually indistinguishable from those of many other conditions affecting the lung. However, alert physicians may be able to make a diagnosis of drug-induced lung disease if they suspect that one or more drugs may be responsible for lung injury, and if they pursue a systematic diagnostic evaluation. Clinical and radiographic data allow the physician to place the patient's lung disease in one of several categories, such as those listed in Table 3-2. A thorough drug history and a broad differential diagnosis are the keys to successful evaluation of the patient with suspected drug-induced lung disease.

The experienced clinician relies on the medical history as the most important step in the diagnosis of drug-induced lung disease. A thorough list of drugs taken by the patient must be obtained. Patients with drug-induced lung disease characteristically complain of dyspnea and cough; in addition, fever due to cytotoxic drugs is present in the majority. However, symptoms are nonspecific and, with the exception of drug-induced bronchospasm and hypersensitivity reactions, do not immediately follow drug use. There is no way to predict which individual patients are predisposed to adverse pulmonary drug reactions. A careful physical examination should be performed, giving specific attention to evidence of lung infiltrates, bronchospasm, pulmonary edema, pleural effusion, and respiratory failure. Patients with interstitial drug-induced lung disease may show typical features such as tachypnea, tachycardia, pan-inspiratory dry crackles (rales) at the lung bases, absence of signs of left ventricular heart failure, and clubbing. Severe pulmonary fibrosis due to drug-induced lung disease may be accompanied by evidence of pulmonary hypertension and cor pulmonale.

After the patient's history has been considered and the physical examination performed, the chest roentgenogram is studied. Correct interpretation of the chest x-ray and correlation with clinical findings are essential in the diagnosis of drug-induced pulmonary disease.[78] Previous chest roentgenograms should always be sought to assure the proper interpretation of new findings. Radiographic findings are rarely specific for a particular cause of drug-induced lung disease, but correlation of the clinical and radiographic findings should allow the clinician to narrow the differential diagnosis.

Selected laboratory studies are then ordered as appropriate in each particular case. In general, laboratory tests do not provide specific proof that lung disease is drug-induced, but they do provide information important to the differential diagnosis. Routine studies should include a complete blood count, a differential white blood count, and a sedimentation rate. An absolute blood eosinophil count and a sputum smear for eosinophils may be helpful if hypersensitivity drug reactions or "pulmonary infiltrate with eosinophilia" (PIE syndrome) are suspected (Table 3-4). Studies of expectorated sputum should include a gram stain for bacterial organisms and stains for acid-fast or fungal organisms, if infection is being considered. In the acutely ill patient, reliance must be placed on the sputum gram stain since aerobic sputum cultures often give misleading results.[79] Cytologic examination of the sputum should be ordered whenever malignant disease involving the lung is suspected. Sputum cytology occasionally yields a diagnosis of non-malignant lung disease. For example, in some viral pneumonias, intracellular inclusion bodies may be identified.

Additional studies designed to rule out lung infection include cultures of transtracheal aspirates, pleural fluid and blood. Serologic studies should be considered if viral pneumonia, fungal infections, or Legionnaires' disease are considered in the differential diagnosis. Both acute and convalescent titers are required in patients with viral pneumonia. Diagnostic intradermal skin testing is helpful in patients with suspected tuberculosis or coccidioidomycosis.

Pulmonary function studies are sometimes helpful in diagnosing suspected drug-induced lung disease. These tests provide objective information about pulmonary function and may allow detection of pulmonary dysfunction before it is clinically evident. These studies also help the clinician understand the mechanisms of the patient's dyspnea and provide a means of following response to therapy. The means of measuring airflow rates, lung volumes, and diffusing capacity are available in most large hospitals. Although some drugs induce bronchospasm with evidence of airflow limitation on pulmonary function tests, the majority of advanced drug-induced lung syndromes have typical restrictive patterns, with reduction of lung volumes and diffusing capacity but preservation of airflow rates. Arterial blood gas analysis is probably the single most valuable test for determining adequacy of respiration. It should be performed whenever there is any suspicion of respiratory failure. Analysis of arterial oxygen tension before and after exercise is particularly helpful in evaluating patients with infiltrative lung disease. Exercise pulmonary function tests are also useful in studying the patient with lung infiltrates.

What is the role of fiberoptic bronchoscopy in the diagnosis of drug-induced lung disease? This versatile procedure has a wide variety of uses in pulmonary medicine. Both solitary masses and diffuse lung infiltrates may be biopsied through the fiberoptic bronchoscope, often with excellent results.[80,81,82,83] It is often possible to obtain adequate specimens of lung parenchyma for histologic study by this technique, thereby saving the patient an open lung biopsy. However, experience with transbronchoscopic biopsy in drug-induced lung disease is limited.[83] Percutaneous small needle aspiration of lung lesions may confirm infectious or malignant disease, but this technique does not provide enough tissue for satisfactory histopathologic diagnosis of drug-induced lung disease.

The role of transbronchial lung biopsy through the fiberoptic bronchoscope versus open lung biopsy in patients with unexplained diffuse lung disease remains controversial.[84,85,86] However, most experienced clinicians recommend thoracotomy with open lung biopsy to obtain adequate tissue for precise pathologic interpretation in patients with diffuse pulmonary disease. Open lung biopsy may be performed through a very short intercostal incision with minimal morbidity.[85,87] Pieces of lung tissue are submitted for appropriate touch preparations, histological studies, and cultures. Special stainings may rule out infection by bacteria, fungi, acid-fast bacilli, and *Pneumocystis carinii.* A search for viral inclusion bodies should be performed.

Histologic features of drug-induced lung disease, like the clinical and radiographic features, are non-specific. They depend upon the particular agent causing the lung infiltrate and the duration of exposure to the offending drug. Electron microscopy and immunofluorescence staining of the biopsy specimen may be valuable in research protocols, but these methods are not widely adaptable to clinical use at the present time.[11] When pathological findings are correlated with clinical information, differential considerations can be ruled out and a specific diagnosis of drug-induced lung infiltrate can usually be made.

A simple but vital method of establishing a diagnosis of drug-induced lung disease is observation of the clinical response upon withdrawal of the suspected offending drug. To rechallenge with the drug may prove helpful, but this is rarely done because of the risks involved. In patients with hypersensitivity-induced lung disease, recurrence of the clinical syndrome upon readministration of the drug is common. Exceptions are patients with methotrexate-induced pneumonitis, who characteristically have no recurrence on rechallenge with the drug.[88]

The diagnosis of drug-induced pulmonary disease is particularly difficult in the patient suffering from diffuse malignant lung disease who has been treated with chemotherapy. Schwarz, Whitcomb, and Goldman have provided a thorough review of this subject.[89] Let us consider a rational approach to the evaluation and management of such a patient. Questions the clinician should ask include the following:

1. How long have the lung infiltrates been present? Old chest x-rays must be examined to exclude chronic disorders such as pulmonary fibrosis, pneumoconiosis, connective tissue diseases and chronic congestive heart failure.

2. What cancer chemotherapy drugs has the patient used? At least eight commonly used chemotherapeutic drugs have pulmonary toxicity (bleomycin, cyclophosphamide, busulfan, methotrexate, mitomycin, chlorambucil, procarbazine, and nitrosoureas.) The patient's pulmonary illness should be compared with the known toxic reaction for the particular drug.

3. Does the patient have a pulmonary infection? Many infectious diseases may mimic drug-induced lung disease, and it is always important to consider these first, since early antimicrobial therapy may be lifesaving. Bacterial pneumonia can be readily diagnosed with appropriate studies, particularly gram stain of a satisfactory sputum specimen. Greater diagnostic skills are required to detect opportunistic lung infection brought about by other causes, such as unusual bacteria (e.g., *Nocardia*), viruses (cytomegalovirus), fungi (e.g., Cryptococcus neoformans, Coccidioides immitis, and Histoplasma capsulatum), and protozoans (*Pneumocystis carinii*). Early recognition and treatment of opportunistic infection are particularly important in the patient who is immuno-compromised by cancer chemotherapeutic agents.

4. Are the lung infiltrates caused by drugs or by the malignancy itself? Both primary and metastatic pulmonary malignancy may mimic drug-induced lung infiltrates, which are usually interstitial and diffuse in nature. Among these neoplastic disorders are alveolar cell carcinoma, lymphoma, and lymphangitic carcinomatosis.[89] Lung biopsy is often required to distinguish drug-induced infiltrate from these malignant disorders.

5. Are iatrogenic causes other than drugs responsible for lung infiltrates? Diffuse pulmonary infiltrates may occur in radiation pneumonitis, oxygen toxicity, embolization due to lymphangiogram contrast material, pulmonary congestion secondary to excessive fluid therapy, leukoagglutinin reactions due to blood transfusions, and pulmonary hemorrhage secondary to drug-induced thrombocytopenia from the use of cytotoxic drugs.[89] Awareness of these iatrogenic disorders should lead to their early recognition.

Management of the patient with established drug-induced lung disease includes discontinuation of the offending drug, replacement of the drug with a safer alternative if necessary, avoidance of further pulmonary insults, and a careful follow-up program, including periodic chest x-rays and pulmonary function studies. Optimal respiratory care should be provided to prevent further deterioration of pulmonary function. Principles of optimal care include clearance of bronchopulmonary secretions, treatment of superimposed bacterial infections, vaccine prophylaxis against viral and pneumococcal infections, judicious use of bronchodilator drugs in patients with obstructive lung disease, treatment of cor pulmonale, and appropriate oxygen therapy in patients with documented hypoxemia. Corticosteroids should be used only in those cases where objective response can be demonstrated by chest x-ray and pulmonary function studies.

In the future we may have more specific markers for lung disease caused by drugs; unfortunately, none are available at the present time. Thus, careful attention to the patient's history, physical examination, chest x-ray, and simple laboratory data must be emphasized as the best approach to the diagnosis of drug-induced lung disease. Pulmonary function studies grade the level of pulmonary insufficiency but are not diagnostic. Open lung biopsy is recommended if a diagnosis of drug-induced lung infiltrate cannot be firmly established on clinical grounds. Appropriate therapy can be considered after numerous other conditions that mimic drug-induced lung disease are systematically excluded.

REFERENCES

1. Seidl LG, Thornton GF, Smith JW, et al: Studies on the epidemiology of adverse drug reactions—III. Reactions in patients on a general medical service. Bull Johns Hopkins Hosp 119:299–315, 1966
2. Kirschner RH, Esterly JR: Pulmonary lesions associated with busulfan therapy of chronic myelogenous leukemia. Cancer 27:1074–1080, 1971
3. Blum RH, Carter SK, Agre K: A clinical review of bleomycin—a new antineoplastic agent. Cancer 31:903–914, 1973
4. Agre K: Bleomycin overview of clinical evaluation in the United States. New Drug Seminar, Bethesda, Maryland, 1974
5. Sostman HD, Matthay RA, Putman EC, et al: Cytotoxic drug-induced lung disease. Am J Med 62:608–615, 1977
6. Patel AR, Shah PC, Phee HL, et al: Cyclophosphamide therapy and interstitial pulmonary fibrosis. Cancer 38:1542–1549, 1976

7. Topilow A, Rothenberg S, Cottrell TS: Interstitial pneumonitis after prolonged treatment with cyclophosphamide. Am Rev Resp Dis 108:114–117, 1973
8. Einhorn L, Krause M, Hornback N, et al: Enhanced pulmonary toxicity with bleomycin and radiotherapy in oat-cell lung cancer. Cancer 37:2414–2416, 1976
9. Samuels M, Johnson D, Holoye P, et al: Large dose bleomycin therapy and pulmonary toxicity. A possible role of prior radiotherapy. JAMA 235:1117–1120, 1976
10. Krous HF, Hamlin WB: Pulmonary toxicity due to bleomycin. Report of a case. Arch Pathol 95:407–410, 1973
11. Bedrossian CWM, Luna MA, MacKay B, et al: Ultrastructure of pulmonary bleomycin toxicity. Cancer 32:44–51, 1973
12. Daskal Y, Gyorkey F, Gyorkey P, et al: Ultrastructural study of pulmonary bleomycin toxicity. Cancer Res 36:1267–1272, 1976
13. Gould VE, Miller J: Sclerosing alveolitis induced by cyclophosphamide: ultrastructural observations on alveolar injury and repair. Amer J Pathol 81:513–530, 1975
14. Rosenow EC: Drug-induced pulmonary disease. Clin Notes Respir Dis 16 (1):3–11, 1977
15. Littler WA, Kay JM, Hasleton PS, et al: Busulphan lung. Thorax 24:639–655, 1969
16. Richman SD, Levenson SM, Bunn PA, et al: $_{67}$Gallium accumulation in pulmonary lesions associated with bleomycin toxicity. Cancer 36:1966–1972, 1975
17. Crittenden D, Tranum BL, Haut A: Pulmonary fibrosis after prolonged therapy with 1,3-bis (2-chloroethyl)-1-nitrosourea. Chest 72:372–373, 1977
18. Holoye PY, Luna MA, MacKay B, et al: Bleomycin hypersensitivity pneumonitis. Ann Int Med 88:47–49, 1978
19. Iriarte P, Hananian J, Cortner J: Central nervous system leukemia and solid tumors of childhood. Treatment with 1,3-bis (2-chloroethyl)-1-nitrosourea. Cancer 19:1187–1194, 1966
20. Refvem O: Fatal intraalveolar and interstitial lung fibrosis in chlorambucil-treated chronic lymphocytic leukemia. Mt Sinai J Med NY 44:847–851, 1977
21. Rubio FA: Possible pulmonary effects of alkylating agents. New Eng J Med 287:1150–1151, 1972
22. Codling BW, Chakera TMH: Pulmonary fibrosis following therapy with melphalan for multiple myeloma. J. Clin Path 25:668–673, 1972
23. Rubin G, Baum P, Vondenberg R: Azathioprine and acute restrictive lung disease. Aust NZ J Med 3:272, 1972
24. Rosenow EC, DeRemee RA, Dines DE: Chronic nitrofurantoin pulmonary reaction. New Eng J Med 279:1258–1262, 1968
25. Bone RC, Wolfe J, Sobonya RE, et al: Desquamative interstitial pneumonia following long-term nitrofurantoin therapy. Am J Med 60:697–701, 1976
26. Stauffer JL: Drug-induced lung disease: the price of progress. Calif Med 119:48–55, 1973
27. Kistler GS, Caldwell PRB, Weibel ER: Development of fine structural damage to alveolar and capillary lining cells in oxygen-poisoned rat lungs. J Cell Biol 32:605–628, 1967
28. Northway WH, Rosan RC, Porter PY: Pulmonary disease following respirator therapy of hyaline-membrane disease. Bronchopulmonary displasia. NEJM 276:257–368, 1967
29. Winterbauer RH, Wilske KR, Wheelis RF: Diffuse pulmonary injury associated with gold treatment. New Eng J Med 294:919–921, 1976
30. Matthew H, Logan A, Woodruff MFA, et al: Paraquat poisoning—lung transplantation. Br Med J 3:759–763, 1968
31. Raffin TA, Robin ED: Paraquat ingestion and pulmonary injury. West J Med 128:26–34, 1978

32. Omaye ST, Reddy KA, Cross CE: Enhanced lung toxicity of paraquat in selenium-deficient rats. Toxicol Appl Pharmacol 43:237–247, 1978
33. Rhodes ML, Patterson CE: Effects of exogenous superoxide dismutase on paraquat toxicity. Am Rev Resp Dis 117(4,Part 2):255, 1978
34. Smith D (Director, Haight-Ashbury Medical Clinic): Personal communication, 1978
35. Jones GR, Malone DNS: Sulphasalazine induced lung disease. Thorax 27:713–717, 1972
36. Davies D, MacFarlane A: Fibrosing alveolitis and treatment with sulphasalazine. Gut 15:185–188, 1974
37. Moore MT: Pulmonary changes in hydantoin therapy. JAMA, 171, 1328–1333, 1959
38. Livingston S, Whitehouse D, Pauli LL: Study of the effects of diphenylhydantoin sodium on the lungs. New Eng J Med 264:648–651, 1961
39. Hazlett DR, Ward GW, Madison DS: Pulmonary function loss in diphenylhydantoin therapy. Chest 66:660–664, 1974
40. Rosenow EC: The spectrum of drug-induced pulmonary disease. Ann Int Med 77:977–991, 1972
41. Grahm JR, Suby HI, LeCompte PR, et al: Fibrotic disorders associated with methysergide (Sansert[R]) therapy for headaches. New Eng J Med 224:359–368, 1966
42. Erwteman TM, Braat MC, vanAken WG: Interstitial pulmonary fibrosis: a new side effect of practolol. Br Med J 2 (6082):297–298, 1977
43. Marshall AJ, Eltringham WK, Barritt DW, et al: Respiratory disease associated with practolol therapy. Lancet 2 (8051):1254–1257, 1977
44. Citro LA, Gordon ME, Miller WT: Eosinophilic lung disease. AJR 117:787–797, 1973
45. Garrell M: Loeffler's syndrome. Report of a case associated with the administration of aurothioglucose (Solganal[r]). Arch Int Med 106:874–877, 1960
46. Cullinan SA, Bower GC: Acute pulmonary hypersensitivity to carbamazepine. Chest 68:580–581, 1975
47. Shear MK: Chlorpromazine-induced PIE syndrome. Am J Psychiatry 135:492–493, 1978
48. Bell RJM: Pulmonary infiltrates with eosinophilia caused by chlorpropamide. Lancet 1:1249–1256, 1964
49. Repo UK, Nieminen P: Pulmonary infiltrates with eosinophilia and urinary symptoms during disodium cromoglycate treatment. A case report. Scand J Respir Dis 57:1–4, 1976
50. Allen RW, Holt AH, Brown MC: Acute pulmonary sensitivity to nitrofurantoin. Am J Roent 104:784–786, 1968
51. Waring FC, Howlett KS: Allergic reactions to PAS. Report of 7 cases including one Loeffler's syndrome. Am Rev Tuberc 65:235–249, 1952
52. Kerchlin S, Loveless MH, Kane EG: Loeffler's syndrome following penicillin therapy. Ann Int Med 38:113–120, 1953
53. Thurston JG, Marks P, Trapnell D: Lung changes associated with phenylbutazone treatment. Br Med J 2:1422–1423, 1976
54. Bayer AS, Targan SR, Pitchon HE, et al: Dilantin toxicity: miliary pulmonary infiltrates and hypoxemia. Ann Int Med 85:475–476, 1976
55. Harper LO, Burrell RG, Lapp NL, et al: Allergic alveolitis due to pituitary snuff. Ann Int Med 73:581–584, 1970
56. Jones SE, Moore M, Blank N, et al: Hypersensitivity to procarbazine (Matulane[r]) manifested by fever and pleuropulmonary reaction. Cancer 29:498–500, 1972
57. Fiegenburg DS, Weiss H, Kirshman H: Migratory pneumonia with eosinophilia associated with sulfonamide administration. Arch Int Med 120:85–89, 1967

58. Ascherl GF, Fulkerson LL, Stein E: Tolbutamide induced diffuse lung disease: case report. Milit Med 141:851–852, 1976
59. Clarysse AM, Cathey WJ, Cartwright GE, et al: Pulmonary disease complicating intermittent therapy with methotrexate. JAMA 209:1861–1863, 1969
60. Filip DJ, Logue GL, et al: Pulmonary and hepatic complications of methotrexate therapy of psoriasis. JAMA 216:881–882, 1971
61. Stutz FH, Tormey DC, Blom J: Nonbacterial pneumonitis with multidrug antineoplastic therapy in breast carcinoma. CMA Journal 108:710–714, 1973
62. Lisbona A, Schwartz J, LaChance C, et al: Methotrexate induced pulmonary disease. J Can Assoc Radiol 24:215–220, 1973
63. Robertson JH: Pneumonia and methotrexate. Brit Med J 12:156, 1970
64. Schwarz IR, Kajani MK: Methotrexate therapy and pulmonary disease. JAMA 210:1924, 1969
65. Green MR: Pulmonary toxicity of antineoplastic agents. West J Med 127:292–298, 1977
66. Finley TN, Aronow A, Cosentino AM, et al: Occult pulmonary hemorrhage in anticoagulated patients. Am Rev Resp Dis 112:23–29, 1975
67. Wiertz LM, Gagnon JH, Anthonisen NR: Intrapulmonary hemorrhage with anemia after lymphography. New Eng J Med 285:1364–1365, 1971
68. Palmer P, Finley T, Drew WL, Golde DW: Radiographic aspects of occult pulmonary hemorrhage. Clin Rad 29:139–143, 1978
69. Jones WN, Trinca CE, Walson PD: Drug-induced systemic lupus erythematosis. Ariz Med 35:16–19, 1978
70. Schwartz C: Lupus-like reaction to phenelzine. JAMA 239:2693, 1978
71. Friou GJ, Quismora FP: Chapter 6, in Alan S Cohen (ed): Laboratory diagnostic procedures in the rheumatic diseases, 2nd ed. Boston, Little, Brown, 1975
72. Woosley RL, Drayer DE, Reidenberg MM, et al: Effect of acetylator phenotype on the rate at which procainamide induces antinuclear antibodies and the lupus syndrome. NEJM 298:1157–1159, 1978
73. Jillsrud PR, Brown LR, Li CY, et al: Pulmonary processes of mature-appearing lymphocytes. Rad 127:289–296, 1978
74. Saltzstein SL, Ackerman LV: Lymphadenopathy induced by anticonvulsant drugs and mimicking clinically and pathologically malignant lympomas. Cancer 12:164–182, 1959
75. Hyman GA, Sommers SC: The development of Hodgkins disease and lymphoma during anticonvulsant therapy. Blood 28:416–427, 1966
76. Brettner A, Heitzman ER, Woodin WG: Pulmonary complications of drug therapy. Rad 96:31–38, 1970
77. Price JE, Rigler LG: Widening of the mediastinum resulting from fat accumulation. Rad 96:497–500, 1970
78. Ansell G: Radiological manifestations of drug-induced disease. Clin Radiol 20:133–148, 1969
79. Barrett-Connor E: The nonvalue of sputum culture in the diagnosis of pneumococcal pneumonia. Am Rev Respir Dis 103:845–848, 1971
80. Ellis JH Jr: Transbronchial lung biopsy via the fiberoptic bronchoscope: Experience with 107 consecutive cases and comparison with bronchial brushing. Chest 68:524–532, 1975
81. Levin DC, Wicks AB, Ellis JH Jr: Transbronchial lung biopsy via the fiberoptic bronchoscope. Am Rev Respir Dis 110:4–12, 1974
82. Hanson RR, Zavala DC, Rhodes ML et al: Transbronchial biopsy bia flexible fiberoptic bronchoscope: Results in 164 patients. Am Rev Respir Dis 114:67–72, 1976
83. Andersen HA: Transbronchoscopic lung biopsy for diffuse pulmonary diseases: Results in 939 patients. Chest 73 (Suppl):734–736, 1978

84. Zavala DC: Transbronchial biopsy in diffuse lung disease. Chest 73 (Suppl):727–733, 1978
85. Ray JF, Lawton BR, Myers WO et al: Open pulmonary biopsy: Nineteen-year experience with 416 consecutive operations. Chest 69:43–47, 1976
86. Andersen HA, Miller WE, Bernatz PE: Lung biopsy: Transthoracic, percutaneous, open. Surg Clin North Am 53:785–793, 1973
87. Hill JD, Ratliff JL, Parrott JCW et al: Pulmonary pathology in acute respiratory insufficiency: Lung biopsy as a diagnostic tool. J Thorac Cardiovasc Surg 71:64–70, 1976
88. Sostman HD, Matthay RA, Putman CE et al: Methotrexate-induced pneumonitis. Medicine 55:371–388, 1976
89. Schwarz MI, Whitcomb ME, Goldman AL: The spectrum of diffuse pulmonary infiltration in malignant disease. Chest 64:88–93, 1973

Martin J. Lipton
Charles B. Higgins
Roger Winkle

4

Drug Hazards in Coronary Arteriography

CONTRAST MATERIAL

The contrast materials currently used for coronary arteriography are monomeric ionic solutions with an osmolarity approximately six times that of normal extracellular fluid. Many experimental studies have shown that the introduction of these materials into the coronary arteries induces a slight inhibition of impulse generation and of conduction through the heart[1,2,3]; a depression in myocardial contraction also occurs.[4,5,6,51] Nevertheless, modern angiographic contrast materials are uncommonly the cause of major complications during or after coronary arteriography. Several large surveys[7,8,9] have revealed that mortality that is directly related to the action of contrast material occurs with a frequency of 0.05 percent. (Non-lethal complications related to contrast material occur with a frequency of 0.90 percent.) Death may result from anaphylaxis, asystole, heart block, ventricular fibrillation, or electromechanical dissociation provoked by the action of the contrast material. Major complications include supraventricular and ventricular arrhythmias, heart block, prolonged hypotension, and renal failure.

The potentially deleterious side effects of contrast material on the heart may be conveniently categorized as follows: inhibitions of the conduction system, elicitation of arrhythmias, depression of myocardial contractile state, and alterations in coronary and peripheral vasoactivity. To a major extent these effects are caused by direct action of contrast materials, but in some instances autonomic reflex responses activated by contrast materials mediate the side effects.[3,21]

Inhibition of the conduction system of the heart. Contrast material infused directly into the artery supplying the sinoatrial node causes sinus bradycardia and asystole.[1,2] This direct inhibition of sinoatrial function is dependent primarily upon the ionic strength of the contrast material and is considerably less for non-ionic material than for monomeric ionic contrast materials (Fig. 4-1). The nonionic material metrizamide, for instance, causes much less of a decrease in heart rate than does the material Renografin 76. To a lesser extent bradycardia ensues by means of a reflex action that can be abolished by cholinergic blockade.[3] Likewise, direct infusion of ionic contrast material into the atrioventricular nodal artery produces a dose-related depression in conduction through the atrioventricular node which, at higher infusion rates, culminates in complete heart

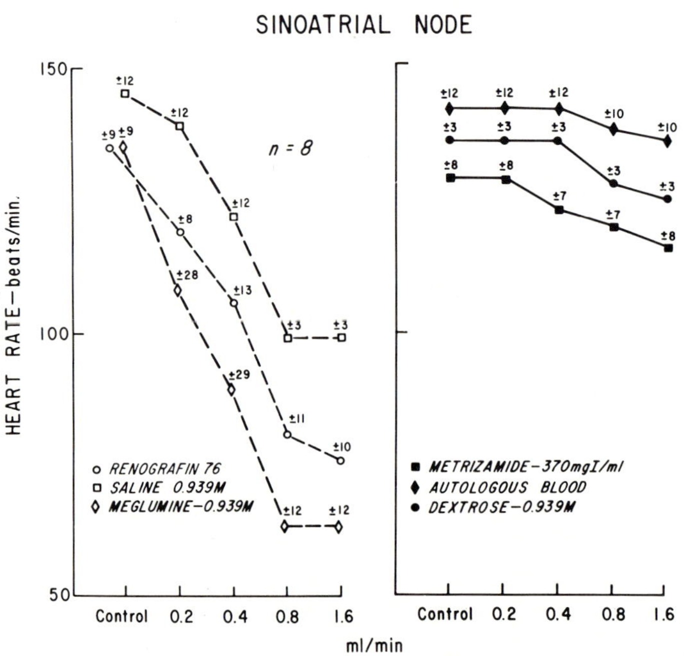

Fig. 4-1. Dose response curves obtained during the infusion of contrast material and various solutions into the artery to the sinoatrial node (left). The solutions (meglumine sodium diatrizoate), Isopaque 370 (calcium sodium meglumine me-material), sodium chloride, and meglumine hydrochloride equiosmolar to Renografin 76 (meglumine sodium diatrizoate). Dose response curves during the infusion of metrizamide (non-ionic contrast material), blood, and dextrose (right). Renografin 76 and the *ionic* solutions equiosmolar to Renografin 76 caused a dose-related inhibition in the sinus rate. On the other hand, metrizamide (*non-ionic*) caused substantially less depression in sinoatrial automaticity. (Reproduced with permission of *Radiology*.)

block. Intraventricular conduction is also inhibited by contrast materials.[10,11,12]

The major mechanism responsible for bradycardia, asystole, and heart block is the direct action of the contrast material on the specialized nodal tissues. Consequently, atropine administration does not preclude this potentially deleterious effect of intracoronary administration of contrast materials.[2]

Repolarization and depolarization abnormalities. Injection of contrast material in experimental animals[11] and man [12,14] routinely produces a shift in the QRS axis, an increase in the duration of the QRS complex, and a reversal or increase in amplitude of the T Wave; these changes are consistent with a prolonged state of myocardial depolarization.[15]

Elicitation of ventricular arrhythmias. Infusion of contrast material into the coronary arteries of dogs provokes ventricular ectopic beats and in some instances ventricular fibrillation.[15-17] The vulnerability to ventricular fibrillation is increased in experimental animals pretreated with digitalis preparations.[16] Non-ionic contrast material (metrizamide) produces less alteration in the QRS complex and T Wave and probably has less potential for inducing ventricular ectopy.[17]

Coronary arteriography is frequently associated with premature ventricular contractions. Ventricular fibrillation occurs with an incidence of 1.28 percent.[7]

Effects on myocardial contractile state. Contrast materials currently used for coronary arteriography produce multiple hemodynamic actions including direct depression in myocardial contractile ability. This has been so for experimental studies in isolated heart preparations[4,51], as well as in situ studies in conscious and anesthetized dogs.[5,6] After injection of contrast material into the coronary artery of the dog, there is initial depression in parameters of the left ventricular contractile state followed by a reflex increase in these parameters (Fig. 4-2). This myocardial depression seems, predominantly, to be a consequence of the high osmolarity of the solution and the content of sodium ions.[4,18] The iodine, containing anion moiety, influences circulatory dynamics to a minor extent. The addition of appropriate concentrations of calcium ions to ionic contrast material reverses or alleviates the myocardial depressing action of the contrast materials (Fig. 4-2).[18] In this regard, some ionic contrast materials lower the concentration of ionic calcium in the coronary circulation by a dilutional as well as a binding effect (Fig. 4-3).[19] This reduction in ionic calcium has been implicated as the cause of electromechanical dissociation and death during coronary arteriography.[20] Newer contrast

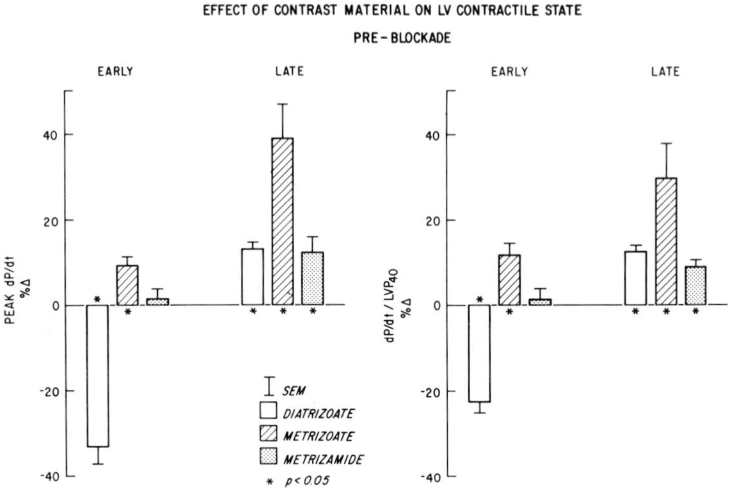

Fig. 4-2. Block diagram contrasts the percent change in parameters of left ventricular contractile state induced by intra-coronary injection of Renografin 76 (meglumine sodium diatrizoate), Isopaque 370 (calcium sodium meglumine mettrizoate), and metrizamide (non-ionic contrast material). Renografin 76 produced a profound depression in contractile state early (1-10 sec.) followed by an adrenergically mediated increase in contractile state (10-20 sec.). Isopaque 370 and metrizamide did not cause any direct depression in LV contractile state initially and did produce the late adrenergically mediated increase in contractile state. Semi-standard error of mean. (Reproduced with permission of *Radiology*.)

materials, which are either non-ionic solutions (metrizamide) and, therefore, less hypertonic (lower osmolarity), or calcium-containing ionic solutions (Isopaque Coronar), produce less or in some studies no myocardial depression (Fig. 4-2).[5]

Transient hypotension almost invariably accompanies injections of contrast material into the coronary arteries. This hypotension is a reflection of two actions of contrast materials: myocardial depression and peripheral vasodilatation. The effect is less severe with the non-ionic and calcium-containing ionic materials.[5] A recent study has suggested that activation of a reflex resembling the Bezold-Jarisch reflex may contribute to the peripheral vasodilatation and hypotension during coronary arteriography.[21] Prolonged hypotension has also been observed after coronary and other types of arteriography, and has been alleviated by volume expansion with crystalloid solutions.[22]

It should be emphasized that, while electrophysiologic and hemodynamic alterations are induced uniformly by injection of contrast material into the coronary arteries, major complications related to contrast mate-

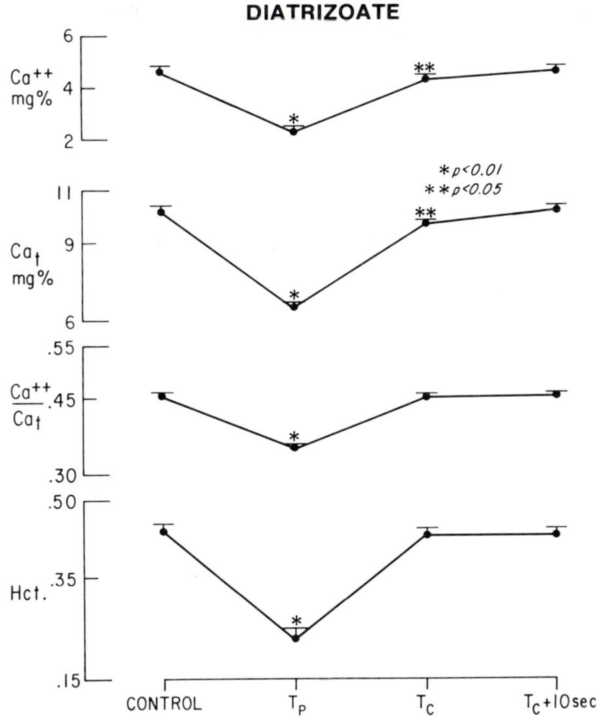

Fig. 4-3. Time sequence of the alterations in coronary sinus ionic calcium (Ca^{++}), total calcium (Ca_t), ratio of Ca^{++} and Ca_t (Ca^{++}/Ca_t) and hematocrit (Hct) induced by intracoronary administration of Renografin 76. The decline in Ca^{++}/Ca_t indicates binding of ionic calcium in addition to the dilutional effect of addition of contrast material to the blood in the coronary circulation. The magnitude of the dilutional effect is reflected by the drop in Hct. Tp = Time of peak coronary sinus opacification; Tc = Time of clearance of opacification of coronary sinus. (Reproduced with permission of the American Heart Association.)

rial are exceedingly infrequent. The current discussion has considered only the usual actions of contrast materials on the cardiovascular system and has not described the so-called allergic or idiosyncratic reactions to contrast material. Allergic or idiosyncratic reactions may rarely occur whenever contrast material is introduced into the vascular system. These reactions seem to be more frequent when contrast material is injected into the venous rather than the arterial side of the circulation.

Finally, expansion of the vascular space by the sheer volume of hypertonic contrast solution has been implicated in producing pulmonary edema.[23] This has been a problem where volumes greater than 200 ml. of contrast material have been administered. It has occurred in patients with apparently normal cardiac function, as well as in patients with heart disease.

DRUGS USED FOR THERAPY AND PROPHYLAXIS

Atropine Sulfate

Although not widely accepted, some coronary angiographers have advocated the prophylactic use of atropine for the prevention of bradyarrhythmias and AV nodal conduction disturbances occurring during coronary arteriography. No large scale trials have evaluated the efficacy of prophylactic atropine for the prevention of these electrophysiologic abnormalities. The experimental and clinical data discussed above suggest that much of the effect of contrast material on the electrical system of the heart is related to its direct effect; its action would probably not be affected by the prophylactic administration of atropine. Although atropine has no apparent role as a prophlyactic agent to be administered prior to coronary arteriography, it can be extremely useful in reversing the hypotension and bradycardia associated with the occasional vasovagal reaction that may occur during this invasive procedure. Atropine may prevent coronary artery spasm, and should therefore be especially avoided as a vaso-vagal prophylactic for patients in whom spasm is a likely diagnosis. The incidence of side effects associated with the dose of atropine is low. It will almost uniformly result in an increase in the heart rate, which may precipitate a bout of angina pectoris, or rarely, a serious ventricular arrhythmia. Other reactions may not manifest themselves immediately in the catheterization laboratory, and may only become apparent after the patient has been returned to the medical ward. These include dry mouth and acute urinary retention. The latter reaction is especially likely to occur in elderly males with symptoms of prostatic obstruction.

Anticoagulants: Heparin and Protamine Sulfate

Early studies[24-26] evaluating the use of the Judkins femoral approach to coronary arteriography indicated that a high rate of femoral thrombosis and systemic embolism (primarily to the coronary arteries) was related to thrombus formed on catheters and guidewires. Subsequently several studies[27-29] have shown that it is possible to achieve a marked reduction in the rate of these complications through the use of sytemic heparinization. These studies have utilized doses of heparin ranging from 3,000 to 10,000 units. Although there is in theory a greater risk that a bleeding complication will arise during the brief period of systemic heparinization associated with performing a coronary arteriogram, studies to date have failed to indicate that this is a serious consideration. It is generally preferred, although not mandatory, that systemic heparinization with protamine sulfate be reversed at the end of the arteriographic procedure, and that this be done prior to catheter removal in order to avoid the occasional hematoma; the dose of protamine can be calculated utilizing the loading dose and half life of heparin, and the duration of the procedure. Potential side effects of intravenous injection of protamine include sudden fall in blood pressure, bradycardia, dypsnea, transitory flushing and a feeling of warmth.[30] In our experience such reactions are extremely infrequent. We have noted the rare occurrence of an apparent anaphylactic reaction following the administration of protamine sulfate. This reaction has occurred only in patients who had previously been treated with protamine containing insulin preparations; therefore, brittle diabetics may become sensitive to protamine and should be treated as special risks.

Nitroglycerin

Nitroglycerin is commonly administered sublingually during coronary arteriography to relieve angina pectoris or reverse coronary arterial spasm, which may occur spontaneously or be pharmacologically provoked. Nitroglycerin may also have some role in reducing the occurrence of spasm caused by the mechanical irritation of the catheter. When used in this manner, nitroglycerin may occasionally provoke transient headaches and/or marked hypotension with associate tachycardia. Nitroglycerin's hemodynamic effects are precipitated by its dilatory action on the venous capacitance of vessels and on the peripheral pooling of blood. In most instances, it is a mild and transient reaction. More severe hypotension can frequently be ameliorated by placing the patient in the Trendelenberg position and administering fluids to maintain circulating blood volume.

Lidocaine

Ventricular arrhythmias may occur during coronary arteriography either spontaneously as a result of the underlying cardiac condition or as a complication of the procedure itself. These arrhythmias commonly include isolated ventricular ectopic beats, ventricular tachycardia and, on occasion, ventricular fibrillation. In general, isolated ventricular ectopic beats occurring during the procedure do not require therapy. However, when they are extremely frequent, as in a bigeminal rhythm pattern, it may be difficult to interpret the left ventricular angiogram that is obtained in association with the coronary arteriography. Under such circumstances it may be desirable to use lidocaine to suppress the ectopic beats. When the ectopic beats during left ventricular angiography are due to mechanical catheter irritation it becomes less clear as to whether lidocaine is therapeutic for eliminating the irritability.

When sustained ventricular tachycardia occurs during coronary arteriography, it is important to assess rapidly the hemodynamic consequences of the rhythm. If the patient is maintaining adequate arterial pressure and not experiencing severe chest pain or showing evidence of decreased cerebral profusion, lidocaine, as an intravenous bolus, may be administered as the initial attempt to terminate the arrhythmia. For sustained ventricular tachycardia associated with marked hemodynamic embarrassment a quick fist "thump" to the chest followed by immediate electrical cardioversion are probably preferable to the administration of lidocaine. Lidocaine should not be used as the immediate therapy for ventricular fibrillation, which is always treated by electrical cardioversion. However, if cardioversion results in only a brief period of normal rhythm that rapidly reverts to ventricular tachycardia or fibrillation, the administration of a bolus of lidocaine is indicated prior to repeating cardioversion. When a patient has experienced sustained ventricular tachycardia or fibrillation, the bolus of lidocaine should be followed by a second bolus as well as maintenance infusion as discussed below.

The usual initial loading dose of lidocaine is 75 to 125 mg. given intravenously over three or four minutes. However, because of the rapid distribution of the drug, plasma concentrations fall rapidly after a single intravenous bolus. Within five to fifteen minutes, the plasma concentrations may fall to subtherapeutic ranges.[31] Thus, if longer protection from lidocaine is desired, it is important to administer an additional small bolus of 25 to 75 mg., (also given slowly over several minutes) approximately ten minutes after the administering of the initial bolus, and to start a constant intravenous infusion of lidocaine at the time of the initial bolus. The usual infusion rate for patients free of hepatic disease or congestive heart failure is 2 to 4 mg. per minute. The use of these doses in most patients will result in therapeutic plasma concentrations of 1 to 6 μg./ml. However, in the presence of congestive heart failure or cardiogenic shock, both the loading dose of lidocaine and the rate of the constant infusion should be markedly diminished to avoid toxic plasma lidocaine concentrations that may result from the reduced volume of distribution in these states.

The side effects of lidocaine are largely restricted to the central nervous system.[31,32] Minor side effects include paresthesia, nausea, somnolence, slurred speech and focal seizures. Grand mal seizures constitute a major adverse reaction and usually occur in association with high plasma concentrations. These high concentrations most frequently occur during rapid intravenous bolus administration, especially in patients with congestive heart failure. Slow administration of the loading bolus and reduction in dose in patients with congestive heart failure should preclude these complications in most patients. Large bolus injections may also result in heart block, sinoatrial arrest, hypotension and respiratory arrest. Under most circumstances, lidocaine does not cause significant hemodynamic alterations.

MECHANICAL HAZARDS

The risk of complications is ever present during invasive procedures and the opportunities for disaster are many. The choice of catheter and injection flow rates remain empirical and are often determined by personal experience and preference. Angiographic contrast medium jet forces and catheter recoil can cause vascular trauma and have recently been analyzed.[33] Appropriate safe injection flow rates can be predicted without sacrificing film quality. However, even when these measures are taken, an injection (hand or mechanical) can be extremely dangerous if the catheter tip position is incorrect. One example that may be fatal is rupture of the coronary sinus by a pressure injection intended for the right ventricle. Fluoroscopy as well as pressure recordings may be used to verify that the catheter is in the right ventricle.[34,35] It is difficult, then, to believe that this complication can occur, and a test injection of a few ml. of contrast medium by hand prior to the angiogram itself will nearly always prevent this kind of disaster. The test injection should be performed while the patient is in precisely the same position and phase of respiration as those to be used for the angiogram. When a second pump injection is made requiring repositioning of either patient or catheter, a second test injection is mandatory and this will usually prevent such complications.

PROCEDURE PLANNING AND ESTABLISHING LABORATORY ROUTINE

Physicians should adopt proven routine patterns for procedures in their laboratories and should be present and scrubbed during necessary trainee supervision. Unfortunately, experience and idiosyncracies vary widely among both hospitals and individual angiographers.

Experienced operators as well as their junior colleagues face unfamiliar situations, and it is during a period or moment of uncertainty that problems are most likely to arise. The angiographer must therefore anticipate such potential hazards. The operator is responsible for assigning the types of medication to be used, the dosages, and the routes of administration. He should personally supervise to ensure proper follow-through. But the importance of developing good habits with frequent emergency drills that involve all members of the catheterization team cannot be sufficiently emphasized.

Pharmaceutical preparations are usually given parenterally for speed and effectiveness during coronary arteriography. It is our routine practice to introduce a small catheter (not a needle) in a peripheral vein at the onset of all coronary arteriograms and to ensure its patency throughout the procedure by slow intravenous drip infusion. Many cardiologists and radiologists do not observe this safeguard, and when right heart catheterization does not precede angiography, parenteral medications may sometimes be administered by direct intra-arterial injection for convenience. This is a dangerous practice. Intra-arterial barbiturates and other preparations such as hydroxyzine hydrochloride (Vistaril) have been known to result in the complete or partial loss of a limb.[36] Van der Port first reported the intra-arterial toxicity of barbiturates in 1942, and it is now known that many other substances, including promazine (Sparine), tubocuracine, strophanthin and amphetamines many also cause toxic reactions when given by direct intra-arterial injection. The mechanism of action was initially thought to be arterial spasm related to high alkalinity, but it is now believed that the major factor is a chemical endarteritis which can result in secondary thrombosis. The selective injection of any drug by way of an intra-arterial catheter results in the delivery of a concentrated solution into the distal capillary bed. The injection, for example, of 5 to 10 mg. of Valium (Diazepam) is usually quite safe when given intravenously, but a similar injection into the aortic root has been known to precipitate cardiac arrest. This sort of complication is fortunately rare, but can be completely avoided.

When right heart catheterization precedes left-sided cardioangiography, as it usually does, then drugs can be administered intravenously. However, the catheter should be withdrawn from the heart and the location of the tip of the catheter checked before any pharmocological preparations are administered. Such injections can be (and have been) given inadvertently into the coronary sinus; if this occurs, a major complication may result. Resuscitative measures including CPR and emergency drug administration can be found in standard texts and will not, therefore, be discussed.

Additionally, each medication should be injected separately from a clean syringe. The tendency to mix drugs in combination (a cocktail approach) should be avoided because various dangerous chemical interactions, including precipitation and/or crystallization of the contrast agent, may occur.

Finally, it is the responsibility of the cardiologist or radiologist to monitor the recovery progress following any angiographic-related complication. One physician who failed to observe this rule was faced with a $750,000 settlement;[37] although an intravenous aramine infusion had been used to treat sudden hypotension, the patient, following recovery to normotensive levels, became hypertensive. Although this episode was only transient, it resulted in intracerebral hemorrhage. Patient management following coronary arteriography does not end when the patient leaves the laboratory, especially when there has been a complication. Monitoring vital signs and documentating details are the responsibilities of the angiographer. The angiographer should always seek the advice of a colleague (when necessary) at the first sign of uncertainty. Impaired renal function is a complication that is diagnosed late in too many patients. Adequate hydration prior to angiography (balanced against the individual patient's cardiac status) will reduce complications. Coronary arteriography is a complex procedure, and physicians performing it will require many qualities including knowledge, patience, and anticipation.

RADIOPHARMACEUTICALS

Radiopharmaceuticals employed in nuclear cardiology are 201 Thallium, 99m-Tc Albumen, 99m-Tc Red Blood Cells, and 99m-Tc Pyrophosphate. These are administered in tracer amounts—rarely micrograms or nanogram units. The quantities are too small to produce allergic or anaphylactic reactions. The only radiopharmaceuticals which may produce adverse reactions involve intra-arterial injections of 131I-MAA or 99m-Tc-MAA, which have been used for estimating myocardial blood flow. The mechanism causing problems is thought to be mechanical occlusion of the capillary vascular bed. Pyrogen reactions are seen extremely rarely, since the pharmaceutical companies provide pyrogen-free preparations.

PROVOCATIVE PHARMOCOANGIOGRAPHY

Coronary arterial spasm has been implicated as an important pathogenetic factor in producing myocardial ischemia in a small group of patients with angina.[38–41] While this pathogenetic mechanism has been most frequently found in patients with rest or variant angina, it has also been noted in patients with crescendo angina and typical exertional angina.[40,41] Spasm has been observed in normal coronary arteries and superimposed on stenoses of coronary arteries. Recently, a variety of drugs have been administered during coronary arteriography in order to provoke coronary arterial spasm in susceptible individuals, thereby documenting spasm as the primary cause of myocardial ischemia in these patients.[39-46]

While the precise mechanism and reason for hypersensitivity of the coronary arteries to vasoconstrictor influences in certain individuals are unclear at this time, several drugs are capable of eliciting localized or diffuse coronary arterial spasm.[39-46] The induced spasm is usually accompanied by angina and electrocardiographic signs of myocardial ischemia. In a few instances, ventricular extrasystoles, ventricular tachycardia, and heart block have ensued.[43,46] While spontaneous spasm during coronary arteriography has resulted in myocardial infarction[47], provocative pharmocoangiography has not to our knowledge caused myocardial infarction. The coronary arterial pathoanatomy should be defined by a baseline coronary arteriogram prior to the provocative arteriogram.

The induced spasm is almost invariably reversed by sub-lingual nitroglycerin. In rare instances reversal of spasm has necessitated intravenous administration of nitroglycerin (direct vasodilator), nitroprusside (direct vasodilator), or phentolamine (direct vasodilator and alpha adrenergic blocker).

A variety of drugs have been used to produce coronary arterial spasm.[39-46] These include: ergonovine maleate, methacholine, methoxamine, epinephrine plus propranolol, and vasopressin. Coronary arterial spasm has also been induced by hyperventilation and the cold pressor test. Besides the potential complications that may arise because of the acute onset of myocardial ischemia, each of these drugs is associated with certain side effects.

The drug most frequently used for provocative pharmacoangiography is ergonovine maleate. In certain susceptible individuals, such as those with Raynaud's disease, the use of ergot compounds has resulted in reversible and irreversible ischemic injuries of the extremities and the parenchymal organs (ergotism).[48,49] These drugs may cause a variety of minor gastrointestinal disturbances, including abdominal cramping, vomiting, retching, and diarrhea.[43,50]

Methacholine has been used mosly by Japanese investigators.[42,44] It has and should be administered subcutaneously; intravenous administration causes an increase in the incidence and severity of side effects, which include syncope, nausea, vomiting, attacks of asthma, hypotension, and heart block.[50] The major contraindications to its use are: asthma, hyperthyroidism, and peptic ulcer disease.[50]

Epinephrine and vasopressin have been used frequently for provocative pharmacoangiography. A complete list of their side effects is available in textbooks of pharmacology.

REFERENCES

1. Higgins CB: Effect of contrast media on the conducting system of the heart. Radiology 124:597, 1977
2. Higgins CB and Feld GK: Direct chronotropic and dromotropic actions of contrast material: Ineffectiveness of atropine in the prevention of bradyarrhythmias and conduction disturbances. Radiology 121:205, 1976
3. Eckberg DL, White CW, Kioschos JM, et al: Mechanisms mediating bradycardia during coronary arteriography. J Clin Invest 54:1455, 1974
4. Wolf GL, Gerlings ED, Wilson WJ: Depression of myocardial contractility induced by hypertonic coronary injections in the isolated perfused dog heart. Radiology 107:655, 1973
5. Higgins CB and Schmidt W: Direct and reflex effects of intracoronary administered contrast materials in the anesthetized and conscious dog. Comparison of standard and newer contrast materials. Invest Radiol, Submitted, 1978
6. Trägårdh B, Lynch PR, Vinciguerra T: Cardiac function during coronary arteriography with calcium enriched diatrizoate and metrizamide. Invest Radiol 11:569, 1976
7. Adams DF, Fraser DB, Abrams HL: The complications of coronary arteriography. Circulation 48:609, 1973
8. Bourassa MG and Noble J: Complication rate of coronary arteriography. A review of 5250 cases studied by a percutaneous technique. Circulation 53:106, 1976
9. Lebowitz WB and Lucia W: Complications of selective percutaneous transfemoral coronary arteriography. Radiology 116:545, 1975
10. Miller D, Lohse J, Wolf G: Slow response induced in canine purkinje fiber by contrast medium. Invest Radiol 11:577, 1976
11. Langou RA, Sheps DS, Wolfson S, et al: Intraventricular conduction during coronary arteriography in patients with pre-existing conduction abnormalities. Invest Radiol 12:505, 1977
12. Sostman HD, Simon AL, Langou RA: Localization of the conduction delay occurring during coronary arteriography. Invest Radiol 12:128, 1977
13. Eie H, Grendahl H, Nordvik A, et al: Electrocardiographic changes during selective coronary angiography. Acta Radiol (Diagn) 12:554, 1972
14. Fernandez F, Scebat L, Lenegre J: Electrocardiographic study of left intraventricular hemiblock in man during selective coronary arteriography. Am J Cardiol 26:1, 1970
15. Simon AL, Shabetai R, Lang JH, et al: The mechanism of production of ventricular fibrillation in coronary angiography. Am J Roentgenol 114:810, 1972
16. Fisher et al: Deleterious synergism of a cardiac glycoside and sodium diatrizoate. Investigative Radiology (In Press), 1978
17. Trägårdh B, Lynch PR, Vinciguerra T: Effects of metrizamide, a new nonionic contrast medium, on cardiac function during coronary angiography in the dog. Radiology 115:59, 1975
18. Salvesen S, Nilsen PL, Holtermann H: Ameliorating effect of calcium and magnesium ions on the toxicity of isopaque sodium. Acta Radiol (Suppl) 270:30, 1967
19. Higgins CB and Schmidt W: Alterations in calcium levels of coronary sinus blood during coronary arteriography in the dog. Circulation (In Press), 1978
20. Caulfield JB, Zir L, Harthorne JW: Blood calcium levels in the presence of arteriographic contrast material. Circulation 52:119, 1975
21. Zelis R, Caudill CC, Baggette K, et al: Reflex vasodilation induced by coronary angiography in human subjects. Circulation 53:490, 1976
22. Obeid AI, Johnson L, Potts J, et al: Fluid therapy in severe systemic reaction to radiopaque dye. Ann Int Med 83:317, 1975

23. Malins AF: Pulmonary edema after radiological investigation of peripheral occlusive vascular disease. Adverse reaction to contrast material. Lancet 1:413–415, 1978
24. Adams DF, Fraser DB, Abrams HL: Complications of coronary arteriography. Circulation 48:609–618, 1973
25. Takaro T, Hultgren HN, Detre KM: An assessment of risks and causes of death in association with coronary arteriography, in JC Norman (ed): Coronary Artery Medicine Surgery–Concepts and Controversies. New York, Appleton Century Crofts, 1975
26. Petch MC, Sutton R, Jefferson KE: Safety of coronary arteriography. British Heart Journal 35:377–380, 1973
27. Wallace S, Medellin H, De Jongh D, and Gianturco C: Systemic heparinization for angiography. Amer J Roentgen 116:204–209, 1972
28. Nelson RM, Osborne AG: Systemic heparinization for percutaneous catheter arteriography. Circulation Suppl II, 42 and 44 (Abstract)205, 1971
29. Walker WJ, Mundal SL, Broderick HG et al: Systemic heparinization for femoral percutaneous coronary arteriography. N Engl J Med 288:826–828, 1973
30. Goodman LS and Gilman A: The Pharmacologic Basis of Therapeutics, 3rd ed, New York, Macmillan, 1974
31. Winkle RA, Glantz SA, Harrison DC: Pharmacologic therapy of ventricular arrhythmias. Amer J Cardiol 36:629–650, 1975
32. Harrison DC, Meffin PJ, Winkle RA: Clinical pharmacokinetics of antiarrhythmic drugs. Progress in Cardiovascular Disease 20:217–242, 1977
33. Lipton MJ, Abbott JA, Kosek JC, Hayashi T, Lee FCS, Bishop E: Cardiovascular trauma from angiographic jets—validation of a theoretic concept in a canine model. Radiology 129:363, 1978
34. Zimmerman HA: Intravascular catherization, 2nd ed, Springfield, Illinois, Charles C Thomas, 1966
35. Ansell G, ed: Complications in Diagnostic Radiology, Oxford, Blackwell Scientific Publications, 1976
36. Klatte EC, Brooks AL, Rhamy RK: Toxicity of intra-arterial barbiturates and tranquilizing drugs. Radiology 92:700–704: March 1969
37. Rubasmen DS, ed: Los Angeles Superior Court Case NWC-43902. Professional Liability Newsletter, California Malpractice Topics 9 No 9, March 1978
38. Prinzmetal M, Kennamer R, Merliss R, et al: Angina pectoris. I. A variant form of angina pectoris. Preliminary Report. Am J Med 27:375, 1959
39. Higgins CB, Wexler L, Silverman JF, et al: Clinical and arteriographic features of Prinzmetal's variant angina. Documentation of etiologic factors. Am J Cardiol 37:831, 1976
40. Wiener L, Kasparian H, Duca PR, et al: Spectrum of coronary arterial spasm. Clinical, angiographic, and myocardial metabolic experience in 29 cases. Am J Cardiol 38:945, 1976
41. Schroeder JS, Bolen JL, Quint RA, et al: Provocation of coronary spasm with ergonovine maleate. New test with results in 57 patients undergoing coronary arteriography. Am J Cardiol 40:487, 1977
42. Endo M, Kanda I, Hosoda S, et al: Prinzmetal's variant form of angina pectoris. Re-evaluation of mechanisms. Circulation 52:33, 1975
43. Higgins CB, Wexler L, Silverman JF, et al: Spontaneously and pharmacologically provoked coronary arterial spasm in Prinzmetal variant angina. Radiology 119:521, 1976
44. Endo M, Hirosawa K, Kaneko N, et al: Prinzmetal's variant angina. Coronary arteriogram and left ventriculogram during angina attack induced by methacholine. N Eng J Med 294:252, 1976

45. Yasue H, Masato T, Kato H, et al: Prinzmetal's variant form of angina as a manifestation of alpha adrenergic receptor-mediated coronary artery spasm: Documentation by coronary arteriography. Am Heart J 91:148, 1976
46. Heupler FA, Proudfit WL, Razavi M, et al: Ergonovine maleate provocative test for coronary artery spasm. Am J Cardiol 41:631, 1978
47. Engel HJ, Page HL, Campbell WB: Coronary artery spasm as the cause of myocardial infarction during coronary arteriography. Am Heart J 91:501, 1976
48. Enge I, Sivertssen E: Ergotism due to therapeutic doses of ergotamine tartrate. Am Heart J 70:665, 1965
49. Robb LG: Severe vasospasm following ergot administration. West J Med 123:231, 1975
50. Goodman LS and Gilman A: The Pharmacological Basis of Therapeutics, 3rd ed, New York, Macmillan, 1974, pp 464–471, 879–886
51. Lipton MJ, Higgins CB, Wiley AA et al: The effect of contrast media on the isolated perfused canine heart. Invest Radiol 13:519–522, 1978

Stephen C. Pardys

5

Drug-Induced Gastrointestinal Disease

A. CLINDAMYCIN-ASSOCIATED PSEUDOMEMBRANOUS COLITIS: A MODEL FOR ANTIBIOTIC-ASSOCIATED COLITIS

Gastrointestinal side effects associated with antibiotic usage are a common phenomenon. Generally, these are non-specific, mildly disabling symptoms such as nausea and cramping and, not infrequently, diarrhea. These symptoms usually subside rapidly when the antibiotic is discontinued. In recent years, however, a more serious, occasionally life-threatening, colonic disorder known as pseudomembranous colitis has been recognized. It has been described in association with the usage of tetracycline,[1] chloramphenicol,[2] ampicillin,[3] lincomycin[4] and, most recently, clindamycin.[5] Clindamycin colitis, because of its greater wealth of literature, will be used as the model.

Clindamycin is a semisynthetic derivative of lincomycin, from which it differs chemically by the substitution of a chlorine atom for a hydroxyl group on the parent compound. This slight modification causes clindamycin to be better absorbed and more potent than lincomycin, thus supplanting it as a first choice treatment in susceptible infections.[6] The primary indication that clindamycin should be used in treatment is the presence of anaerobic bacterial infections caused by certain species of *Bacteroides* not sensitive to penicillin, especially *B. fragilis*. Its use is also indicated in infections caused by susceptible gram-positive organisms resistant to the penicillins and erythromycins, and in patients who cannot tolerate these drugs. It is administered orally, intramuscularly, and intravenously; the development of pseudomembranous colitis has occurred with each route, although the oral route seems to have the largest number of associated cases.[7] In addition, there appears to be no correlation between antibiotic dosage and the occurrence of colitis.[7] Of additional unique interest is the fact that the disorder affects the colon almost exclusively, with only rare small bowel involvement.

Clinical Features

GENERAL SYMPTOMS

The initial features of pseudomembranous colitis are basically non-specific and include fever, cramping, and abdominal pain, with or without the onset of diarrhea (although intractable diarrhea frequently develops).

PROCTOSCOPIC FINDINGS

When pseudomembranous colitis patients are examined proctoscopically, a characteristic mucosal appearance is present, consisting of an erythematous, friable surface covered with small (1 to 5 mm.), raised, yellow-white plaques, often separated from each other by intervening hyperemic mucosa, but occasionally confluent, especially in the later stages of the disorder. Copious amounts of thick mucus are often found which usually must be removed before the characteristic plaques can be seen. When pseudomembrane formation is present, ulcers are not.[8] This helps to distinguish it from other forms of antibiotic-associated colitis, which may reveal ulceration, friability, and hemorrahage suggestive of idiopathic ulcerative colitis and/or ischemic colitis. Crypt abscesses, seen in idiopathic ulcerative colitis, are not seen in antibiotic-associated colitis. When rectal biopsy is obtained in pseudomembranous colitis, the pseudomembrane is noted to be composed of fibrin and inflammatory cells which arise on top of a mucosal ulceration. The surrounding mucosa is intact, but filled with a mixed inflammatory infiltrate.[9,9a] If the entire plaque surface is not obtained by the biopsy forceps, the diagnostic features can be missed.

Recently, six patients were reported who had either normal or only edematous rectal mucosa, and the diagnosis of antibiotic-associated colitis was made by colonoscopy in five of them. One patient did not have any pseudomembranes; the diagnosis was made by positive stool toxin.

RADIOLOGICAL FINDINGS

Radiological studies are not required in making the diagnosis of pseudomembranous colitis. Frequently the radiological findings are non-specific but occasionally characteristic radiological features are noted

(Figs. 5-1–4). Also helpful in the diagnosis of more severe cases are plain films, which demonstrate markedly edematous and distorted haustral markings, an increase in the overall thickness of the colon wall, and moderate to severe distension involving nearly the entire colon.[10] Air contrast barium enema is preferable to a routine study because it affords a better evaluation of the mucosal surface, and can demonstrate the

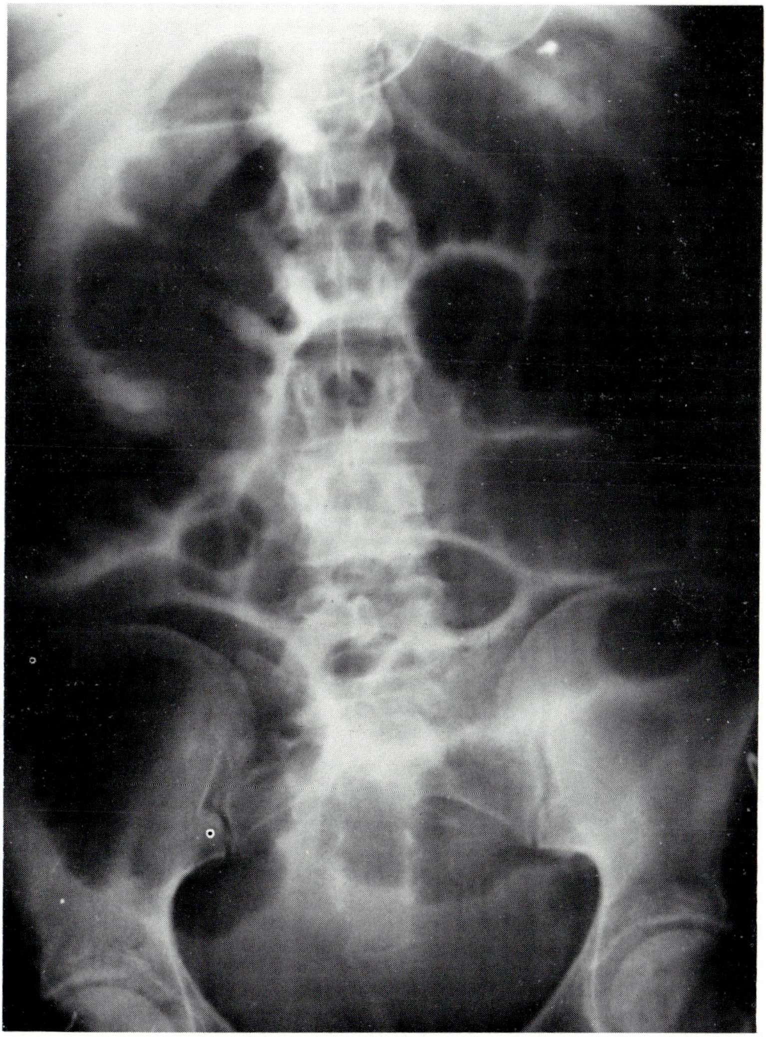

Fig. 5-1. Plain film of abdomen demonstrating severe pancolonic distension with edema and distortion of haustral markings.

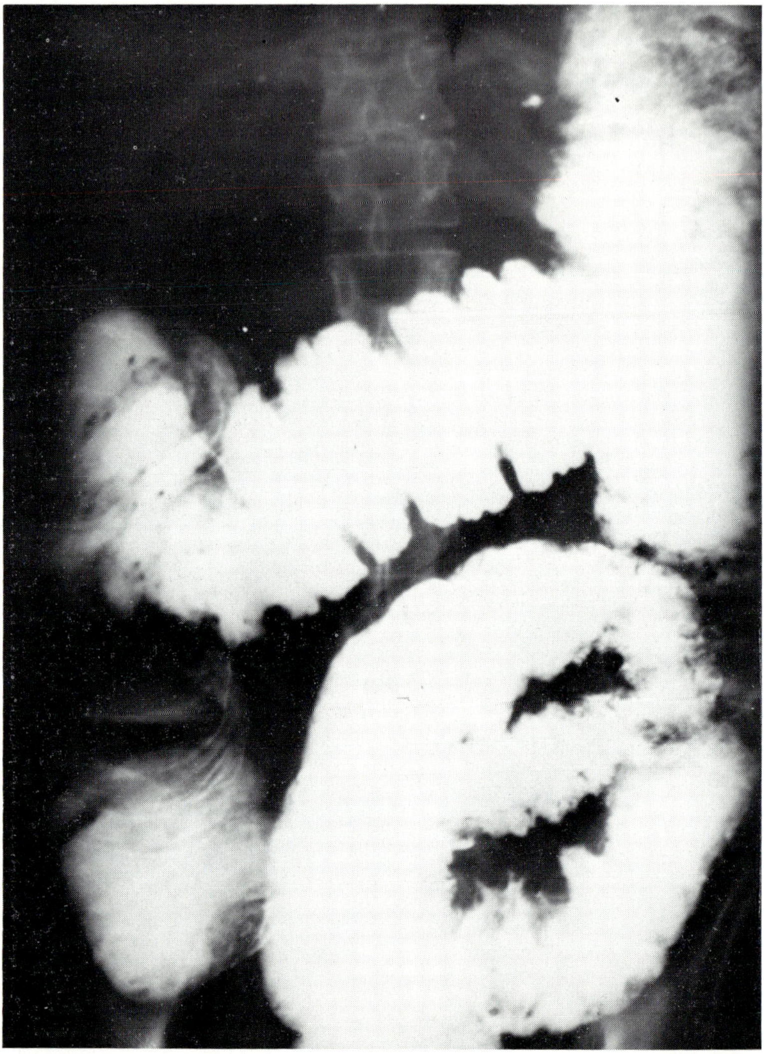

Fig. 5-2. Barium enema demonstrating marked mucosal irregularities involving the entire colon.

mucosal plaques in profile.[11] This may not be possible if there is a great deal of tenacious mucus in the lumen, however. Occasionally, small mucosal irregularities which may simulate ulcers, but which actually represent the pseudomembranous plaques, can be seen. These findings are different from those of ischemic disease, which usually involves only limited segments of the colon, and those of ulcerative colitis, which

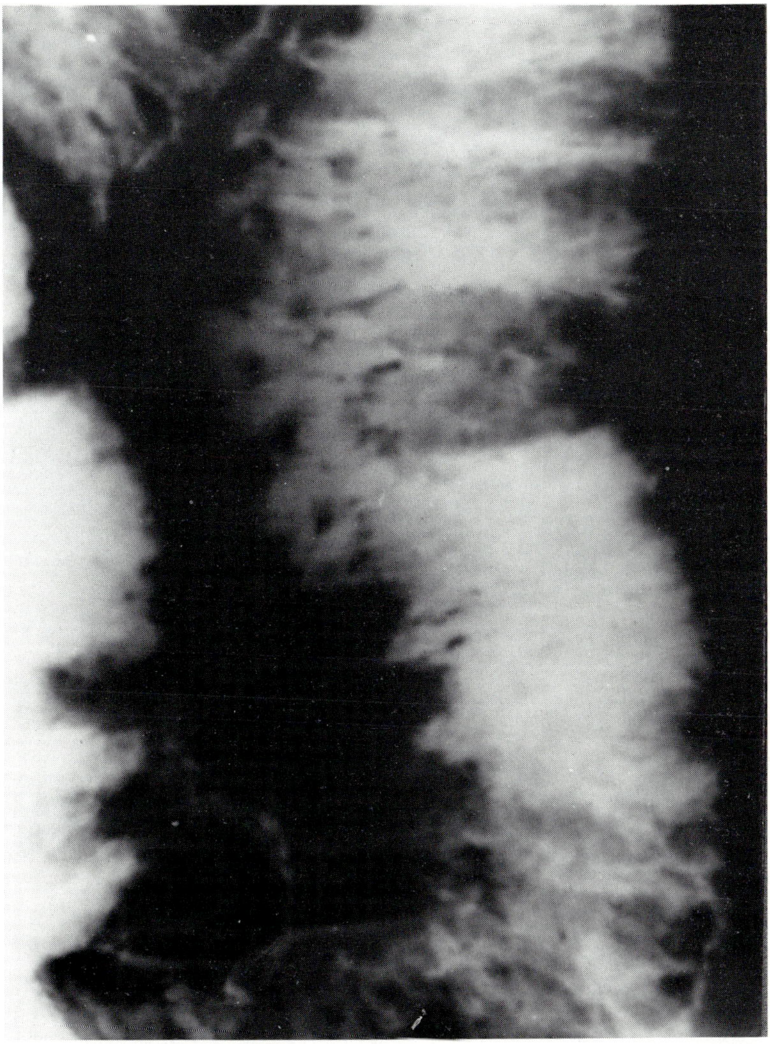

Fig. 5-3. Spot film of descending colon in the same patient as Fig. 2 demonstrating that the mucosal irregularities appear to be raised and flat without obvious ulcerations.

usually presents more gaseous distension and a thin colonic wall with occasional pseudopolyp formation.

If the diagnosis is suspected clinically, proctoscopic evaluation should be diagnostic and radiological studies would be unnecessary. This would be beneficial to the patient in terms of comfort and lower costs, and would prevent the risks of toxic megacolon and perforation which could

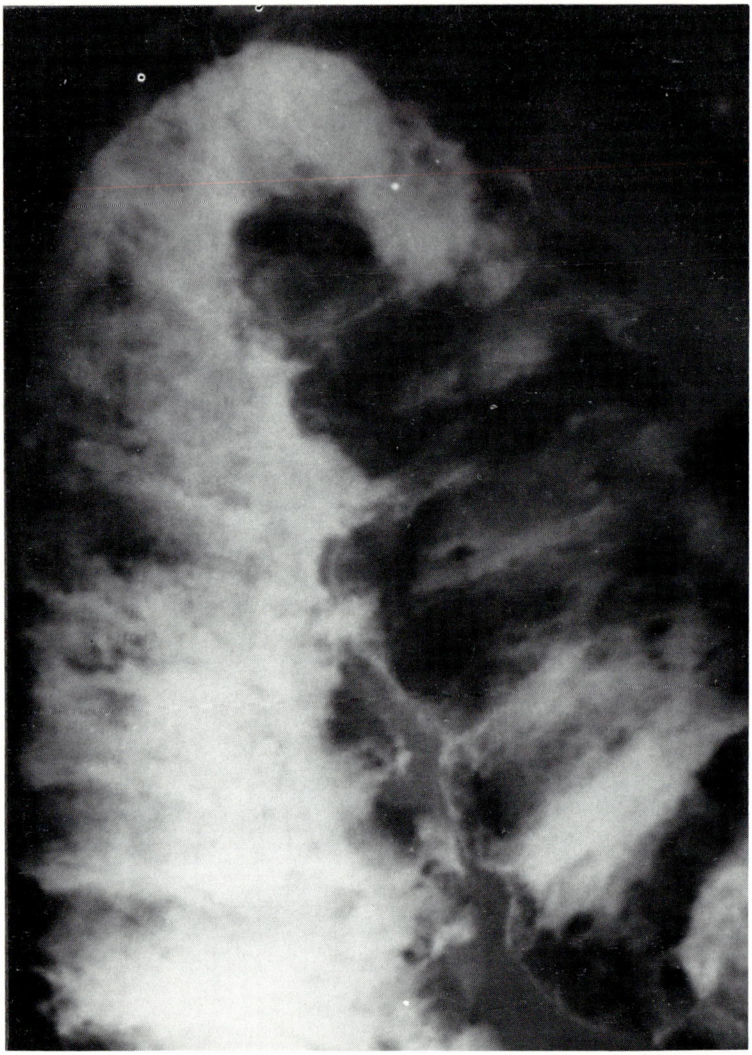

Fig. 5-4. Spot film of ascending colon and proximal transverse colon in the same patient as Fig. 2.

be present in the more severe cases characterized by submucosal involvement.[12]

AGE AND SEX

A greater proportion of females than males have been reported with this disorder. Age does not appear to be a very relevant factor, with the exception that the condition is rare in the pediatric population. Older patients may be at greater risk because of other underlying conditions, such as congestive heart failure, shock and surgery, that contribute to the development of pseudomembranous colitis without antibiotic association.

CLINICAL COURSE

The diarrhea usually starts within a week of therapy and is usually mild to moderate, although severe cases with development of marked hypoalbuminemia, dehydration, hypotension, and electrolyte imbalance have been reported.[7] Cases in which the diagnosis was suspected and made earlier in the course of the illness rarely developed into severe problems. The diarrhea may begin to improve during the first week, but usually lasts at least two to three weeks. Occasionally, symptoms fail to develop until after the antibiotic therapy has been discontinued. The stool is not grossly bloody and is usually negative for occult blood. Most cases resolve spontaneously, but there is an overall mortality of approximately 15 percent when the larger series are combined.[13] Fewer cases of severe disease have been reported in the literature in recent years.

Incidence

The incidence of clindamycin-associated colitis seems to be determined by several variables. These include not only the lower incidence associated with failure to perform sigmoidoscopy in certain centers, but also a geographical variability in the distribution of cases, as well as a temporal variability within the same institution.[14] The manufacturer reported an incidence of one in 50,000 to 100,000 treatment courses.[15] However, when reports of the centers with the largest numbers of cases are examined, this figure does not hold up.

In a prospective study of 200 consecutive patients treated with clindamycin in Barnes Hospital, St. Louis, Missouri, the incidence of patients who developed diarrhea was 21 percent.[7] Pseudomembranous colitis was found in seventy-eight percent of those who were proctoscoped—an incidence of ten percent of all patients treated with clindamycin. None of these patients had a fulminant course resulting in death. A retrospective study in the Dallas area reported an incidence of one in 5,000 to 10,000.[16] The University of Oregon Medical School reported on six cases recognized in a six month period. Two of those patients subsequently expired;[17] both had serious underlying disorders. Michael Reese Hospital in Chicago, Illinois reported that there were no obvious episodes of colitis during the first twenty months of clindamycin usage at that institution. In the ensuing two months, however, nine patients (17 percent) developed colitis, eight percent of whom had documented pseudomembranous changes. These figures are similar to those in the St. Louis series.[14] Four of these patients died, all of whom had serious underlying disorders. A study of 1,000 consecutively-treated patients at Stanford revealed only a 6.6 percent incidence of diarrhea, of which only 0.3 percent were severe, protracted cases.[18] In a later study by the Barnes Hospital group of 47 cases, 74 percent were not associated with serious underlying disease.[19] When all of the above studies are examined, it is interesting to note that the vast majority of cases of the disorder occurred in 1974. The reason for this is not readily apparent and has led to an impression of a possible "epidemic" nature.

Etiology

The cause of clindamycin-associated colitis is currently unknown, although several experiments performed over the past two years, which will be discussed subsequently, have revealed some fascinating results suggesting a particular bacterium as the culprit.[20-24] Several major theories were previously advanced. One is that the antibiotic and/or its metabolites has a direct toxic effect on the gut. No studies have been reported as yet to confirm this theory. Another theory is that changes in bacterial flora are responsible for the condition, or that it is due to superinfection by pathogenic bacteria.

Because of the previously known entity staphylococcal enterocolitis, attempts were made to culture staphylococcal organisms in the stools of affected patients. No unusual staphylococcal counts were discovered. A blind prospective study was undertaken to assess the hypothesis that alterations in the microbial flora of the colon were responsible. All of the patients whose stools were tested were receiving clindamycin, and all had diarrhea secondary to the use of the drug. There was a striking decrease, both qualitatively and quantitatively, in the anaerobes present in patients with diarrhea and pseudomembranous colitis. In patients with diarrhea but without pseudomembrane formation, there was a decrease in quantity, but an essentially normal qualitative mixture. The third group of patients were no longer symptomatic, had resolving pseudomembranous colitis, and had large numbers of anaerobic organisms similar to those found in normal fecal cultures. No other information was gleaned.

In a subsequent study, a filterable, heat-labile toxin was described as being present in the feces of five patients with pseudomembranous colitis but absent from control cases.[21] This toxin was believed to be of bacterial origin, and in later studies was found to be neutralized by *Clostridium sordellii* antitoxin.[22] Attempts to culture *C. sordellii* in the stools of affected patients, however, were not successful.

Studies were performed on rabbits given clindamycin by nasogastric tube in doses comparable to those used in man.[23] At autopsy the major gross pathological finding was limited to massive dilatation of the cecum with watery stool. Light microscopy demonstrated necrosis of the surface epithelium, which suggested a cytotoxic process. Aerobic and anaerobic cultures of the cecal contents were obtained, and no change was noted in total anaerobe counts in the clindamycin-treated rabbits when compared with controls. When selective culture media for *Clostridia* were used, however, a marked increase in clostridial species was demonstrated. Of additional interest was that none of the rabbits given vancomycin concurrently with the clindamycin developed fatal colitis, and cecal contents showed a decrease in clostridial species.

After several laboratories reported that stools from patients with antibiotic-associated colitis contained a cytopathic toxin inactivated by clostridial antitoxins, a study was performed on the stools of 38 patients with this disorder to detect clostridia which produce a cytopathic toxin in vitro. *Clostridium difficile* were recovered from six of eight specimens that were positive in the tissue culture assay.[24] One hundred nine clostridia strains were tested in the tissue culture assay and *C. difficile* was the only species to produce a cytopathic toxin. In each test, this cytotoxicity was neutralized by *C. sordellii* antitoxin. These studies do not prove that this organism is the sole cause of colitis, but they certainly represent a strong, important contribution.

There have also been recent electron microscope studies of mucosal biopsies in patients with clindamycin-associated pseudomembranous colitis in which virus-like particles were demonstrated.[25,26] Whether these are artifacts of tissue processing or actually infective viral bodies has not yet been resolved.

Treatment

The successful treatment of antibiotic-associated colitis depends primarily on early recognition of the disorder followed by immediate discontinuation of the drug. Most cases with prolonged symptoms or more severe sequelae occurred when the diagnosis was made later in the course of the illness, or when the antibiotic was continued in the face of persistent diarrhea.[7] Corticosteroids have been used but without documented effectiveness. There is controversy over the use of antiperistaltic agents, such as Lomotil, that may either prolong the course of the illness, as has been suggested in infectious diarrheas, or precipitate the development of toxic megacolon, as has been suggested in acute flares of chronic idiopathic ulcerative colitis.[27] Lomotil has been used with apparent success, however, without contributing to further difficulties.[7] Cholestyramine, a resin compound of great symptomatic benefit in patients with bile salt-induced diarrhea, has also been utilized and several cases of apparent benefit have been described.[28] Larger studies of benefit confirming this have not subsequently been described. Based upon evidence gathered from recent animal studies that demonstrates the apparent effectiveness of protection attainable by co-administration of vancomycin, it has been suggested that patients with antibiotic-associated colitis be treated with oral vancomycin in doses of 500 mg. every six hours.[29] Further trials with this therapy will be needed to prove its efficacy. In patients with more severe cases, relevant supportive measures may be needed to maintain adequate intravascular volumes, such as those of colloid and blood. The most severe cases may require surgical intervention and varying degrees of colectomy. Even following subtotal colectomy, some cases have persisted with a proctitis severe enough to require proctectomy.[30] A recent study performed on hamsters provided hopeful results suggesting that prior treatment with *Clostridium sordellii* antitoxin would provide passive immunization from colitis after clindamycin challenge.[31] In addition, unlike the case of vancomycin, where relapses were observed after treatment had been discontinued, no relapses have been observed with this method.

Summary

The development of antibiotic-associated colitis may be triggered by the use of several different antibiotics, but the disorder has been reported most frequently in association with the use of clindamycin. Clindamycin associated colitis often has a specific colonic mucosal pattern characterized by the formation of pseudomembranes which may be visualized by proctoscopy, the choice diagnostic procedure. Radiologic studies may also be diagnostic, but, with the exception of plain films, are often unnecessary if skillful sigmoidoscopy is performed. Generally, the disorder is self-limited, and resolves completely when the antibiotic is discontinued. Occasionally a more serious form develops which can be fatal or require surgical intervention. The disorder is not antibiotic dose-related, but occurs more frequently when the oral route is utilized. Although the etiology is not certain, recent studies suggest that a toxin liberated by *Clostridium difficile* may be the cytopathic agent. Because of some apparent cyto-protective effect produced by vancomycin, it is currently felt that patients with antibiotic-associated colitis should be treated with oral vancomycin in doses of 500 mg. every six hours.

REFERENCES

1. Klotz AP, Palmer WL, Kirsner JB: Aureomycin proctitis and colitis—a report of 5 cases. Gastroenterology 25:44–47, 1953
2. Reiner L, Schlesinger MJ, Miller GM: Pseudomembranous colitis following aureomycin and chloramphenicol. Arch Pathol 54:39–67, 1952

3. Schapiro RL, Newman A: Acute enterocolitis. Radiology 108:263–268, 1973
4. Benner EJ, Tillman WH: Pseudomembranous colitis as a sequel to oral lincomycin. Am J Gastroenterol 54:55–58, 1970
5. Cohen LE, McNeill CJ, Wells RF: Clindamycin-associated colitis. JAMA 223:1379–1380, 1973
6. AMA Drug Evaluations (ed. 3). Littleton, Mass, PSG Publishing, 1977
7. Tedesco FJ, Barton RW, Alpers DH: Clindamycin-associated colitis: a prospective study. Ann Intern Med 81:429–433, 1974
8. Tedesco FJ, Stanley RJ, Alpers DH: Diagnostic features of clindamycin-associated pseudomembranous colitis. N Engl J Med 290:841–843, 1974
9. Sumner HW, Tedesco FJ: Rectal biopsy in clindamycin-associated colitis. Arch Path 99:237–241, 1975
9a. Tedesco FJ: Antibiotic-associated pseudomembranous colitis with negative proctosigmoidoscopy examination. Gastroenterology 77:295–297, 1979
10. Stanley RJ, Melson GL, Tedesco FJ, et al: Plain-film findings in severe pseudomembranous colitis. Radiology 118:7–11, 1976
11. Stanley RJ, Melson GL, Tedesco FJ: The spectrum of radiographic findings in antibiotic-related pseudomembranous colitis. Radiology 111:519–524, 1974
12. Tully LE, Feinberg SB: A reappearance of antibiotic-induced pseudomembranous enterocolitis. Radiology 110:563–567, 1974
13. Alpers DH: The pseudomembranous enterocolitides, in Sleisenger MH, Fordtran JS (eds): Gastrointestinal Disease (2nd ed). Philadelphia, WB Saunders Co, 1978
14. Kabins SA, Spira TJ: Outbreak of clindamycin-associated colitis. Ann Intern Med 83:830–831, 1975
15. The Upjohn Company: Letter to Physicians. 16 August 1974
16. Ramirez-Ronda CH: Incidence of clindamycin-associated colitis. Ann Intern Med 81:860, 1974
17. Keefe EB, Katon RM, Chan TT, et al: Pseudomembranous enterocolitis—resurgence related to newer antibiotic therapy. West J Med 121:462–472, 1974
18. Swartzberg JE, Maresca RM, Remington JS: Gastrointestinal side effects associated with clindamycin. Arch Int Med 136:876–879, 1976
19. Tedesco FJ: Clindamycin-associated colitis: review of the clinical spectrum of 47 cases. Amer J Dig Dis 21:26–32, 1976
20. Marr JJ, Sans MD, Tedesco JF: Bacterial studies of clindamycin-associated colitis. Gastroenterology 69:352–358, 1975
21. Larson HE, Price AB: Pseudomembranous colitis: presence of clostridial toxin. Lancet 2:1312–1314, 1977
22. Bartlett JG, Chang TW, Gurwith M, et al: Antibiotic-associated pseudomembranous colitis due to toxin-producing clostridia. N Engl J Med 298:531–534, 1978
23. Katz L, LaMont JT, Trier JS, et al: Experimental clindamycin-associated colitis in rabbits: evidence for toxin-mediated mucosal damage. Gastroenterology 74:246–252, 1978
24. Bartlett JG, Moon N, Chang TW, et al: Role of Clostridium difficile in antibiotic-associated pseudomembranous colitis. Gastroenterology 75:778–782, 1978
25. Steer HW: The pseudomembranous colitis associated with clindamycin therapy—a viral colitis. Gut 16:695–706, 1975
26. Lusk RH, Fekety FR, Silva J Jr, et al: Gastrointestinal side effects of clindamycin and ampicillin therapy. J Infec Dis 135, Suppl:S111–119, 1977
27. DuPont HL, Hornick RB: Adverse effects of Lomotil therapy in shigellosis. JAMA 226:1525–1528, 1973
28. Burbidge EJ, Milligan FD: Pseudomembranous colitis. Association with antibiotics and therapy with cholestyramine. JAMA 231:1157–1158, 1975

29. DuPont HL: Etiology of antibiotic-associated colitis. Gastroenterology 75:913–914, 1978
30. Goodacre RL, Hamilton JD, Mullins JE, et al: Persistence of proctitis in 2 cases of clindamycin-associated colitis. Gastroenterology 72:149–152, 1977
31. Allo M, Silva J Jr, Fekety R, et al: Prevention of clindamycin-induced colitis in hamsters by Clostridium sordellii antitoxin. Gastroenterology 76:351–355, 1979

B. ORAL CONTRACEPTIVES AND INTESTINAL ISCHEMIA: CAUSE OR COINCIDENCE

The use of oral contraceptives has been associated with an increased incidence of vascular problems in younger women. Most common among these problems have been venous thrombotic disease of the lower extremities, pulmonary embolism, and cerebral vascular accident,[1] and while their incidence is very low, they do occur at a statistically-significant higher rate in women on oral contraceptives.[2] Since 1963 a number of cases have been reported in which vascular problems of the intestinal tract occurred in women taking oral contraceptives.[3–11] These cases have included superior mesenteric vein thrombosis, superior mesenteric artery thrombosis, and celiac artery thrombosis with subsequent ischemic problems of the small intestine, as well as less well-defined lesions associated with ischemic colitis. Hepatic vein thrombosis has also been described.[12–14] The age range of the patients was from 20 to 45 years, and in none of them had there been any evidence of disorders associated with a risk of intestinal vascular problems such as atherosclerosis, vasculitis, shock, hernia incarceration, malignancy, previous abdominal surgery, or hyperviscosity disorders. Is this association between intestinal vascular disease and the use of birth control pills real or merely coincidental?

Colonic Ischemia

All of the cases of large–bowel ischemic disease had a typical presentation of cramping lower abdominal pains and hematochezia. Proctosigmoidoscopy and stool evaluations ruled out diagnoses of idiopathic ulcerative colitis, Crohn's disease, and bacterial or parasitic infections, and subsequent barium enemas showed the classical radiographic findings of "thumb printing" due to submucosal edema, hemorrhage, and luminal narrowing (Fig. 5-5). Ischemic colitis is a dynamic process that can either progress to bowel infarction or resolve with either complete healing or stricture formation (Fig. 5-6). None of the patients died, but stricture developed in some cases and in one case, partial colectomy was required because of infarction. Aside from the lower age factor, other differences between these patients and typical cases of ischemic colitis include lesion

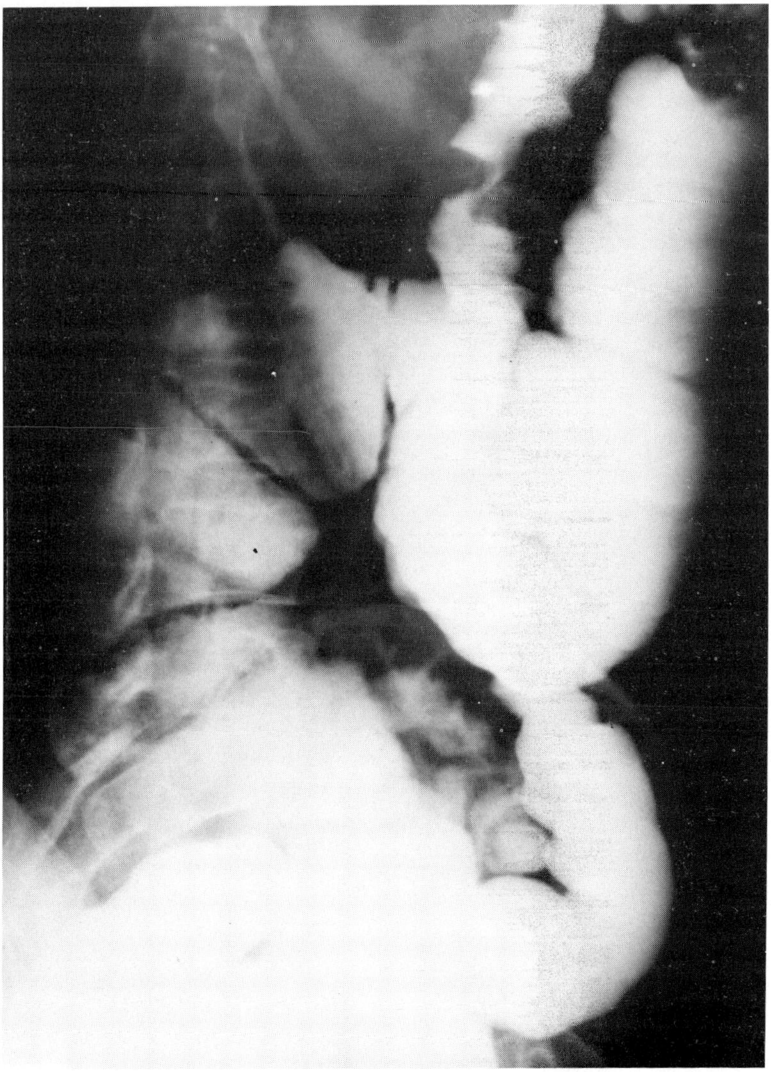

Fig. 5-5. Barium enema demonstrating "thumbprinting" and narrowing in the splenic flexure region.

location and sex. Patients with ischemic colitis are usually males over 60 years of age, whereas these patients were all females under 45 years of age. The lesion is usually on the left side of the colon in the "watershed" area—the segment of the colon where the origin of the blood supply changes (i.e., the recto-sigmoid and the splenic flexure), whereas in some of the newer patients, the right side of the colon was the affected region.

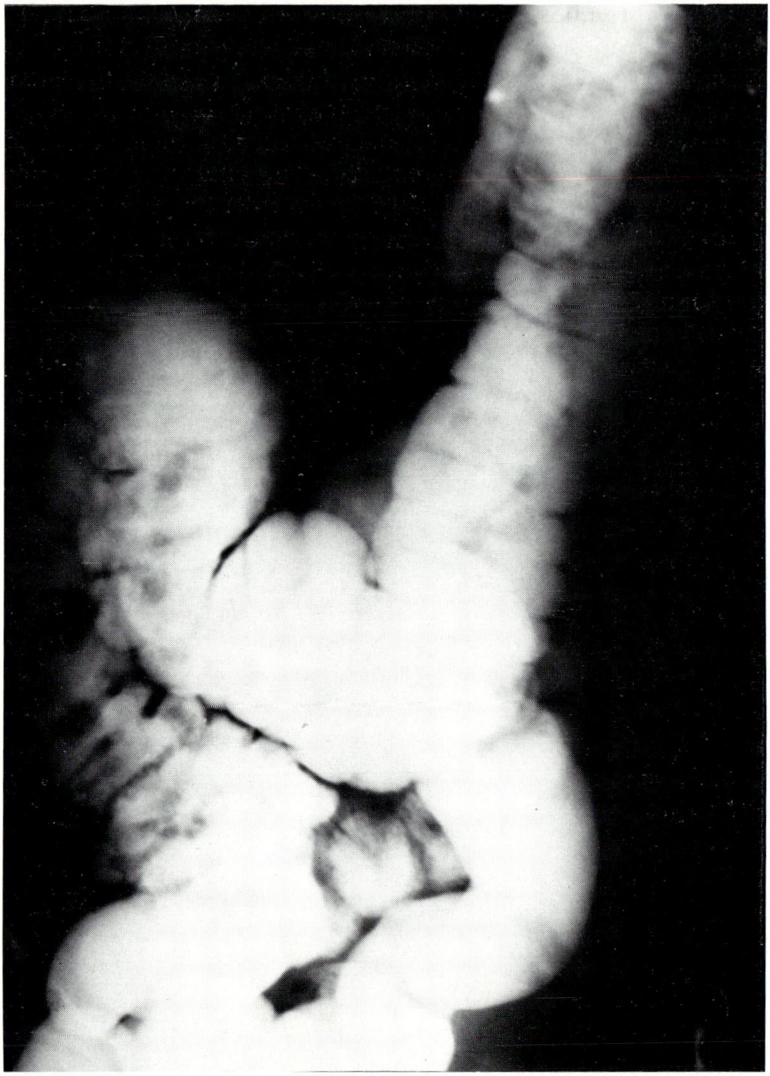

Fig. 5-6. Barium enema five months later on the same patient as Fig. 5 showing complete resolution of the radiographic abnormalities in the splenic flexure region.

Small Intestinal Ischemia

In the reports describing small intestinal ischemia, patients did not fare as well as those with ischemic colitis. The details of 18 previously reported cases accumulated by Hoyle et al.[10] and three personally-studied cases indicated six instances of superior mesenteric artery thrombosis, ten cases of superior or other mesenteric vein thrombosis, one case of celiac artery thrombosis, and one case where a specific vascular lesion was not described because the patient recovered fully after cessation of contraceptive intake. Of these 21 cases, 19 developed intestinal infarction and ten patients died. In almost every case laparotomy was performed, sometimes more than once, and the resectioning of large portions of jejunum and ileum was often required. The clinical presentation also differed from that of colonic ischemia, with the initial symptoms often being somewhat vague. Abdominal tenderness was the usual common complaint, but it often lasted for several weeks with non-specific findings, and rarely presented with signs of intestinal hemorrhage. Plain films usually demonstrated some small bowel distension, but barium x-ray studies were hardly ever obtained in these patients since the acuteness of their condition led to early laparotomy. A small bowel series performed on one patient during early symptoms revealed findings consistent with small intestinal ischemia that, however, reversed after cessation of the use of oral contraceptives.

Other Features

The duration of use of oral contraceptives did not appear to be a relevant factor in the development of small or large bowel ischemic problems. Some of the women had been on the pills for only a few weeks, while others had been using them for several years. Most of the pills contained at least 0.5 mg. of estrogen, but the problem appeared to be non-specific with regard to combination with progestogen or the use of sequential preparations.

Three cases of small intestinal ischemia were not entirely free of possible predisposing causes of thrombosis in that they were blood group A, Rh positive. In addition, all three were smokers and two were hypertensive. None of these, nor any of the other patients were observed to have any specific coagulation disorder, however.

Cases of transient hemorrhagic colitis consistent with a picture of ischemic colitis have also been reported in young adults, both male and female, in whom no obvious predisposing cause was present.[15-16] (The females had not used birth control pills.) These cases demonstrated that the ischemic colitis syndrome presented in young adults who were not using oral contraceptives.

SUMMARY

An association between the use of oral contraceptives and the development of both small and large intestinal ischemia has been suggested. The number of such reported cases (approximately 40), however, is very small when considered in light of the millions of women who have used and are using oral contraceptives. No specific coagulation disorder has ever been characterized and a causative role has not been established. Nevertheless, the marked debility suffered by women who had developed small intestinal infarction, and the improvement that seemed to follow cessation of the use of oral contraceptives, especially in cases of colon involvement, suggest that clinicians and patients alike should be alert to the possibility of this association, and that the use of oral contraceptives should be stopped in any woman who develops unexplainable abdominal pain or rectal bleeding.

REFERENCES

1. Inman WHW, Vessey MP, Westerholm B, et al: Thromboembolic disease and the steroidal content of oral contraceptives: A report to the Committee on Safety of Drugs. Br Med J 2:203–209, 1970
2. Oral contraception and increased risk of cerebral ischemia or thrombosis, Collaborative Group for the Study of Stroke in Young Women. N Engl J Med 288:871–878, 1973
3. Reed DL, Coon WW: Thromboembolism in patients receiving progestational drugs. N Engl J Med 269:622–624, 1963
4. Kilpatrick ZM, Silverman JF, Betancourt E, et al: Vascular occlusion of the colon and oral contraceptives—possible relation. N Engl J Med 278:438–440, 1968
5. Brennan MF, Clarke AM, Macbeth WAAG: Infarction of the midgut associated with oral contraceptives. N Engl J Med 279:1213–1214, 1968
6. Welin G, Persson T: Oral contraceptives and thrombosis of coeliac artery. Lancet 2:1348, 1968
7. Hurwitz RL, Martin AJ, Grossman BE, et al: Oral contraceptives and gastrointestinal disorders. Ann Surg 172:892–896, 1970
8. Cotton PB, Thomas ML: Ischaemic colitis and the contraceptive pill. Br Med J 3:27–28, 1971
9. Medical Staff Conference, University of California, San Francisco: Ischemic disease of the colon and oral contraceptives. West J Med 126:378–385, 1977
10. Hoyle M, Kennedy A, Prior AL, et al: Small bowel ischaemia and infarction in young women taking oral contraceptives and progestational agents. Br J Surg 64:533–537, 1977
11. Nothmann BJ, Chittinard S, Schuster MM: Reversible mesenteric vascular occlusion associated with oral contraceptives. Am J Dig Dis 18:361–368, 1973
12. Ecker JA, McKittrick JE, Failing RM: Thrombosis of the hepatic veins. Amer J Gastroent 45:429–443, 1966
13. Somayaji BN, Eeles GH, Paton A, et al: Budd-Chiari syndrome after oral contraceptives. Br Med J 1:53–54, 1968
14. Rothwell-Jackson RL: Budd-Chiari syndrome after oral contraceptives. Br Med J 1:252, 1968
15. Dudley HAF, Faris I: Ischaemic colitis without predisposing cause. Br Med J 3:637–638, 1971
16. Clark AW, Lloyd-Mosten RH, Sadler MR de C: Ischaemic colitis in young adults. Br Med J 4:70–72, 1972

C. John Rosenquist
Sam Silverman

6

Radiographic Studies of Animal Models for Evaluation of Drug- and Occupationally Induced Diseases

With the rapid development and expansion of our industrialized society in the last 100 years, many new diseases have been recognized to have resulted from occupational or environmental exposure to hazardous materials. Increasing levels and varieties of environmental pollutants have been responsible for numerous newly described health problems. In addition, as the number of different therapeutic drugs has increased, new toxic effects have been discovered that are caused by ingestion of these agents. Occupational and environmental pollutants, radiation hazards, and exposure to a multitude of therapeutic drugs, have all produced new and complex clinical problems that have been evaluated in a variety of ways. Methods for studying these conditions have included epidemiologic surveys, studies of individuals exposed to environmental or drug hazards, and studies of animals either exposed incidentally in their environment or intentionally in laboratory experiments.

The use of animal models has played a significant role in developing diagnostic methods, treatment, and prevention of many drug- and occupationally induced conditions. These animal studies may be grouped into two broad categories. First, certain laboratory experiments have shown that the effects of radiation, a certain drug, or an environmental or occupational hazard, are magnified in particular animal groups. Many thousands of such experiments have been performed on numerous species in order to evaluate the somatic, genetic, carcinogenic, or teratogenic effects of a particular agent. It is not our intent to review these investigations, but rather to discuss one such experiment in which radiological methods were used to evaluate the harmful effects of a commonly used steroid, triamcinalone. The second category of animal study that may be useful in studying drug- or occupationally induced diseases is that in which the effects of a particular agent or environmental pollutant are first noted in an animal in its natural environment. Although information gathered from this second category has not been as extensive as that obtained from experimental animal studies, many diseases have been discovered or further understood through such information. We will discuss two models in which conditions noted in the animals under study closely resemble those in humans. One investigation concerns the toxic effects of small amounts of polychlorinated biphenyls. This is an environmental pollutant that has been noted in many parts of the world and has been found to produce toxic effects in many animal species as well as humans. The second animal study involves the toxic effects of vitamin A and a derivative of vitamin A, Retinoic acid, both of which also have important implications for humans.

These particular animal models were chosen not only for their important relationships to man, but also because radiographic techniques were helpful in evaluating the problem in both of them. X-ray studies have several unusual features that are useful. First, an abnormality may be observed radiographically over an extended period of time in a noninvasive manner. Second, certain changes, especially in osseous structures, can be demonstrated quite effectively by x-ray studies. Finally, radiographic studies provide a reproducible method for measuring changes that occur during an investigation. The studies described in this chapter will illustrate these points.

TERATOGENIC EFFECTS OF TRIAMCINALONE ON THE SKELETON

Triamcinalone is a synthetic adrenocorticosteriod which has had widespread use in humans as an anti-inflammatory agent and in replacement therapy for adrenal insufficiency as well as control of allergic conditions. Although many adverse effects of this drug have been observed, only recently have the teratogenic effects been evaluated.[1] Because of their close phylogenetic relationship and similarities in placentation, nonhuman primates were utilized in this radiographic investigation of the teratogenicity of corticosteroid compounds.

Radiographic studies have demonstrated a variety of teratogenic craniofacial anomalies in primates. The dosage required to produce specific defects such as cleft palate varies within and among species of experimental animals. Radiological evaluation is a valuable investigative technique for the diagnosis of skeletal anomalies and in the elucidation of their pathogenesis. This is especially true with regard to oralfacial and craniofacial anomalies. Physical evaluation is sufficient to diagnose only the presence of severe anomalies. Without post mortem analysis, examination is of limited value in identifying the anatomical defect responsible for the observed anomaly. Furthermore, internal defects such as tooth bud abnormalities, malrotation of cranial planes or angles, and ossification abnormalities frequently remain undiagnosed without radiographic techniques. Conventional radiography assists the investigator in describing many of the skeletal defects and is an effective method of following the development of the abnormality throughout the maturation process (Fig. 6-1 A, B). Since many cranial and oral–facial defects originate on the internal surfaces of the skull and are complex in nature, supplemental techniques are required to further investigate these anomalies. Radiographic cephalometric analysis, the evaluation of precise measurements made from radiographs, offers the investigator a technique that enables him to document the presence of the defect, quantitate its severity, and study its pathogenesis during maturation. Although some teratogenic

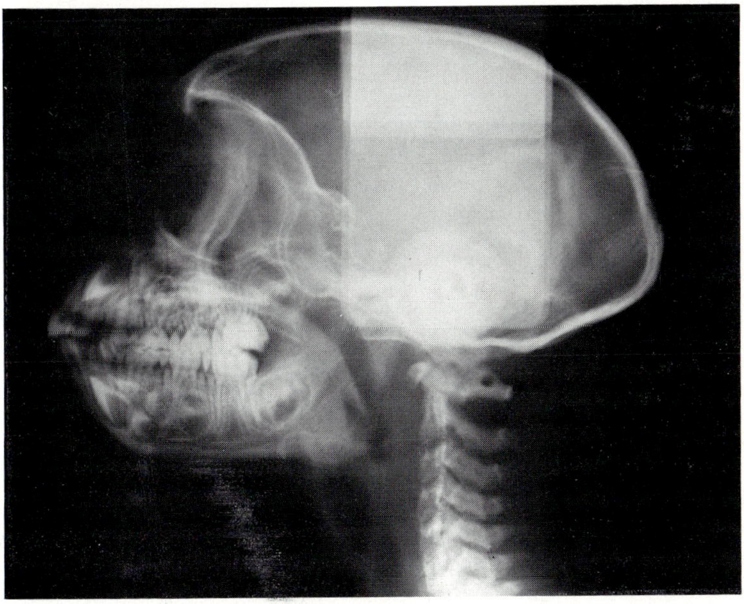

Fig. 6-1A. Lateral view of skull of normal rhesus monkey.

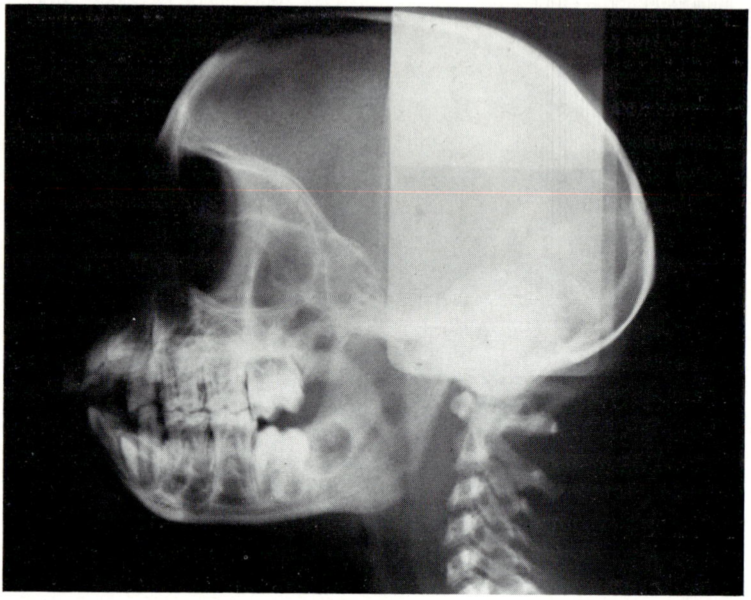

Fig. 6-1B. Lateral view of skull of rhesus monkey exposed to triamcinolone in utero. Multiple craniofacial abnormalities include increase in height of cranial vault, prominence of the frontal bone, mandibular retrusion, abnormal tooth development, and depression of the nasal bridge. By using cephalometric studies it is possible to quantitate these changes and follow their progression.

defects are obvious, many are difficult to diagnose without cephalometric analysis or sacrificing the animal. Some defects become more severe during maturation and would be overlooked if experimental animals were terminated and examined immediately post partum. Radiographic techniques are noninvasive and therefore well suited for long term teratological studies.

Contrast radiography is also useful in some teratological investigations, especially those involving soft tissue structures. Choanal atresia, similar to the condition seen in humans, has been studied radiographically in primates exposed to triamcinalone during gestation. The obvious mandibular defects were diagnosed prior to radiography, but the cartilaginous nature of the defect precluded its diagnosis without contrast radiographic procedures (Fig. 6-2).[2]

Nonhuman primates are common test animals in drug toxicity studies and are useful in studying craniofacial and oral–facial anomalies. The utilization of radiographic techniques, especially cephalometric analysis, is essential in complete teratologic investigation. The documentation of

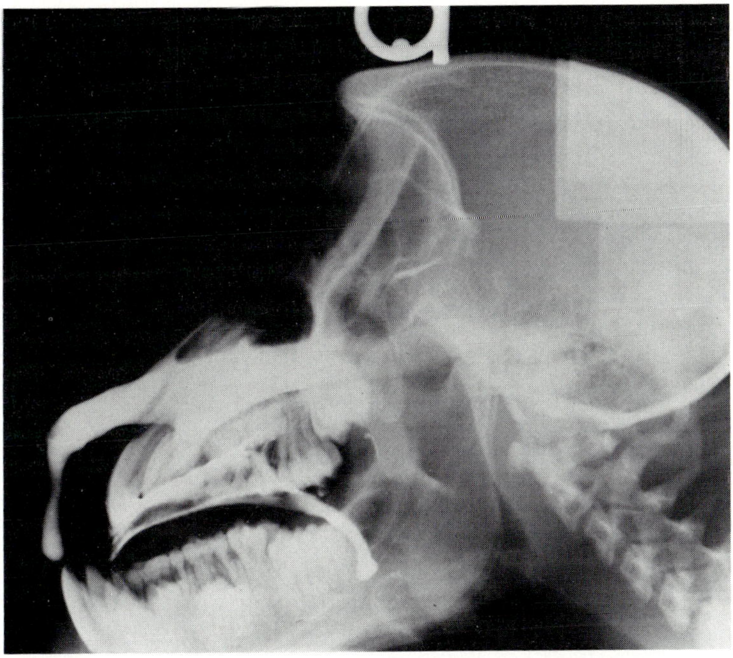

Fig. 6-2. Lateral view of skull of baboon. Contrast material has been placed in the nasal cavities and demonstrates complete obstruction of the nasopharynx. The abnormality is similar to choanal atresia seen in humans.

triamcinalone induced teratologic defects relies on the utilization of radiological examination. The information obtained in these studies may be important in extrapolating experimental results to human clinical situations.

RADIOGRAPHIC STUDIES OF HYPERVITAMINOSIS A

Radiographic studies in several animal species and man have been helpful in furthering our understanding of hypervitaminosis A. Ingestion of foods excessively high in vitamin A or vitamin A concentrates may cause acute or chronic hypervitaminosis A in humans and animals. Seal liver and polar bear liver ingested by arctic eskimos and Australian pioneers have been documented to produce the acute vitamin A toxicosis.[3,4] Skeletal abnormalities are not associated with the acute vitamin A toxicosis. Chronic toxicosis is more frequently encountered in children than adults and is associated with skeletal abnormalities. Excessive periosteal new bone formation, growth retardation, calvarial thickening, metaphyseal cupping, and rarefaction of long bone cortices have been identified radiographically in individuals with chronic hypervitaminosis A. Congenital defects have been reported in a small number of children whose mothers ingested large doses of vitamin A concentrates during pregnancy.

Spontaneous and experimentally induced chronic hypervitaminosis A with accompanying skeletal changes similar to those described in humans have been described in several animal species.[5,6,7] The majority of experimental work deals with cats and pigs.[8,9] Raw liver and vitamin A supplemented diets containing 17-35 μgm/gm body weight of vitamin A produced skeletal changes within ten months in newly weaned kittens. Skeletal changes were not produced in kittens fed diets containing 15 μgm/gm body weight. In cats the skeletal lesions were predominantly severe exostoses of the cervical and thoracic vertebrae. The exostoses progress to produce cervicothoracic spinal fusion. Periosteal new bone formation is also noted in the shoulder and elbow joints; complete arthrodesis may occur. (Examples of changes noted in the adult cat are shown in Fig. 6-3 and 6-4.) The sternabrae and costochrondral junctions

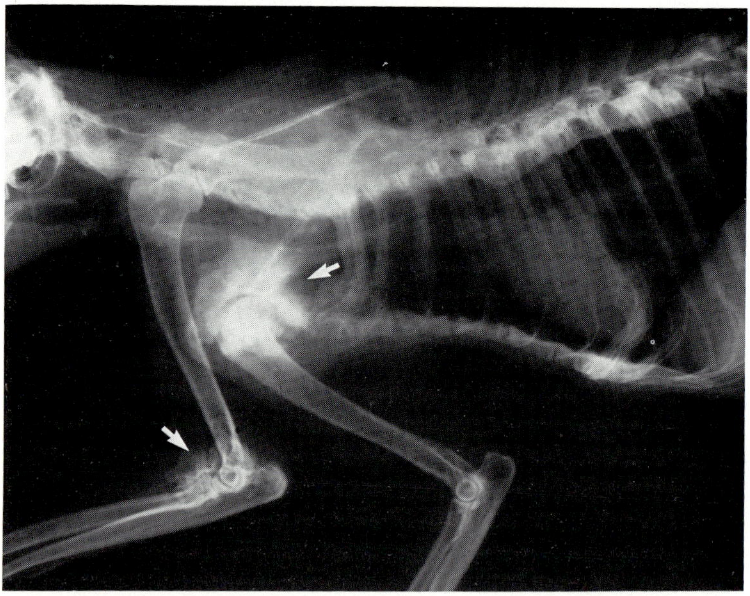

Fig. 6-3. Lateral view of the cervical and thoracic spine in adult cat with hypervitaminosis A. There is sclerotic reaction of the vertebrae ajacent to the interspaces, and extensive new bone formation is seen surrounding the cervical and thoracic vertebral bodies. Narrowing and irregularity of the shoulder joint and one elbow joint are also seen with surrounding new bone formation (arrows).

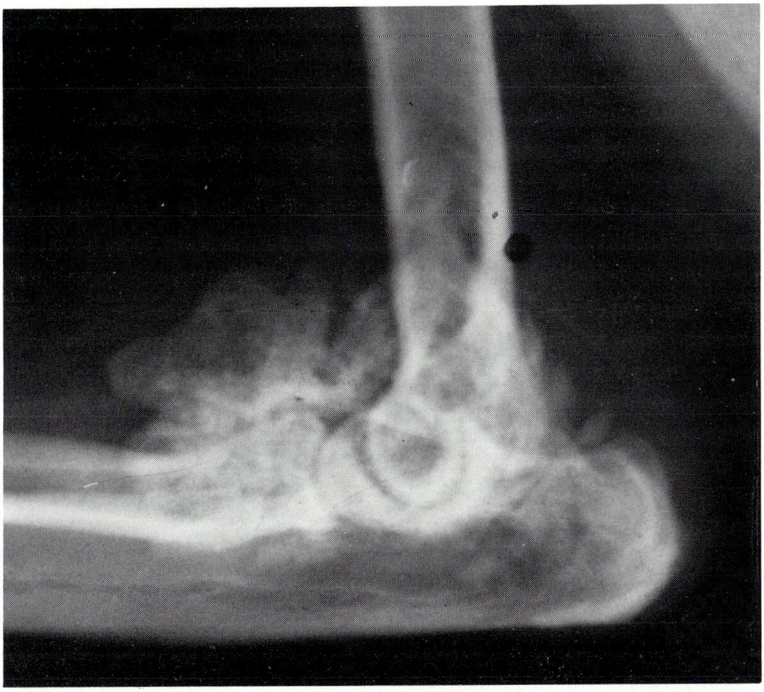

Fig. 6-4. Lateral view of elbow in adult cat with hypervitaminosis A. There is narrowing and irregularity of the joint with sclerosis of the surrounding bone. Extensive new bone formation is seen surrounding the joint.

are variably affected with similar exostosis. Although skeletal changes do occur in the lower extremities, they are less common. The bone marrow in the affected bones is commonly fibrotic and acellular. In immature animals growth retardation and cortical thinning are identified in chronic hypervitaminosis A.

Experimental work in cats demonstrated that two mechanisms were responsible for the skeletal changes produced by hypervitaminosis A.[8] Appositional bone growth is reduced due to suppressed osteoblastic activity. The haversian canals are enlarged, and the number of osteoblasts reduced. These changes are reversible after discontinuation of the excessive vitamin A. Enchondral ossification is disrupted by degenerative changes in the physeal cartilage. These changes are more permanent than the appositional changes and, depending on their severity, result in permanent growth retardation and deformities. Premature epiphyseal fusion is commonly noted in immature animals with chronic hypervitaminosis A.

Retinoic acid, a vitamin A derivative, is teratogenic in nonhuman primates. The congenital defects primarily involve the soft tissues, but craniofacial skeletal anomalies and appendicular skeletal anomalies have been reported. These data suggest the implications of vitamin A supplementation to pregnant women and require further study.

In conslusion, several species of commonly available laboratory animals have been observed to produce lesions similar to those seen in humans with hypervitaminosis A. These animal studies have helped elucidate the pathophysiology of skeletal defects and the need for further study in the potential teratogenicity of vitamin A derivatives.

STUDIES OF TOXIC EFFECTS OF POLYCHLORINATED BIPHENYLS IN THE RHESUS MONKEY

In recent years it has become apparent that there is a worldwide contamination of water supplies and food by small amounts of polychlorinated biphenyls (PCBs).[10] This is a group of organic compounds consist-

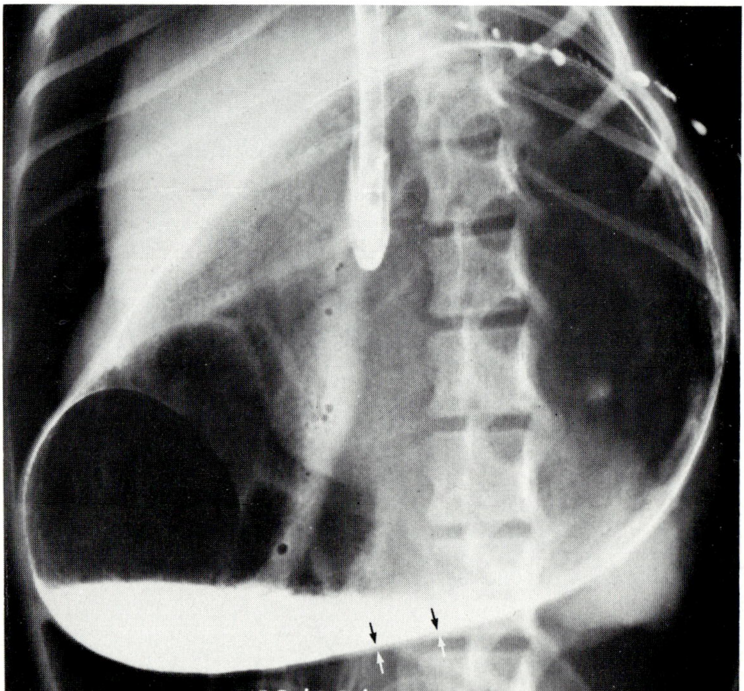

Fig. 6-5A. AP radiograph of the normal stomach in the rhesus monkey. CO_2 has been injected into the peritoneal cavity and air and barium have been injected into the stomach. The mucosal and serosal surfaces of the stomach are smooth and the gastric wall measures 1-2 mm in thickness (arrows).

ing of multiple isomers of chlorinated phenyl rings. These compounds are highly stable under many conditions including high temperatures, and have had numerous industrial uses because of these characteristics. As one might expect, contamination is greatest in water supplies of industrialized countries; however, small amounts of PCBs have been found in such isolated areas as the Yukon River. Since the discovery of the harmful effect of PCBs their use has been curtailed, although significant levels of the material remain in the water supplies and soil in many parts of the world.

Deleterious effects of PCBs have been noted in both animals and man. Several industrial accidents have resulted in ingestion of significant amounts of PCBs by groups of people.[11] Some of the toxic effects noted incluce skin eruptions and hyperpigmentation, edema, vomiting, diarrhea, and weight loss. Toxic effects in animals have been discovered both by study of animals in their natural environment and by laboratory investigations. The findings described above in humans have also been reported in animals that received small amounts of PCBs in their food.

One of the toxic effects noted in rhesus monkeys is an unusual type of gastric hyperplasia that develops when the animals are fed small amounts

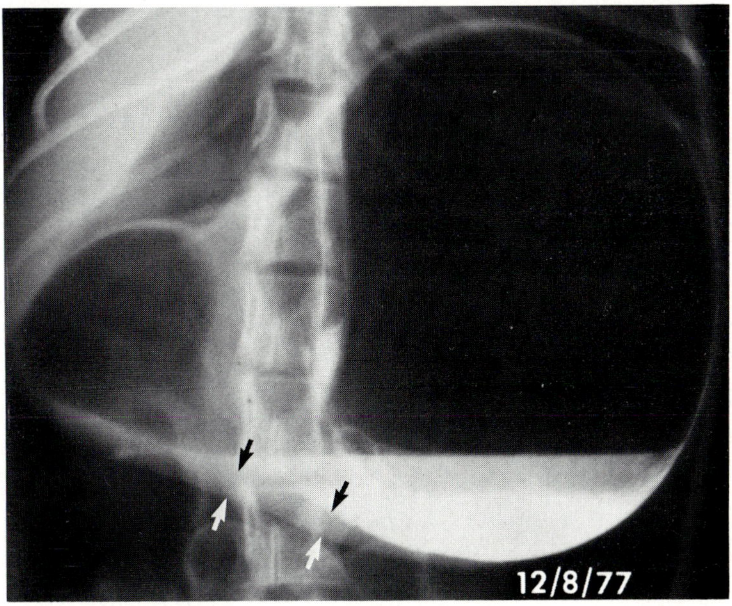

Fig. 6-5B. AP radiograph of stomach approximately 1 month after receiving an isomer of PCB. The gastric wall remains smooth but has increased in thickness to 4mm (arrows).

of PCBs.[12] These lesions develop after a period of one to several months and involve the mucosa and submucosa of the stomach with marked submucosa glandular hyperplasia which may extend to the serosa. Despite the invasive characteristics of the lesions, they probably represent hyperplasia and not malignancy; no evidence of metastatic lesions has been found in these animals.

Radiographic studies have provided a useful method for detecting and following the progression of these gastric lesions.[13] A double contrast barium study of the stomach combined with injection of CO_2 into the peritoneum enables one to visualize radiographically the gastric wall thickness and mucosal surface. Fig. 6-5 (A,B,C) shows the typical features of the stomach as the lesion develops. With this radiographic technique the gastric wall normally measures one to two millimeters in thickness and has a smooth mucosal surface (Fig. 6-5A). One month after receiving an isomer of PCB (3,4, 3′, 4′, tetrachlorobiphenyl) an area of thickening is noted along the greater curvature of the stomach (Fig. 6-5B). Finally, after three months of receiving PCB's, marked progression of the

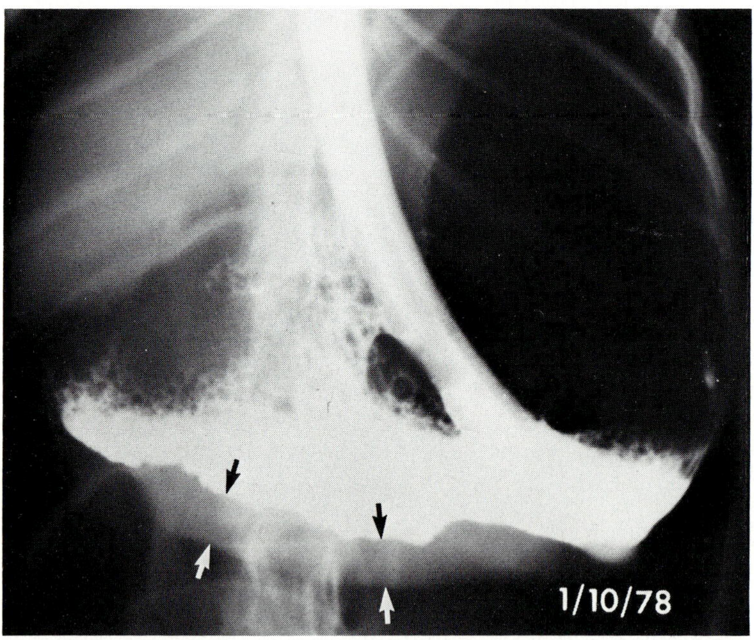

Fig. 6-5C. AP film of stomach after 2 months of PCB isomer ingestion. There is now marked thickening of the gastric wall with irregularity of the mucosal and serosal surfaces (arrows). This is typical of the lesions which develop in rhesus monkeys given small amounts of PCBs.

lesion has occurred along the greater curvature. There is more thickening of the gastric wall, and both the mucosal and serosal surfaces are irregular (Fig. 6-5C). Histologically, these lesions demonstrate a disorderly growth of the mucus glands which extends deeply into the thick edematous submucosa. Cysts may be formed in the submucosa.

No similar gastric lesions have been reported in people exposed to PCBs; however, no survey of possible gastric abnormalities has been conducted in such individuals. Experiments in other animals (dogs, rats) have failed to produce this type of gastric abnormality. The condition known as heterotopic submucosal gastric cysts has been described in humans and has similar histologic patterns. There is, however, no known association of this condition with PCB ingestion.

REFERENCES

1. Hendrick AG, Sawyer TG, Terrell TG, Osburn BI, Hendrickson RV, Steffek AJ: Teratogenic effects of triamcinalone on the skeletal and lymphoid systems in nonhuman primates. Fed Proc 34(8):1661–1665, 1975
2. Silverman S, Mertan DF, Anderson JH, Hendrick AG: Radiographic diagnosis of choanal atresia induced prenatally with triamcinalone in the baboom (Papiocynocephalus). Journal of Medical Primatology 6:284–297, 1977
3. Rodahl K, Moore T: The Vitamin A content and toxicity of beaver and seal liver. Biochem J 37:166–168, 1943
4. Cleland JB, Southcott RV: Illnesses following the eating of seal liver in Australian waters. Med J Aust 56(1):760–763, 1969
5. Seawright AA, English PB: Deforming cervical spondylosis in the cat. J Path Bact 88:503–509, 1964
6. Fry PD: Cervical spondylosis in the cat. J Small Animal Practice 9:59–61, 1968
7. Seawright AA, English PB, Gartner RJW: Hypervitaminosis A and deforming cervical spondylosis of the cat. J Comp Path 77:29–39, 1967
8. Wolke RE, Eaton HD, Nielsen SW, Helmholdt CF: Qualitative and quantitative osteoblastic activity in chronic porcine hypervitaminosis A. J of Pathology 92(4):677–686, 1969
9. Clark L: Hypervitaminosis A: A Review. Aust Vet Journal 47:568–571, 1971
10. Kolbye AL: Food exposure to polychlorinated biphenyls. Environ Health Perspect 1:85, 1972
11. Kuratsune J, Yoshimura T, Malsuzaka J, Yamaguchi A: Epidemiologic study of yusho, a poisoning caused by ingestion of rice oil contaminated with a commercial brand of polychlorinated biphenyls. Environ Health Perspect 1:119, 1972
12. Allen JR, Norback DH: Polychlorinated biphenyl-antriphenyl-induced gastric mucosal hyperplasia in primates. Science 179:498, 1973
13. Silverman S, Rosenquist CJ, McNully WP: Radiographic study of gastric hyperplasia induced by polychlorinated biphenyls in the rhesus monkey. Invest Radiology Jan-Feb, 1979

PART 2

Irradiation-Induced Disease

J. H. E. Carmichael
C. K. Warrick

7
Management of Radiation Hazard: The Place of the Ten Day Rule

In this century medicine has advanced remarkably in its efforts to cure disease and to halt the onward progress of degenerative processes. Nevertheless, while considerable emphasis and effort devoted to curative medicine and the halting of the onward progress of diseases are indispensable, an equally vigorous effort must be made in preventive medicine. The introduction of vaccination against smallpox by Jenner in the early 1800s was the first successful technique in preventive medicine, and its influence is still being felt today. But it took nearly 180 years to eradicate a disease that in Jenner's time was realized to be easily preventable by a very safe technique. In many other areas since then, and particularly in the last 35 years, there have been considerable advances in preventive medicine.

Radiology may relate to preventive medicine in two ways. The first is its role in surveys that help to detect disease at an early stage—mammography is one such field. The second is how radiology may be employed with the least possible harm due to radiation itself. Germane to this discussion is the place of the "Ten Day Rule."

ICRP publication No. 26[1] is currently the definitive document in terms of radiation protection in broad principle. One of its main features is the principle of "optimization." This is the assessment of any practice whereby one may balance the positive features on the one hand against the negative on the other to arrive at an equation that will determine whether there is net benefit or net detriment. One inconvenience here is that the units of this equation are not necessarily the same; mathematical processes, therefore, are often performed with difficulty. The equation is quoted in paragraph 73 of ICRP publication No. 26, and the net benefit is defined as the gross benefit less the sum of the basic production cost, the cost of achieving a selected level of protection and the cost of the detriment involved in the operation or in the production use and disposal. Cost as used here includes social as well as purely economic costs. It is here that the concerned doctor may find difficulty in putting a value on a particular practice and where two equally concerned doctors may arrive at different conclusions.

Mammography is a valuable technique of keen interest to the general public. Examined on a benefit detriment analysis basis, the benefits must be, primarily, the earlier detection of breast cancer and a higher cure rate and, secondarily, an increase in the time between diagnosis and death in those patients who are not cured. In opposition, the following detrimental aspects must be considered. First, we have to be certain that early detection of breast cancer does in fact increase the cure rate or enhance the *quality,* not merely the *quantity* of life in patients who are not cured. The quality of the additional years of life may be so poor that we would have been better not to have given them to the patient at all. There is some evidence that mammography increases neither the cure rate nor the quantity and quality of life in those who are not cured. This is a significant factor to pose against the benefit and is noted prior to even considering the question of radiation hazard.

The positive yield in mammography surveys performed in well women clinics has been as low as one positive in 2,000 cases. Observer fatigue and error at this level can be high. A survey conducted by George et al.[2] showed, in fact, that radiological error in such cases was as great as that of non-medical observers such as nurses who were trained to look at mammograms. The quantity of radiation exposure needed to achieve this one positive in population dose terms would be quite high. If one rad per projection in mammography is achieved, then the examination was probably performed as well as could have been expected; therefore, to produce one positive case in 2,000, an exposure of 8,000 man rads would be needed assuming two projections per breast. If routine mammography in a well women clinic was begun under the age of 30—which many concerned women might well consider highly desirable—then the total dose over the years would accumulate very considerably. A concerned woman might well feel that a need for two examinations per year from the age of 28 was indicated. By the age of 40, 24 examinations would have been conducted, giving a dose of 96 rads to the breast tissue (48 rads per breast). This dose in itself might be considered sufficient to cause a higher incidence of breast cancer in those who received it; there is evidence that irradiation of the female breast for purposes such as fluoroscopy during the treatment of pulmonary tuberculosis causes an increased incidence of breast cancer.[3]

ICRP 26 regards the breast as the second most radiosensitive tissue after the gonads. It could, then, be said that irradiation of the breasts of women under the age of 40, for example, might be contraindicated as a general screening technique. Evidence suggests that, when exposure begins after the age of 45, the risk of breast cancer drops considerably. It might be suggested, therefore, that mammography as a screening procedure be reserved either for those over the age of 50[4] or for those in the high risk group. Let us look at this latter section.

Based on either family history or parity and related factors, certain patients can always be classified as being "high risk." We may say, therefore, that this group should be subjected to mammography as a screening procedure (even if the general population is not) in spite of the fact that the breast is the second most radiosensitive tissue. Might not the subjection to radiation of those breasts, which are at a high risk of developing carcinoma, prove in itself to be the trigger that will produce a higher incidence of carcinoma than those high risk breasts would otherwise have developed? The evidence is difficult to evaluate, but the hypothesis must be put forward both to members of the medical profession and to concerned potential patients.

On a benefit/detriment analysis, therefore, an argument could well be made in favor of restricting routine mammography *as a screening procedure* to those over the age of 45, but using it in patients of any age where there are symptoms or clinical signs that raise a doubt either in the mind of the clinician or the mind of the patient and in which mammography may well provide the answer—in the form of either reassurance or the need to pursue an active clinical course. If we add to the above the suggestion by George et al.[2] to train intelligent women in the correct method of self-palpation of the breast then we might expect a considerable reward. If the results of such self-examination equal the yield of mammography, self-palpation should be used in mammography's place since it is in no way detrimental.

Another factor to confront in a discussion of mammography is the analysis of techniques available and the yield that may likely be obtained from them. In mammography, for any given radiation dose, a maximum of possible information may be obtained. In a recent survey, White et al.[5] at St. Bartholomew's Hospital, London, investigated the information yield as measured by a phantom in nearly 70 centers performing mammography. The results of the survey showed that four choices of technique were available. On the one hand, either a tungsten target or a tube with low inherent filtration and a molybdenum target could have been used; on the other, either xerography or rare earth screens with appropriate film in a vacuum pack. In terms of radiation dose and information yield the best choices were the use of a tungsten target with xerography and the use of a molybdenum target with rare earth film and screen. The yield in these two was similar, although the radiation dose involved was marginally lower in the tungsten/xerography combination. The dose rate was somewhat higher using a tungsten target and rare earth film and screen and the information yield was poorer. The radiation dose using a molybdenum target and xerography was extremely high and the information yield poor. But until these techniques were assessed by a suitable phantom in terms of radiation dose and information yield, radiologists lacked vital information. Certain departments were giving much higher radiation doses to the breast than were necessary—in some cases unacceptable doses reaching as high as 3.5 rads per projection. Furthermore, because the information yield was poor, some departments were undoubtedly giving false negative information when they should have been providing positive information. This is perhaps the most dangerous aspect of this work. Therefore, in terms of optimization and reducing radiation hazard, testing of this nature has shown that certain practices are unacceptable from several points of view and that only two techniques are, in fact, acceptable. Analyses such as that of White et al. may alert radiologists to unexpected aspects of their work and help them to keep in mind that radiation is a weapon to be used with care.

How much more difficult, therefore, is the decision to use radiation in the case of a female patient, when we must consider not only the patient's health, but also that of a fetus which she may be carrying?" We have already discussed benefit/detriment analysis as it applies to other situations in radiology, but in this case our equation is further complicated.

Concern was shown in the early 1950s about possible damage resulting from irradiation of the female during the period of organogenesis. In 1952 and 1955 the Russells[6,7] described damage to mouse and rat fetuses resulting from irradiation during this period. They then extrapolated their work to the human and recommended that irradiation of the uterus in women of childbearing age be carried out in such a way that there was no possibility of damage to a fetus during the period of organogenesis. Conception is likely to occur 14 days after the onset of a menstrual period, in which case organogenesis will commence about 23 days after the first day of the menstrual period. This is five days before the expected date of the next period. Therefore, the first few days of organogenesis in any pregnancy will occur at a time when the mother cannot know that she is pregnant. If we irradiate a patient prior to the onset of her period during this second half of the menstrual cycle, we may be irradiating a pregnancy during the period of implantation and the early days of organogenesis. The Russells, therefore, recommended that irradiation be restricted to two weeks following the first day of the last menstrual period. This was then slightly modified to give a greater safety margin and it was generally recommended that irradiation of the female pelvis in women of reproductive capability be restricted to within ten days of the first day of the last menstrual period. The Russells were the originators of what later became known as the "Ten Day Rule." The recommendation that, in women of childbearing capacity, non-urgent diagnostic radiographs of the abdomen be confined to the pre-ovulatory phase of the menstrual cycle (i.e., the ten days following the onset of the last menstrual period) was made by the International Commission on Radiological Protection in 1964.[8]

It is unfortunate that the phrase "Ten Day Rule" incorporates the word "rule," for it has led to the involvement of the legal profession in what *should* be purely medical decisions based on the circumstances of individual cases. The authors have made a recent attempt to assess the evidence in the British Journal of Radiology[9] and have made a plea that the word "rule" be dropped and replaced by the word "principle." This proposed modification stresses the advisory nature of the recommendation rather than any mandatory aspect. Nevertheless, it must be said that the rule was contained in the British Code of Practice for the protection of Persons against ionising radiation arising from Medical and Dental Use[10] and that it was endorsed by the working party of the U.K. Law Commission on Damage to the Unborn Child.[11]

Advice on the implementation of the Ten Day Rule has been given by Warrick[12] and by the Royal College of Radiologists.[13] Application of the Ten Day Principle would mean that non-urgent radiography involving the abdomen and nearby structures—in particular, the pelvis and hips—of women between the ages of 15 and 50 should be carried out only in the first ten days of the menstrual cycle. In practice there are many reasons why the principle may be ignored. The patient may well be able to give an assurance that there is no possibility of pregnancy and that there will be none until after the examination has been completed. The patient may have had a hysterectomy or a tubal ligation and, although pregnancies have been reported after the latter procedure, in practice, one must assume that there cannot be a pregnancy. Again it would seem reasonable to accept the patient's assurance that adequate contraceptive measures are being taken and have been proved to be adequate by usage over a period of not less than, say, three months.

If, after all of the above are taken into account, there is still a risk of pregnancy, it would seem reasonable to defer the examination until the next suitable period *unless there is medical urgency*.

It is perhaps advisable to list the types of examination with which the Ten Day Principle is concerned. They include straight abdomen, intravenous urography, barium meal, barium enema, cholecystography and cholangiography, venography of the pelvic veins, radiculography and straight radiography of the pelvis, hips, sacro-iliac joints and lumbar spine.

It is not necessary to apply the Principle to radiography elsewhere. In particular, even in *early* pregnancy it would seem that there should be no limitation of chest radiography on radiation protection grounds. But in *late* pregnancy, when the fetal gonads and body are high in the maternal abdomen, it is much less desirable to conduct chest radiography. However good the physician's intentions regarding the adequate use of beam limiting devices may be, there is too much risk in late pregnancy of fetal irradiation resulting from chest radiography for the procedure to be used with regularity and freedom.

Mass miniature radiography should be avoided in pregnancy if possible. There are three reasons for this; first, the poor diaphragm collimation, which would lead to a greater area of radiation than necessary; second, the higher skin dose; and third, as pregnancy advanced, poor collimation would lead to significant irradiation of the fetus, and in particular of the fetal gonads, at an earlier stage of pregnancy than would conventional radiography with good collimation. Taking into account all of these factors, however, the potential fetal dose in early pregnancy is still insufficient to justify enforcing the Ten Day Principle in mass miniature radiographic examinations.

Recently the American College of Radiology, the National Council on Radiation Protection and Measurements (in Report No. 54: 14), the U.S. Department of Health, Education and Welfare (Food and Drug Administration, 1976), and scientific workers at certain universities in the United States[15,16] have been examining the justification for, and the implications of the Ten Day Principle, and have come to the conclusion that restricting radiation to the first 10 to 14 days of the menstrual cycle is irrational and might even be disadvantageous.

NCRP Report No. 54 uses the phrase, "elective examination," defining it as an examination that does not contribute to the diagnosis or treatment of a woman in relation to her immediate illness.[14] This phrase deserves very careful examination. What is its true meaning, and in what circumstances would a radiological examination that did not contribute to the diagnosis or treatment of a patient be used? The report further suggests that ICRP agrees with this concept, but there is no phrase of this nature in any ICRP report and it would be unwise to think that this statement has gained international acceptance.

NCRP No. 54 proposes that only these elective examinations be postponed.[14] Brown et al. employ a similar approach, stating that, "planned scheduling should only be undertaken for radiological examinations of the abdomen that are not concerned with the current illness."[16]

Again one must ask, what examinations are likely to be performed that are not concerned with the current illness? Clearly, there is a differing outlook between American and British practice. Judging from the tenor of the American reports and papers quoted above, very little would be postponed. One could question what in fact the authors mean by examinations that may be postponed. Possibly they refer to examinations required by insurance practices and similar investigations. These are of course used much more widely in America than elsewhere, but their worth is questioned in WHO publication No. 611,[17] which discusses the use of radiation in research and other areas. We do not mean to suggest that this WHO publication forbids such examinations, but it does recommend that they be performed as infrequently as possible.

Over the past several years, British practice has been to postpone more and more examinations so that, in many departments in the U.K. the trend is already well toward postponement, rather than performance of examinations that would fall outside the Ten Day Principle period. The point is always made that medical urgency must override the Ten Day Principle, but we must try and define urgency in this respect. Surely, an examination may be considered urgent if the health of the patient will suffer significantly should it not be performed. Let us, therefore, quote some of the circumstances where the health of the mother may be affected if an examination is postponed. Renal colic would require an immediate straight abdomen film and probably an immediate pyelogram if a suspected calculus was seen on the straight film. Bowel obstruction would also require an immediate radiological investigation, as would any suspected carcinoma.

On the other hand, the postponement of certain examinations would not significantly affect the health of the patient. Suspected peptic ulcers require a barium meal, but whether it is done today or in three weeks is probably immaterial, for the patient's history is commonly either clear cut or so indefinite that there is no risk of mistaking a simple indigestion for a malignant one. The investigation of low back pain will require films of the lumbo-sacral spine and possibly sacro–iliac joints. But the vast majority of such patients will have had their symptoms for a considerable time and, therefore, the radiological investigation of their spine may be postponed until the next menstrual cycle.

It is likely that the different patterns of health care in the USA on the one hand and UK on the other influence radiological practice. In the UK it is usual for patients to be seen at a clinic by appointment after having placed their names on a list and waiting between a few weeks and a few months, depending on the urgency of the case. The referring physician in collaboration with the clinic decides in view of limited resources, which patients need to be seen immediately and which can wait. The majority of those waiting the longer period will need radiological investigation; as these patients have already been deemed non-urgent, it seems reasonable that their radiological investigation be regarded as non-urgent and, therefore, that it be scheduled after the onset of the next menstrual cycle.

In the U.S.A. the trend is for a patient to be seen and fully investigated in a much shorter period of time. As there are approximately twice as many radiological investigations per thousand inhabitants per year in the United States as in the UK, it may well be that the threshold for referral in the USA is lower than elsewhere. Certainly, the United States has one of the highest rates of radiological examination in the world. This low threshold, combined with the usual American business-like approach to a problem, seems to account for the more rapid referral and investigation. In summary, this differing outlook between members of the medical profession in the UK and the United States—doctors of different backgrounds—is probably a good example of concerned professionals putting a value on a particular procedure and working out the benefit/detriment equation to arrive at two different answers.

Incorporated in NCRP No. 54 is the concept that the health of the mother and of the embryo or fetus are synonymous. This cannot always be so; at times either the mother's or the fetus' health must take precedence. A parallel can be drawn from clinical medicine. We discussed above differing attitudes in peptic ulcer investigation. If a peptic ulcer is known to be present then surgery is often advised. Such an operation would be elective, and would be performed at a time convenient to both doctor and patient. If the patient were known to be pregnant, no elective operation for peptic ulcer would be undertaken unless there were some suspicion of pyloric stenosis or malignant change in an ulcer. The health of the fetus would take precedence over the mother's eventual need of an operation. Equally, the health of the fetus may need to take precedence over the need of the mother with regard to the desirability of a radiological examination.

Brown et al. of the University of California discussed the quantitative and qualitative risks of radiation during pre-conception and pregnancy.[16] Their outlook is very much influenced by the work of Graham,[18] who reported data suggesting that the ripening follicle may be as adversely affected by radiation exposure as the fertilised ovum. In both his view and that of Brown, the follicle ripens between the first and tenth days after the onset of menstruation. This is true of the experimental animals in Graham's work, but it is not necessarily true of humans; the data have not been confirmed. If it were true, irradiation within the one to nine day period before conception might cause damage, but not necessarily to the extent that the damaged ovum would be lost by abortion. Irradiation during days 14 to 23 of the menstrual cycle—in other words, the preimplantation period of days one to nine post-conception—would probably produce a damaged zygote that would be lost by abortion. Zygotes that do survive are likely to be normal since irradiation at this stage is thought to have an all or none effect. Both the Russells[6] and Rugh[19] imply that there may be a threshold effect of the order of ten rad. Irradiation below these doses might not lead to damage. Nevertheless, none of the experimental work has so far been definitive. Brown et al. suggest that days 14 to 28 of the menstrual cycle would be the safest on the grounds that irradiation on days 1 to 10 might damage the ripening follicle while irradiation after this would have an all or none effect leading to either abortion or normality.

This all depends on one's interpretation of Graham's work. Baker[20] and Beaumont[21] have suggested that extrapolation to the human cannot be assumed. Both radiation responses and patterns of oogenesis vary according to species. In the human the oocyte is probably in a resting phase until 36 hours prior to ovulation,[22] at which time the so-called LH surge begins. Mandl[23] states that radio–sensitivity increases by a factor of ten as the cell passes to metaphase one. The second division is completed in the fallopian tube. Therefore, it would seem logical to suggest that in the human, the period of increased sensitivity only begins 36 hours prior to ovulation. We have already stressed that the Ten Day Principle allows about four days for either early ovulation, or these 36 sensitive hours; the practice of the Ten Day Principle covers both of these periods and would appear to give a sound scientific basis to those who currently observe the Principle.

A recent UNSCEAR publication[24] suggests that if irradiation occurs within the 9 to 40 days following conception, there is some risk of resulting malformation. This period is 23 to 54 days after the first day of the last menstrual period assuming ovulation on about the fourteenth day. The importance of this period is that the first five days fall immediately prior to the next expected menstrual period. This is the time when the patient cannot know that she is pregnant. She will not know until she realizes that she has missed a menstrual period. Most women would probably assume for the first two or three days after missing a period that this was just a menstrual irregularity; therefore, any irradiation up to that time would involve the first seven or eight days of the period of organogenesis. What is the risk in this? Again, quantification is difficult, but extrapolation of the Russells' data suggests a figure of 1 per 2,000 per rad.

Irradiation during the fetal period (from day 65 onwards) carries a risk of malignancy in childhood estimated at 1 per 2,000 per rad.[25] Brown et al. comment that risk involved in a radiological examination at this stage of pregnancy is no more or less than the risk involved at any other stage of pregnancy.[15,16] We would not disagree; however, inherent in the principle of scheduling is the expectancy that, if pregnancy does intervene, the examination will be postponed until after the end of the pregnancy.

Numerous types of examinations fall into the "postponable" category. Many investigations of indigestion, back pain, or mild bowel irregularity would undoubtedly be postponed in the U.K. if the patient were found to be pregnant. In U.K. practice, though, there would be no suggestion that an examination be postponed until later in a pregnancy, for in all likelihood the examination would be delayed until after the end of the pregnancy. Brown et al. would extend this to the period of preconception, but we have stated that we disagree with this concept.[16]

Is there a safe period during which radiography of the lower abdomen of a woman of reproductive capacity can be carried out? The American College of Radiology would seem to indicate that there is not. They stress that the possibility of pregnancy should always be considered before abdominal radiography is carried out in women of childbearing age, but again they recommend that scheduling be undertaken only for radiological examinations that are not concerned with the patient's current illness. Surely, examinations that are not concerned with current illness should be minimized or eliminated.

In matters of doubt such as this, workers turn obviously to international recommendations. But the clearest possible advice is not always obtainable or completely understood through the printed word in the form of an international recommendation. Many workers will seek some phrase or sentence that agrees with their own pre-conceived ideas; none of us are immune to this. Let us examine the most recent pronouncement in ICRP 26, paragraph 206: "Because of the risk of radiation injury to any embryo or fetus, the possibility of pregnancy is one of the factors to be considered in deciding whether to make a radiological examination involving the lower abdomen in a woman of reproductive capacity." This portion of the paragraph mirrors international thinking. The paragraph then goes on, "Although such an examination is least likely to pose any hazard if carried out during the ten day interval following the onset of menstruation (this is the Ten Day Principle) attention should always be paid to details of radiological technique that would ensure minimisation of exposure to any embryo or fetus that may be present, whether or not the woman is known to be pregnant." It is this latter phrase which concerned doctors may interpret so as to reach a different conclusion. It may indicate to some that a technique that will ensure minimal dose is more desirable than observing the Ten Day Principle. To others it may indicate that the Ten Day Principle is the main recommendation and that this last phrase is a safety mechanism so that if either knowingly or unknowingly a fetus is irradiated, then the dose will at least be less than it might have been. We believe that the latter is the correct interpretation, and therefore conclude that the Ten Day Principle should be followed.

The scientific evidence has been examined, and a case has been made on scientific grounds for following the Ten Day Principle. This is a practice of preventive medicine, never to be considered as clear cut as therapeutic medicine. It has been stressed that minimization of harm to the fetus is the aim, and this is certainly primary; but it must be remembered that if a fetus were irradiated unknowingly, there would likely be considerable mental distress to the mother. The general public is well aware of the risks of childhood cancer or fetal abnormality following irradiation of the maternal abdomen. Minimization of the psychological trauma to a mother in such a situation is, therefore, a further aim of the preventive medicine role of the Ten Day Principle.

Nevertheless, there must be no confusion between what is recommended to prevent the irradiation of a possible fetus and the course of action that may need to be taken if a fetus has been irradiated knowingly or unknowingly. This situation, where the possibility of abortion exists, is entirely beyond the scope of this paper.

Still controversial is whether the Ten Day Principle should be applied to radio–pharmaceutical investigations.[26,27] A research group at the UK Medical Research Council Isotope Advisory Panel[28] advised that the Ten Day Rule be considered only for patients who, during the investigation, were likely to be given gonad doses in excess of 50 millirads and in whose cases the radio–pharmaceutical employed was likely to have an effective half–life of less than ten days. In conventional diagnostic radiology the radiation problem is simple; it is short and definitive in its time of delivery. In radio–isotope radiation this of course is not so, and clear cut advice cannot be given. Langmead[29] suggests that it would be logical to advise the patient to attempt to avoid pregnancy for a period after the administration of the isotope and suggests that this period be approximately three to four effective half–lives of the radio–pharmaceutical concerned. Langmead further states that, even if conception were to take place before the end of the recommended period, the total fetal dose would be less than that in a situation where the patient was not advised. He agrees that the gonad dose of 50 millirads is reasonable, but the evidence and the recommendations are not yet definitive. The doses involved in the diagnostic use of radioactive isotopes are small, but certainly it would seem reasonable to examine each patient's situation and attempt a reasonable assessment of the gonad dose after the administration of the particular isotope. The recommendation in this respect might be considerably stronger if the isotope were being given for therapeutic purposes.

Whatever decision a radiologist or clinician may make with respect to a given patient will obviously be very personal; nevertheless, by presenting the evidence, by discussing the arguments for and against the Ten Day Principle and by making more doctors aware of the problem, we may rest assured that whatever decision is made will have been carefully considered and in the best interests of the patient.

REFERENCES

1. ICRP: Recommendations of the International Commission on Radiological Protection, Publication No 26, para 206. Oxford, Pergamon Press, 1977
2. George WD, Gleave EN, England PC et al: Screening for breast cancer. Br Med J 2:858–860, 1976
3. Boice JD Jr, Monson RR: Breast cancer in women after repeated fluoroscopic examinations of the chest. J Nat Canc Inst 59:823, 1977
4. Shapiro S: Cancer 39: 2772, 1977, quoted in Bailar John C III, International symposium on the late biological effects of ionising radiation, Vienna, March 15, 1978
5. White DR et al: personal communication
6. Russell LB, Russell WL: Irradiation hazards to the embryo and fetus. Radiology 58:369, 1952
7. Russell LB, Russell WL: Hazards to the embryo and fetus from ionizing radiation. Proceedings of the First International Conference on the Peaceful Uses of Atomic Energy Vol XI. Geneva, 1955, pp 175–178
8. ICRP: Recommendations of the International Commission on Radiological Protection, Publication No 6, para 69. Oxford, Pergamon Press, 1964
9. Carmichael JHE, Warrick CK: Radiology now—the ten day rule—principles and practice. Br J Radiol 51:843–6, 1978
10. HMSO: Code of practice for the protection of persons against ionizing radiation arising from medical and dental use. London, HMSO, 1972
11. Law Commission: Injuries to unborn children, Working Paper No 47. London, Law Commission, 1973
12. Warrick CK: The ten day rule. Br J Radiol 47:293, 1974
13. Royal College of Radiologists: Recommendations on the implementation of "The Ten Day Rule." Br J Radiol 49:201–202, 1976
14. NCRP: Report No 54, Medical radiation exposure of pregnant and potentially pregnant women, 1977. Washington D.C., National Council on Radiological Protection and Measurement
15. Brown RF: Prepared remarks for the October 10, 1976 ACR press conference. Wall Street Journal, October 21, 1976
16. Brown RF, Shaver JW, Lamel DA: A concept and proposal concerning the radiation exposure of women. Univ of Calif RHSEP Pub No 874, 1976
17. World Health Organization: Use of ionising radiation and radionuclides on human beings for medical research, training and non-medical purposes. Technical Report Series No 611 (Geneva), 1977
18. Graham S, Levin ML, Lilienfield AM, et al: Preconception and postnatal irradiation as related to leukaemia. National Cancer Institute Monograph No 19:347–371, 1966
19. Rugh R: Proceedings of the Ninth Annual Hanford Biology Symposium—chairman's remarks. US Atomic Energy Commission, Division of Technical Information AEC Symposium Series 17:381–391, 1969

20. Baker TG: The radiosensitivity of mammalian oocytes with particular reference to the human female. Am J Obst Gyn 110:746–761, 1971
21. Beaumont HM: Proceedings symposium on effects of low radiation doses on the maturation of the developing human ovum and foetus. Br J Radiol 41:714–722, 1968
22. Edwards RG: Mammalian eggs in the laboratory. Scientific American 215:72–80, 1966
23. Mandl AM: The radiosensitivity of oocytes at different stages of maturation. Proceedings of the Royal Society (London) Series B 158:119–141, 1963
24. United Nations Scientific Committee on the Effects of Atomic Radiation: Sources and effects of ionizing radiation. New York, United Nations, 1977 pt II sec C.32
25. Stewart A, Kneale GW: Radiation dose effects in relation to obstetric x-rays and childhood cancers. Lancet 1:1185–1188, 1970
26. Bligh AS, Davies ER, McCready VR, et al: Report of working party of MRC isotope advisory panel on the application of the ten day rule in radiopharmaceutical investigations. Br J Radiol 52:81–82, 1979
27. Croft DN, Maisey MN: Statements of the MRC isotope panel. Br J Radiol 51:58–59, 1978
28. Ellis RE, Nordin BEC, Tothill P, Veall N: The application of the "Ten Day Rule" in radiopharmaceutical investigations: Report of a working party of the MRC isotope advisory panel. Br J Radiol 40:200–202, 1977
29. Langmead WA: The application of the "Ten-day Rule" in radiopharmaceutical investigations. Br J Radiol 50:840, 1977

J. H. E. Carmichael

8
Management of Radiation Hazard: Radiology in Late Pregnancy and the Neonate

Observance of the "Ten Day Rule" will usually preclude irradiation of an early pregnancy. The principle and practice of this rule have been discussed elsewhere.[1] If care is taken to avoid irradiation of an early pregnancy, should not similar care be taken to reduce radiation in late pregnancy and the neonatal period? Although there is no risk of fetal abnormality, the danger of later childhood cancer does persist.[2]

It must be acknowledged that the radiation dose per examination in late pregnancy has diminished appreciably since the 1956 work of Alice Stewart.[2] Several factors have been responsible for this reduction. The awareness of the hazard has led to the desire to reduce the number of films per examination from a common figure of four to one or two. There have also been recent advances in radiographic technique, particularly the use of rare earth screens, which have further reduced the dose. Nevertheless, it is quite likely that an element of risk is still present; therefore, diagnostic x-rays in late pregnancy and the neonate should be kept to a minimum. In 1976 Carmichael and Berry[3] published a survey they had carried out at eight different hospitals in the U.K. These were all maternity units of widely differing natures, representing several different forms of obstetric practice. The survey was based on 12 months of figures gathered in 1974 and early 1975. The figures showed that an average of 22.7 percent of delivery patients had an abdominal x-ray for obstetric reasons late in their pregnancies. There was a wide variation in the figures: one department was as low as 8.6 percent, while the percentages at two others were over 34. In the area of the survey over 90 percent of all deliveries were in hospitals. In one district the percentage was over 98. Since the problem cases as well as a considerable majority of the uncomplicated cases were being delivered in hospitals, one could have expected that the percentage of patients requiring abdominal x-rays in late pregnancy would have fallen over the years. By the time 98 percent of the deliveries were made in the hospital, the percentage should have been expected to have dropped appreciably. Therefore, one hospital having figures going back 25 years was examined closely. It was observed that in 1953, 30 percent of deliveries were examined radiologically; by 1955 the figure was 39.7 percent. At this stage the impact of the early work of Alice Stewart began to be felt and the percentages dropped to 24 in 1957, 14.5 in 1959, and 11 in 1961. This situation might have been considered satisfactory, but for the fact that by 1974 the figure had risen to 23 percent. The impact of Alice Stewart's work had undoubtedly worn off, and a new generation of obstetricians was disregarding her warning. There were grounds for believing that this trend—a drop to the early 1960s followed by a rise to the 1970s—was typical of practice throughout the U.K.

One realizes that the quality of obstetric work has improved, and that radiological demands have, perhaps, increased with the passage of time. The aim of radiology in obstetrics should be to produce a higher percentage of live children, while minimizing trauma to the mother. Therefore, we might expect to find that, as the percentage of abdominal radiology in late pregnancy dropped to the figure of 11 in 1961, there would have been some rise in the perinatal mortality rate (still births plus deaths under one week). If we examine the U.K. perinatal mortality rate we find that in the 1960s there was no such rise. In fact the rate per thousand births has dropped steadily from 38.2 in 1951, to 36.2 in 1957, 32 in 1961, 26.9 in 1965, and 22.3 in 1971. It might be inferred from these figures that radiology was not contributing at all to the safe management of labor, nor was it helping in the slightest to produce an increased percentage of live children. This surely would be an exaggerated reaction, but it might well be true that only part of the radiology performed during late pregnancy had contributed to safe management. It might, therefore, be postulated that the 11 percent rate of 1961 represented the hard core of cases requiring abdominal radiology. This, of course, might well accord with the figure quoted originally, where one hospital managed to reduce its rate to 8.6 percent. It must be admitted that, with planned induction, there has been a greater demand for accurate maturity and the assurance that there is no fetal abnormality. Nevertheless, this should not account for the very sharp rise that has occurred.

It is obvious that the use of radiology varies widely from place to place; this is undoubtedly as true in the U.S. as it is in the U.K. That it is possible in the U.S. to achieve a low percentage became clear when Hobbins and Taylor[4] at Yale indicated that their current irradiation of the abdomen in late pregnancy was less than nine percent. The point they brought out was that the proper use of ultra sound helped to reduce the demand for x-rays. They suggest that the failure to provide proper ultrasonic facilities leads directly to fetal irradiation in 14 percent of the population, when it could be avoided. (That is, the average of 22.7 percent comprises 14 percent in whom the irradiation could be avoided—by the use of ultra sound—and just under nine percent in whom it could not.) Nevertheless, it has to be pointed out that one of the hospitals quoted in 1974 with a rate of abdominal examination of 34.3 percent was, at that time, making full use of an ultra sound service under the direction of a nationally recognized ultra sound obstetrician. Therefore, although the argument of Hobbins and Taylor might well be valid, it must be stated that the presence of adequate ultra sound does not necessarily reduce the demand for abdominal irradiation. One can suggest that it *should* do so, admitting, however, that this is not always in fact the case.

As a follow-up, the department discussed above was re-examined. The total number of deliveries in the earlier series was 4,049; in the later series (1977) it was 3,856. It is reasonable to assume, therefore, that the type of work had not changed at all in this time. The total number of antenatal patients x-rayed for obstetric reasons was 1,573—a percentage of 40.8. Thus, in three years there had been significant *rise* in the percentage of obstetric cases x-rayed, in spite of the use of ultra sound in the hands of an extremely able and committed obstetrician. The assumption must surely be made, therefore, that in spite of the availability of ultra sound services, many obstetricians were not willing to rely (as they should have) solely upon ultra sound, but were using it with irradiation as an auxiliary weapon. It is precisely this attitude that leads to the perpetuation of high x-ray percentages such as those quoted above. Physicians must aim to limit the number of obstetric x-rays to under ten percent of deliveries. The use of ultra sound as a proper service should be as widespread as possible. Pregnancies should be examined early enough to establish maturity definitively and to rule out most fetal abnormality; ultra sound should then be used in later pregnancy, following a definitive examination, at which time it will give a tremendous amount of extremely accurate information—probably more accurate than that obtainable with radiology.

If we consider the care required in the irradiation of the maternal abdomen in order to avoid unnecessary exposure of a fetus before birth, we should also consider the case of the neonate, since the dangers of radiating a fetus four weeks prior to delivery and those of radiating the four-week neonate are probably very similar. What, then has been the experience of neonatal units regarding radiology and the new-born? Carmichael and Berry in their paper quoted above went on to give evidence from one hospital that indicated that approximately ten percent of all live babies were examined within the first month of life. In another hospital 340 babies, or 6.9 percent, were x-rayed. (There had been nearly 5,000 deliveries.) The number of films taken of these 340 new-born was 1,641—an average of 4.8 films per child. Eleven of these 340 had had 25 or more films taken and were obviously the severely ill congenital cardiac patients. If each of these 11 babies averaged 50 films, then the remaining 329 averaged 3.6 films each—a disturbingly large number.

These figures relate to 1974 and 1975. Let us look at the 1977 figures of the hospital quoted above. Of 3,856 deliveries, 1,573 (40.8 percent) were irradiated ante-natally. Of the children born during this period, 722 (18.7 percent) were x-rayed in the neo-natal period. It would be reasonable to assume that 40.8 percent of these were irradiated ante-natally also. Thus, 59.2 percent (427) would have been irradiated for the first time post-natally. To summarize, the total irradiated in the few weeks either side of delivery was 1,573 + 427 = 2,000. This equates to 51.9 percent of all children born at the hospital—a truly remarkable figure.

This chapter is entitled, "Management of the Radiation Hazard." It is our duty to realize the potential problem in this field and to do everything possible to reduce the number of radiological examinations. Now that the magnitude of the problem has been indicated, surely concerned Doctors will resolve it. A hazard is certainly present, and it is my belief that it can in part be avoided by a truly careful assessment of the *need* to obtain information by either ionizing or non-ionizing radiation.

REFERENCES

1. Carmichael JHE, Warrick CK: Radiology now: the ten day rule—principle and practice. Br J Radiol 51:843–6, 1978
2. Stewart A, Kneale GW: Radiation dose effects in relation to obstetric x-rays and childhood cancers. Lancet, 1:1185–88, 1970
3. Carmichael JHE, Berry RJ: Diagnostic x-rays in late pregnancy and the neo-nate. Lancet, 1:351–2, 1976
4. Hobbins JC, Taylor KJW: Diagnostic x-rays in pregnancy. Lancet, 1:739, 1976

Albert A. Moss

9

Radiation Injury to the Gastrointestinal Tract

Most forms of medical or surgical therapy entail calculated risks of harm that must be weighed against the potential for benefit. Modern radiation therapy has the capacity to cure certain patients with malignant tumors and to increase the survival time for many others. To reach a maximum benefit/risk ratio, radiotherapy must be employed aggressively. Care must be exercised, however, if the complication rate is to be kept at a minimum. The optimum therapeutic balance is difficult to achieve, and in order to fully eradicate malignancies some radiation injury to normal structures is unavoidable. Radiation injury to the gastrointestinal tract is not an infrequent consequence of abdominal and pelvic radiation therapy, and often produces acute and chronic disability.

HISTORICAL ASPECTS

The radiotherapist has long been aware that damage to the gastrointestinal tract may occur as a consequence of radiation therapy (Table 9-1). In 1897, two years after the discovery of the x-ray, the first case of intestinal damage caused by roentgen ray exposure was reported by Walsh[1] and deaths were reported following radiation therapy by Edsall in 1906.[2] In 1917 Franz and Orth[3] reported the first fatality resulting from a radiation injury to the gastrointestinal tract, which was documented with autopsy evidence. In succeeding years there was a gradual increase in the understanding of the damage that could be done to the intestinal tract by irradiation (Table 9-1). Von Franque[4] noted that radiation therapy could

Table 9-1
Historical Aspects of Radiation Injury to the Gastrointestinal Tract

Author	Date	Contribution
Walsh[1]	1897	Clinical evidence of enteritis
Edsall[2]	1906	First deaths
Franz, Orth[3]	1917	First autopsy
Von Franque[4]	1918	Diarrhea, severe colic, skin
Heck[5]	1920	damage intestinal cutaneous fistula 16 months after radiation
Haendly[6]	1921	Analysis 127 cases-gross and microscopic analysis
Mathias[7]	1922–23	Intense intestinal damage in region of bowel fixed by adhesions
Fisher[8]	1922	Intestinal necrosis, rectovaginal, mesocolic fistulae
Schwarz[9]	1923	Sigmoid ulceration and fibrosis
Sarders[10]	1924	Stenotic ileum, intestinal endoarteritis and enophlebitis obliterans
Elliott, Jenkinson[11]	1934	Gastric ileal ulceration analysis 422 cases-5 cases benign stricture sigmoid colon
Newell, Crossen[12]	1935	Rectal stricture
Todd[13]	1938	Rectal pseudotumor
Warren, Friedman[14]	1942	Pathology, pathologic diagnosis of radiation induced gastrointestinal injury
Mulligan[15]	1942	Summary of radiation induced gastrointestinal injury

lead to ulceration of the mucosa of the colon and small intestine and in some areas cause necrosis of the intestinal wall. Perforation, fistulae, abscesses, peritonitis and hemorrhage were commonly reported complications of abdominal radiation therapy.[5–11] Newell and Crossin[12] documented five instances of rectal stricture occurring as a complication of pelvic irradiation, and Todd[13] was the first to call attention to the rectal pseudotumor which occurred following radiation treatment of cervical cancers. In 1942, Warren and Friedman published as classic paper on the pathology of radiation-induced gastrointestinal lesions[14] and Mulligan[15] summarized the experience up to that time.

In addition to the occurrence of gastrointestinal injury following radiation therapy, the nature of the equipment previously available precluded the delivery of high tumor doses deep within the abdomen without causing significant skin damage. Using megavoltage therapy, the problem of excessive skin exposure is avoided, but the increased radiation dose which may be delivered to abdominal and pelvic neoplasia increases the chance of damage to portions of the gastrointestinal tract positioned close to the radiation field. Thus, despite tremendous advances in radiation therapy, equipment, and technique, gastrointestinal damage remains a sequelae in a small but significant percentage of patients undergoing abdominal or mediastinal radiation therapy.

OCCURRENCE

The incidence of radiation injury to the bowel has been reported to range from less than one percent to 23.9 percent of all patients receiving radiation therapy for neoplasms of the abdomen or pelvis.[16–24] The great variation in reported incidence depends in part on what is meant by "injury." While minor symptoms due to radiation effects on the rectum and bladder occur in most patients during and immediately following radiation therapy to the pelvis, serious complications of pelvic irradiation occur in only one to two percent of all patients.[17,22–24]

Treatment for carcinoma of the cervix is responsible for approximately 75 percent of radiation-induced gastrointestinal injury.[25–27] Radiation injury to the rectum and sigmoid colon is most frequently reported, while radiation damage to the small intestine, stomach and esophagus is less frequent.[20,28–32] Rather than reflecting differing sensitivity to radiation exposure, the different incidence rates are more likely a factor of the infrequency with which the upper abdomen is treated.[31]

ETIOLOGIC FACTORS IN RADIATION INJURY

The radiation dose and technique of radiation therapy are major factors affecting the incidence of radiation-induced gastrointestinal injury.[19,22,24,33,34] Pelvic radiation exposures over 5,500 R predictably result in rectal injuries.[14,19,24] Accidental overdose and misplacement of radium account for a small percentage of gastrointestinal injuries. Individual factors of obesity, age and race do not appear to be significant,[25] but individual idiosyncrasies in tolerance to radiation exposure vary greatly and cannot be predicted.[24] Decosse[25] reported a higher incidence of gastrointestinal complications in patients with small cell carcinoma of the uterus, and a history of prior surgery, either pelvic or abdominal, has been reported to result in a higher incidence of radiation enteropathy.[20,34–36] A controlled retrospective study by LoIudice et al.[37] confirmed these findings. In his study of 24 patients with radiation injury,

75 percent had had prior surgery, while only 11 percent of patients receiving identical radiation therapy but without gastrointestinal injury had had previous surgery.[37]

It is postulated that the high incidence of radiation gastrointestinal injury in patients with prior surgery results because of fixation of bowel loops by post-operative adhesions. Bowel loops so immobilized may receive very high doses of radiation, and chances for injury increase. A similar increase in radiation enteritis has been noted in patients with pelvic inflammatory disease[24] and in patients with large, bulky tumors.

PATHOLOGY AND PATHOLOGIC DIAGNOSIS

Radiation injury to the gastrointestinal tract produces changes in connective tissues of the mucosa submucosal, vessels, muscle layers, and serosal or adventitial tissues.[14,38-40] Fibrosis and scarring with thickening of the bowel wall (without ulceration) has been termed "sclerosis" by Warren and Freidman[14] and may be severe enough to result in bowel stricture.

Following radiation injury, the bowel wall is found to be thickened and indurated, with telangiectasiae present on the serosal surface. The mesentery attached to the bowel is frequently involved in a similar fashion[14] and the mucosa is frequently ulcerated.[41] The ulcerations may range from shallow superficial lesions to deep, punched out penetrating ulcers. An inflammatory response to penetrating ulcerations consisting of fibrinopurulent membranes, adhesions, and even necrosis may be evident. Fistulae and strictures are common sequelae of ulcerating radiation injury to the bowel.

Histopathologic changes may be found in connective tissue, blood vessels, mucosa, and muscle of tissues damaged by radiation. Early reactions in connective tissue are characterized by edema, frequently with an exudate of fibrin and precipitated protein. As the injury advances, hyalinization of collagen fibers occurs and collagen bundles become enlarged and glossy. Superficially, the hyalinized connective tissue may resemble amyloid. The edema and hyalination of the connective tissue increase the thickness of the bowel wall with the most marked changes occurring in the submucosa and subserosa. The fibroblasts have large, distorted processes with enlarged, bizarrely shaped nuclei containing prominent nucleoli and chromatin surrounded by a pale cytoplasm giving the cells an "owl's eye" appearance.

Edema followed by hyalination is found in the wall of the small arteries, but sclerosis is more pronounced in the veins; obliterative endophlebitis is usually present. Severe changes are characterized by fibrinoid necrosis, thrombosis, vascular sclerosis and telangiectasia of the lymphatic vessels.

The mucosa is markedly altered by irradiation. Ulceration and/or atrophy of the mucosa is common. Goblet cells are large and full, indicating mucous stasis with overproduction. Muscle fibers show edema, vacuolation, degeneration and atrophy. Interstitial fibrosis and hyaline degeneration of muscle fibers are also noted. The necrotic tissue present in ulcerations sometimes has a homogeneous acidophilic structure similar to that produced by a cautery.

The primary pathological criteria most important to diagnosis of radiation intestinal injury are hyalination of the connective tissue, abnormal fibroblasts, telangiectasia and hyaline degeneration of vessel walls. Secondary diagnostic features are endothelial and muscle changes and phlebosclerosis. Epithelial changes are found in any process that damages the mucous membrane and is a nonspecific feature of radiological injury.

CLINICAL PROFILE OF RADIATION INJURY

Esophagus

Relatively little has been written about the effects of radiation on the normal esophagus. Most patients receiving mediastinal radiation for bronchogenic carcinoma tolerate their therapy well and have no clinical complaints referable to the esophagus. However, Goldstein et al.[31] reported 30 patients who complained of persistent dysphagia or substernal burning following radiation therapy of 4,500–6,000 rads to the mediastinum over a six to eight week period. Seaman and Ackerman[29] noted esophageal symptoms in 20 patients following mediastinal radiation. Nielsen,[42] Fried,[43] and Phillips et al.[44] all described instances of radiation-induced esophageal stricture causing dysphagia.

Patients with radiation esophagitis usually complain of mild to moderate substernal burning following the ingestion of solid or liquid food. Rarely does the pain radiate to the chest, neck or post-auricular region. The discomfort may last for several minutes after each swallow, and in Seaman's[29] patients the onset of symptoms varied from the twelfth to thirteenth day after the onset of radiation and continued for several weeks after completion of treatment. In most patients the symptoms were mild, caused no interference with nutrition and gradually disappeared.

In a minority of patients with radiation esophagitis, the symptoms may be more severe, sometimes persisting for months after therapy is completed. Twenty-five percent of cases described by Seaman and Ackerman[29] and 16.7 percent of those described by Goldstein[31] developed permanent esophageal stenosis. Strictures occurred three to 18 months post-therapy[31] and required esophageal dilatation. Tracheo-esophageal fistula may also result following mediastinal radiation.

Pathologically, there is an initial destruction of the esophageal epithelium, which regenerates rapidly after cessation of radiation. In chronic radiation esophagitis the esophageal epithelium may appear relatively normal at esophagoscopy, despite prominent changes in the submucosa. Edema and fibrosis of the submucosa and muscular layers are prominent and cellular disruption of muscle may be present. Vascular damage is minimal, suggesting that damage is secondary to a direct radiation effect upon muscle and connective tissues.

Stomach and Duodenum

The effect of radiation therapy on the normal stomach and duodenum has not been the subject of many publications. In 1954 Friedman[45] reported radiation injury to the stomach in a group of patients receiving supervoltage therapy to the para-aortic lymph nodes for testicular carcinoma. Recently, Goldstein et al.[31] described an 8.3 percent incidence of radiation injury to the stomach and duodenum in 121 female patients receiving total abdominal para-aortic lymph node irradiation of 5,000 rads.

A variety of clinical manifestations occur after radiation injury to the stomach and duodenum.[31] Following low doses of radiation (less than 4,000 rads) patients may experience symptoms of dyspepsia and gastritis characterized by vague abdominal pain. These patients usually recover completely without treatment. The clinical syndrome of radiation dyspepsia or gastritis may occur from one month to four years after irradiation[45] and spasm or fixed narrowing of the gastric antrum may be found at endoscopy.

At radiation doses above 4,500 rads, gastric ulceration may occur. The mean time of ulcer formation is five months (range one to six months);[31] patients complain of abdominal pain which is typically unrelenting and not related to meals. Ulcers are most frequently located on the posterior antral wall and show little if any tendency to heal on medical therapy. Above 5,000 rads, gastric injury is common and reached 64 percent in the series reported by Roswit et al.[32]

Gastric ulceration with perforation or obstruction is more frequent as radiation doses increase above 5,000 rads. Acute, severe life-threatening gastric complications usually occur one to two months following radiation therapy. Patients have symptoms of intractable pain, hemorrhage and vomiting. Surgical intervention is needed to prevent perforation, massive hemorrhage, or death.

Radiation injury to the duodenum is most severe in the descending duodenum with post bulbar ulceration and stricture formation being sequelae of radiation dosages above 5,000 rads. Patients complain of abdominal pain, and vomiting is common as the duodenum becomes stenotic. Radiation-induced duodenal ulcers show little evidence of healing even with adequate medical care.[31,32]

The gastric and duodenal epithelial, vascular, and connective tissues in the submucosa are directly damaged by radiation. The epithelium sloughs and regenerates, but progressive connective tissue fibrosis and vascular sclerosis may occur. The stomach and duodenum are not more resistant to radiation exposure than other parts of the intestinal tract. The low incidence of significant radiation injury to the gastroduodenal area probably reflects the low frequency with which the stomach and duodenum are present within the usual pelvic or abdominal radiation fields. Preexisting vascular disease, atherosclerosis, diabetes or hypertension do not appear to alter patient tolerance for gastroduodenal radiation.[31]

Small Bowel

Radiation injury to the small bowel is not an uncommon sequelae to abdominal or pelvic irradiation. Roswit et al.[32] indicated the small bowel to be the most radiosensitive of the gastrointestinal viscera. Were it not for the constant movement of small bowel loops during radiation therapy, there would undoubtedly be an even higher incidence of small bowel injury following abdominal irradiation.

Two distinct clinical phases are identifiable in patients suffering small bowel injury following radiation therapy. The occurrence of acute radiation enteropathy is heralded by the onset of severe diarrhea while therapy is in progress. Associated clinical symptoms may be abdominal pain, nausea, and vomiting. Diarrhea is a very common clinical manifestation of radiation treatment of the abdomen, and in most cases is self-limiting. Less frequently, the acute episode may be more severe and present with bloody diarrhea and marked abdominal pain; the abdomen may become distended, simulating an intestinal obstruction. Rarely, acute intestinal necrosis is produced, and peritonitis, perforation and/or fistula formation occur. At 4,500 rads a one to five percent risk of ulceration is present. The risk increases to 25 to 50 percent at doses of 6,000 rads.[32]

The intestinal injury in acute radiation enteropathy depends upon dose. Initial changes are inhibition of mitosis with degeneration and necrosis of crypt epithelial cells. Endothelial cell damage, edema, hyperemia and neutrophilic infiltration rapidly occur. The crypt cell population rapidly decreases, the villi are shortened and the bowel surface is flattened. If the radiation dose is sublethal there is recovery of crypt cells and the epithelial surface is repaired. Large doses of radiation produce vascular damage leading to ulceration and infarction.[32]

Laboratory studies in patients having acute radiation enteritis have shown abnormalities of serum protein, fats, electrolytes and glucose.[46,47] Reeves demonstrated low blood levels of ^{131}I-glycerol trioleate and high fecal fat in 77 percent of patients receiving 2,500 to 3,000 rads of pelvic or abdominal radiation.[48] Duncan and Leonard,[47] using ^{131}I-labeled PVP, documented intestinal protein leakage with clinically employed radiation dosages, and Lipkin et al.[49] showed protein synthesis to be inhibited in the mouse.

The exact cause for diarrhea following abdominal radiation is unclear, but is thought to be due in part to the effect of irradiation on ileal function.[30,50] In some patients decreased bile salt absorption in the ileum occurs following irradiation.[50] The passage of excessive amounts of bile salts into the colon produces diarrhea as large amounts of water and electrolytes are secreted by the colon mucosa.[50,51] This clinical state is termed "cholerheic enteropathy." It occurs during or shortly after irradiation is complete and responds to cholestyramine, a nonabsorbable anion-exchange resin which binds bile salts, making them inactive in the colon.[50]

The cholyl-glycine breath test[30,40] is a quantitative method of studying the degree of ileal dysfunction present following radiation therapy. A dose of 1.5 to 5 μCi of cholyl–glycine–1–^{14}C ethanol is ingested, and breath samples are obtained 2, 4, 5, 8, 12, 18 and 24 hours later and analyzed for $^{14}CO_2$. Total $^{14}CO_2$ excreted in 24 hours is expressed as a percentage of administered dose. The appearance of elevated levels of ^{14}C-labeled carbon dioxide in the breath indicates ileal dysfunction and abnormal contact between bacteria and bile salts.[30]

Recently, Mennie et al.[52] successfully treated post-radiation diarrhea with acetylsalicylate—a prostaglandin inhibitor. This indicates that prostaglandin release from irradiated small intestine may be a contributing factor in the production of diarrhea following radiation therapy.

Chronic small bowel injury usually manifests itself six months to five or more years after therapy. When intestinal symptoms begin so long after therapy, there may be a great problem in differential diagnosis. Clinically, patients complain of intermittent colic, diarrhea, obstipation, vomiting, anorexia, abdominal pain and fatigue.[30] While acute small bowel obstruction, enteric fistula, and intestinal infarction are possible late complications of radiation therapy, patients most frequently suffer from chronic bowel dysfunction, low grade obstruction, recurrent cramps, diarrhea and rapid motility.[30] Chronic malabsorption may lead to a megaloblastic anemia, vitamin, fat, protein, fluid and electrolyte loss, and may make the patient a nutritional cripple.

Radiation-induced damage to the vasculo-connective tissues is thought to be the basis for late clinical intestinal syndromes. Slow occlusion of vessels with fibrosis produces partial vascular obstruction within one to five years.[40] The rate at which these changes occur is a function both of radiation dose and the rapidity with which the dose was administered. The larger mesenteric arteries are usually spared, but diffuse abnormalities in microvascular structures within the bowel wall are found.[53]

Colon and Rectum

Radiation injuries may involve all portions of the colon, but damage to the rectum and sigmoid colon are most frequent due to the greater frequency with which pelvic irradiation is employed for cervical or ovarian carcinoma. As in other areas of the bowel, colonic radiation injury produces a varied clinical picture depending upon the time after radiation and the amount and method of radiation administration.

Acute radiation proctitis is the most common radiation injury to the colon, occurring in 12 percent of patients having pelvic irradiation.[24] The symptoms occur within the first three to nine months post irradiation and consist of pain, diarrhea, tenesmus and rectal bleeding. The symptoms are usually self-limited and respond to medical therapy consisting of a low residue diet, antispasmotics, stool softener, sulfonamides and steroid enemas.[23,54,55]

Proctoscopic examination reveals friable, red mucosa which is bleeding or bleeds easily. The abnormality may be diffuse or involve only a portion of the rectal mucosa. Symptoms usually subside in four to 16 weeks, and few patients require hospitalization. Proctitis is rare when total dosage is 4,000 rads or less, but increases as dosage climbs above 6,000 rads. The most severe damage typically occurs in the anterior rectal wall at the level of the posterior fornix.

Radiation-induced rectal ulceration causes symptoms which are similar to those found in uncomplicated proctitis, but the symptoms are more severe and persistent. The onset of symptoms occurs from nine to fourteen months following radiation therapy, and the diagnosis is confirmed by proctoscopy or barium enema. The incidence of rectal ulceration is negligible below 5,000 rads, approximately five percent above 5,500 rads, and at 8,000 rads, rises to 25 to 50 percent. A rectovaginal fistula is the most common serious injury to follow pelvic irradiation, and usually develops at a site of rectal ulceration. Rectovaginal fistulae occurred in 0.3 percent of 2,765 patients treated for cervical carcinoma.[32] Symptoms are characterized by the onset of a vaginal discharge with pain and bleeding in the perineal area. The fistula most frequently occurs 6–10 cm. from the anus.

Pelvic irradiation may produce a proctosigmoiditis having a clinical picture similar to that of radiation proctitis. Rectal bleeding, pain on defecation, constipation, abdominal cramps, and mucous discharge are not frequently produced. Sigmoidoscopy reveals mucosal edema, friability and spasm.

The late complications of rectal or sigmoid radiation injury are rectal or sigmoid stenosis and/or stricture formation.[13,24,28,39,54] Symptoms from stenosis or stricture formation may begin 6 to 18 months following completion of therapy and may start with bleeding and/or diarrhea.[24] Obstructive symptoms appear gradually and are usually subacute in nature. Proctosigmoidoscopy or colonoscopy demonstrates an area of scarring and narrowing with localized ulcerations. Clinically, the scarring and fibrosis may make differentiation from recurrent tumor very difficult. Physical examination also may be unable to distinguish pelvic fibrosis secondary to irradiation from the frozen pelvis of recurrent carcinoma.

Late complications of radiation injury to the sigmoid are fistula formation and, rarely, the development of adenocarcinoma secondary to radiation therapy.[25,56–58]

Radiation-induced cystitis is common during and shortly after irradiation. Dysuria, spasm, increased frequency, and hematuria may be present, and on cystoscopy there is evidence of cystitis with or without ulceration.[33] Bladder ulcerations have been reported[33,59] but are infrequent. When they occur they are usually located in the trigone region and only rarely in the bladder dome.

RADIOGRAPHIC MANIFESTATIONS OF RADIATION INJURY

Esophagus

The initial radiological abnormality demonstrable on barium study of the radiation-damaged esophagus is altered esophageal motility. The primary esophageal wave is interrupted at the site of irradiation. Tertiary nonpropulsive peristaltic waves are seen distal to the irradiated segment. Goldstein et al.[31] also noted a failure of the distal esophageal sphincter to relax and a delay in esophageal emptying in some patients. Morphologically, the esophagus may be normal at this stage and the motility abnor-

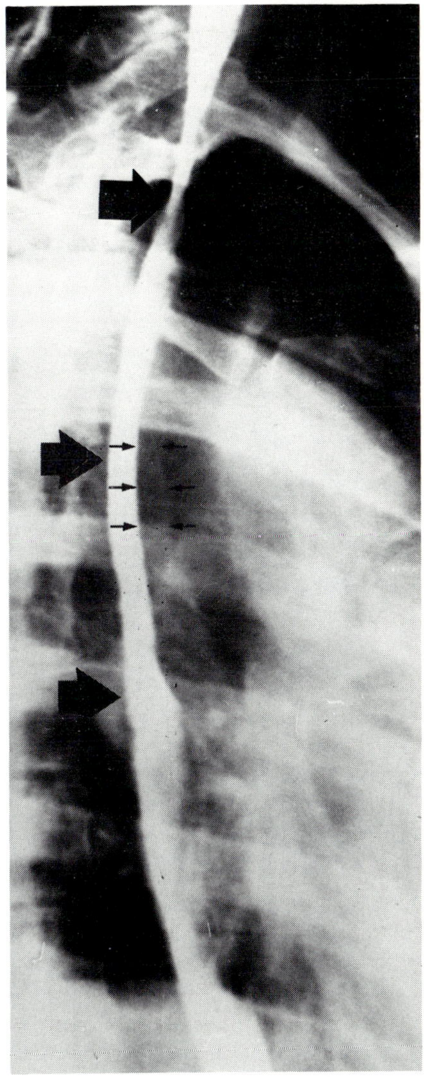

Fig. 9-1. Radiation-induced esophageal stenosis: A 32-year-old female who received 6,000 rads to the upper mediastinum as treatment for metastatic squamous cell carcinoma two years ago. An esophagogram shows the esophagus to be narrowed (large arrows). The margins of the stenosed esophagus are smooth and tapered. The thickened esophageal wall (small arrows) is also demonstrated.

malities may appear very subtle and undetectable unless a careful esophageal examination is performed with the patient in the prone or supine position.

While radiographic studies of the esophagus are often normal in radiation-induced acute esophagitis,[29,31] occasionally, a thickening of esophageal folds and/or fine serrations may be detected by barium esophagography. Double contrast esophagography should be performed to detect these early epithelial esophageal abnormalities. The esophago-

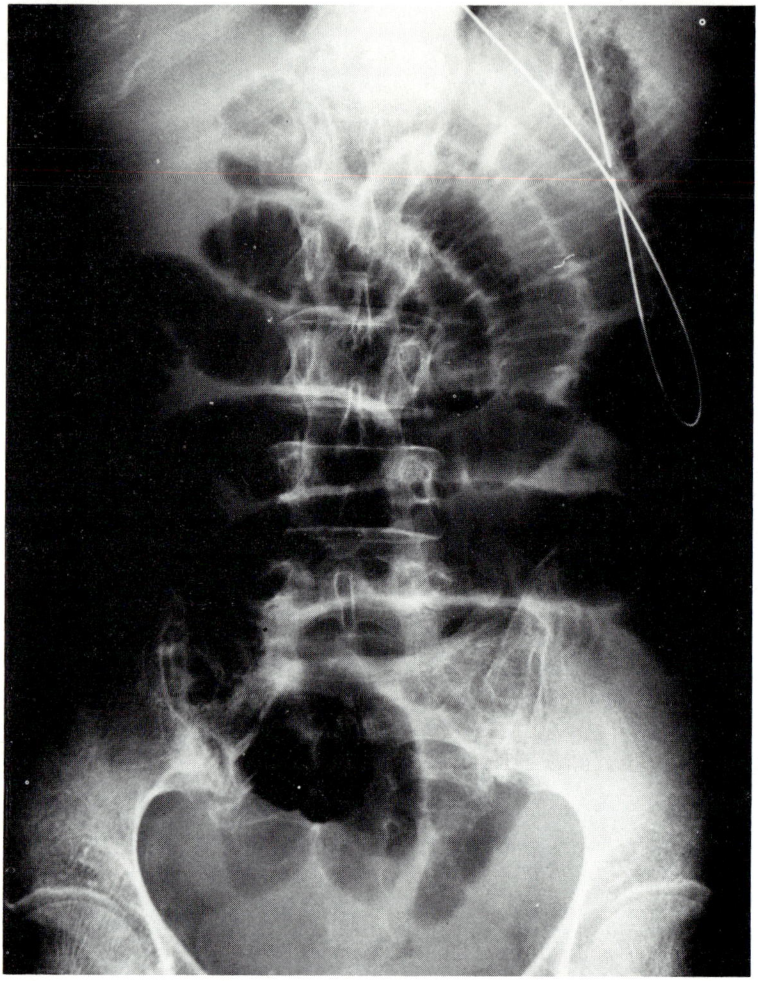

Fig. 9-2A. Acute radiation enteritis appearing as a small bowel obstruction: A supine abdominal radiograph shows dilated loops of small bowel without any gas in the colon.

gram usually reverts to normal within three to six months as the epithelial injuries heal and the patients become and remain asymptomatic. The radiologic differential diagnosis in patients with radiation-induced acute esophagitis is reflux esophagitis and superinfection.

Occasionally, radiation therapy produces damage to the vascular and connective tissues of the esophagus; the changes of chronic radiation esophagitis ensue.[29,31] The most frequent radiological finding is the development of a constrictive narrowing of the esophagus, usually first

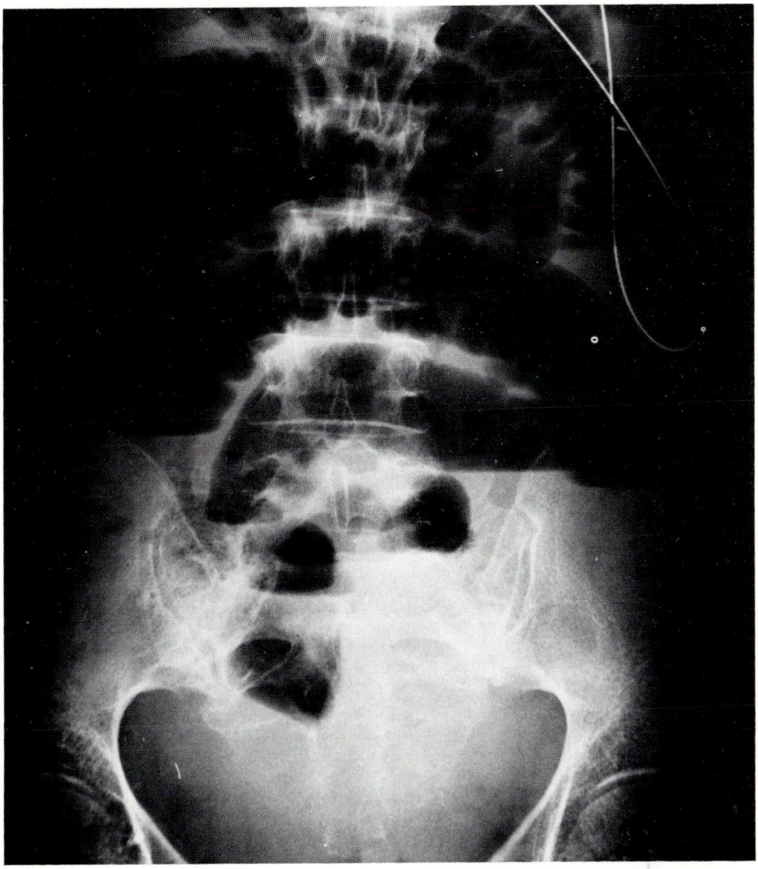

Fig. 9-2B. An erect abdominal radiograph demonstrates air fluid levels in the small intestine and no air in the rectum or sigmoid colon. Acute radiation ileitis was found at laporotomy.

detectable three to eight months following therapy. The strictured area is the result of submucosal edema and fibrosis. The abnormal area always lies within the radiation field and appears benign on barium examination. The strictured region is focal in nature and usually has smoothly tapered margins without associated irregularity or mucosal destruction (Fig. 9-1). Angulation of the esophagus near the focal stricture may occur. It is postulated that the esophageal angulation is the result of radiation changes to the mediastinum with resultant fibrosis of adherent mediastinal structures. Frank esophageal ulceration and tracheo-esophageal fistula have been reported, but are exceedingly rare unless very large radiation exposures are given.

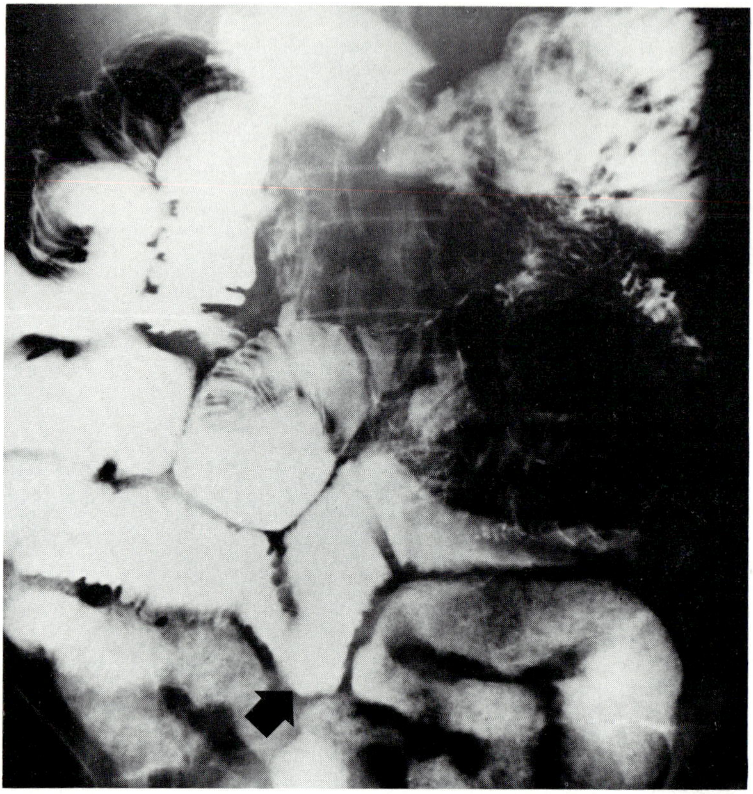

Fig. 9-3. Acute radiation enteritis: A small bowel examination reveals 1) dilated loops of jejunum and ileum, 2) excess secretions in the ileum producing a granular, smudged appearance to the barium and 3) angulation (arrow) of the small intestine.

Stomach

The stomach tolerates radiation doses employed in clinical practice remarkably well because of its thick muscular coat and rapidly replicating mucosal lining. As in other areas of the gastrointestinal tract, the frequency and severity of lesions are related to dose.

At 4,500 rads or less symptoms of gastritis and dyspepsia are frequent; the stomach, though, is usually radiographically normal but may demonstrate reduced motility or spasm in the irradiated area.[31,32] As radiation exposure increases to between 4,500 and 5,000 rads, radiation-induced gastric ulceration occurs typically in the posterior wall of the antrum or prepyloric region. The ulcerations are virtually identical radiographically to benign peptic ulcers. However, healing is either extremely slow or does not occur at all.[31,32] Most gastric ulcers occur months after

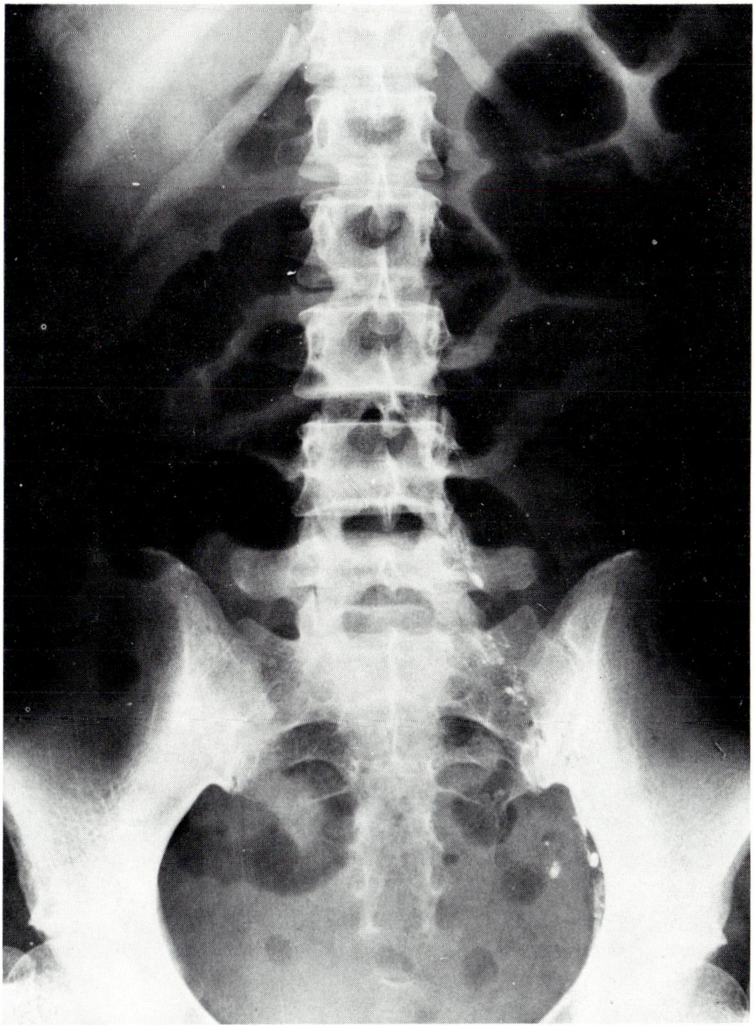

Fig. 9-4A. Radiation enteritis simulating a partial small bowel obstruction: A 60 year old female one year following 5,000 rads of radiation therapy having symptoms of bloating and abdominal pain. A plain abdominal radiograph reveals dilated small bowel loops in the upper abdomen with a paucity of gas in the large colon.

completion of radiation therapy, but when radiation exposures exceed 6,000 rads, acute severe radiation-induced ulceration, which may lead to perforation, may occur.[32,45,60]

Narrowing and stiffening of the gastric antrum is a sequelae of radiation therapy which appears similar to an infiltrating gastric malignancy. Peristaltic activity is absent; superficial ulcerations and thick folds may be

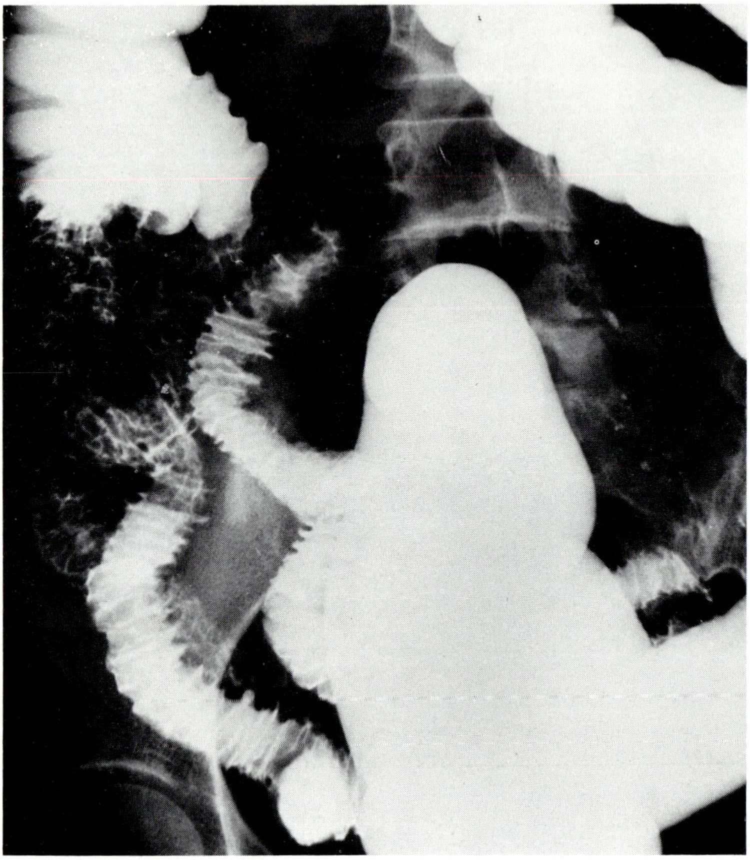

Fig. 9-4B. A barium enema demonstrates the folds of the terminal ileum to be thickened, straightened and rigid. The margins are spiculated. In some areas it has a picket fence appearance.

present. The narrowing may be severe enough to result in gastric outlet obstruction.

Duodenum

Radiation injury to the duodenum occurs in patients receiving radiation therapy to the para-aortic lymph node chain or right retroperitoneal region. Roswit et al.[32] reported the duodenum to have the least tolerance to radiation exposure of any segment of gastrointestinal viscera. However, rather than representing an actual difference in radiation tolerance, the apparent duodenal sensitivity probably reflects its fixed position and

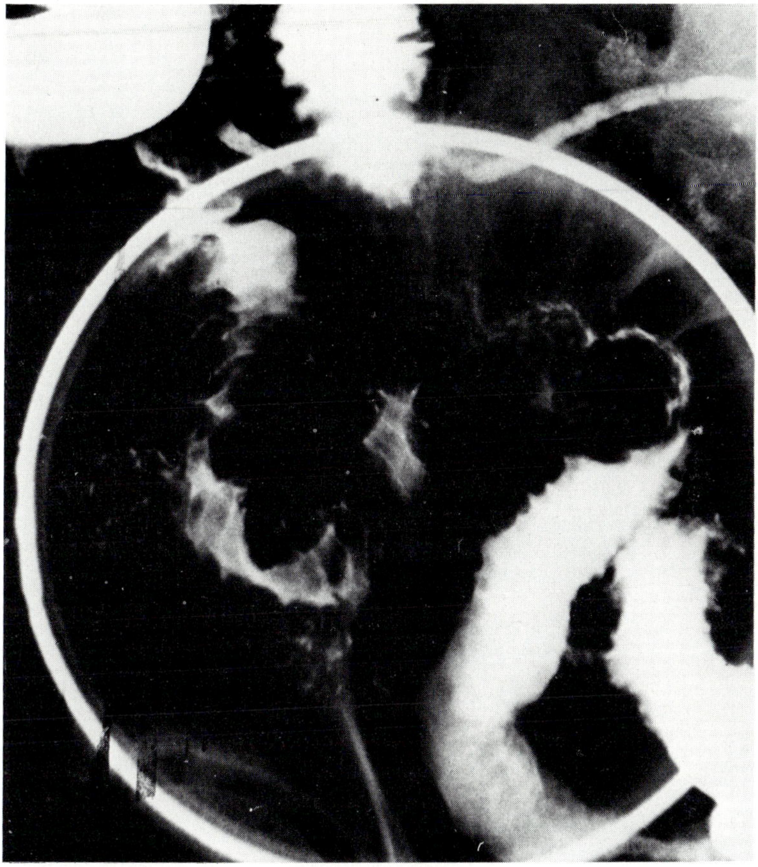

Fig. 9-5. Chronic radiation damage to the terminal ileum two years after radiation therapy with 6,000 rads for uterine cancer. The terminal ileum is rigid and the folds are thickened, the loops of bowel are separated and the intestinal lumen is narrowed.

limited mobility. Injuries are infrequent if exposure is below 4,000 rads and increases with increasing dosages. Diffuse thickening of the duodenal fold pattern has been termed radiation duodenitis.[31] While duodenitis may occur without ulceration, radiation-induced ulceration in the pyloric channel, duodenal bulb or second portion of the duodenum are frequently demonstrated. The ulcers do not respond to conventional medical therapy and, as the acute inflammatory reaction subsides, strictures may be formed. Duodenal strictures have been noted as early as one month after radiation therapy but more usually present three to eight months after completion of irradiation.

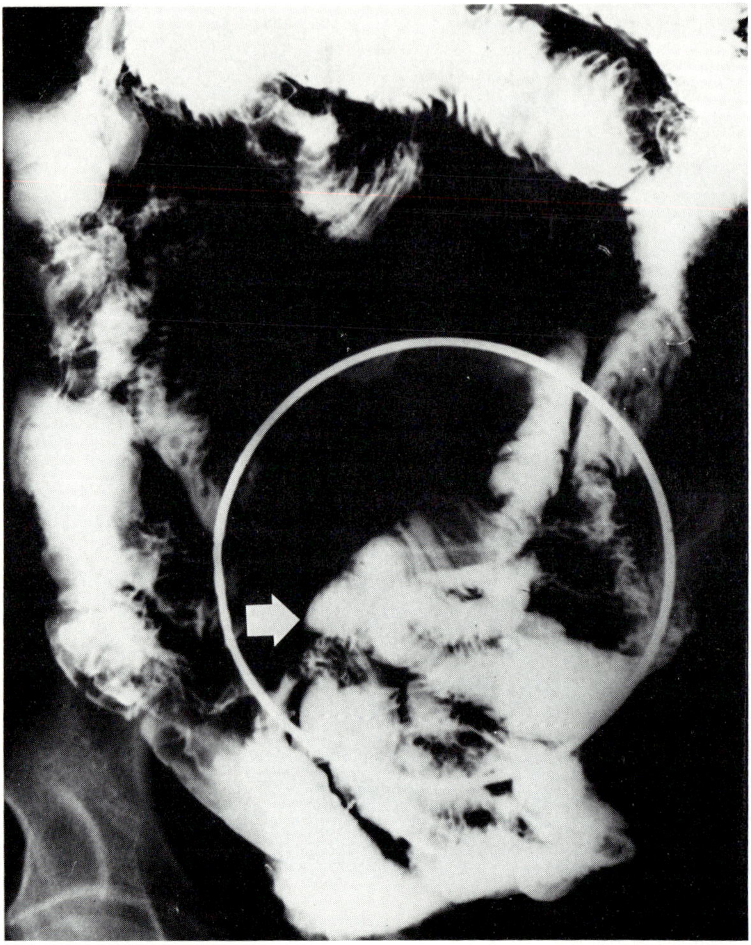

Fig. 9-6. A small bowel examination reveals fixation of the small intestine. The small bowel is sharply angulated (arrow) and kinked due to adhesions and radiation induced fibrosis.

The stomach is frequently irradiated with the duodenum, and radiographically demonstrable lesions of the stomach and duodenum frequently occur together.

Small Bowel

Radiological manifestations of radiation injury to the small intestine are multiple and reflect the underlying pathophysiology induced by radiation treatment. While radiographic appearances of the small bowel at

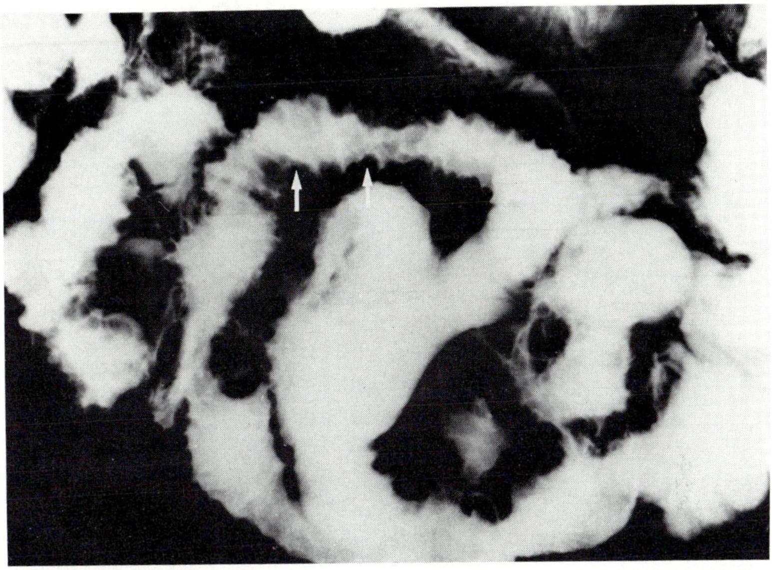

Fig. 9-7. Intestinal damage four years after radiation therapy. Diffuse small bowel thickening, bowel separation and focal areas of narrowing are shown on a small bowel examination. Submucosal thickening may produce nodular contour defects (arrows) which simulate metastatic disease.

times correlate with a patient's clinical state, the radiographic features more likely underestimate the extent and severity of radiation-induced injury and correlate poorly with the patient's clinical status.

The findings of radiological examinations done during the course of radiation therapy have rarely been reported. The abdomen may be distended by dilated, atonic loops of small bowel in a pattern that simulates a partial small bowel obstruction (Figs. 9-2A and B). Barium studies may also reveal a dilated small bowel with excess secretions (Fig. 9-3). Patients with acute radiation enteritis usually respond to conservative therapy, and follow-up radiographs are normal.

Chronic radiation injury to the small bowel is produced by the late effect of fibrosis, vascular injury, adhesions and arteritis. As these processes progress, a variety of intestinal abnormalities are produced which may eventually become disabling.

Chronic radiation enteritis may produce mucosal atrophy, superficial ulceration and even penetrating ulceration.[31,32] Except when deep penetrating ulcers are present, conventional barium examinations usually fail to detect the superficial ulceration commonly seen at autopsy. Perhaps a more widespread use of double contrast small bowel examinations will detect these subtle mucosal abnormalities.

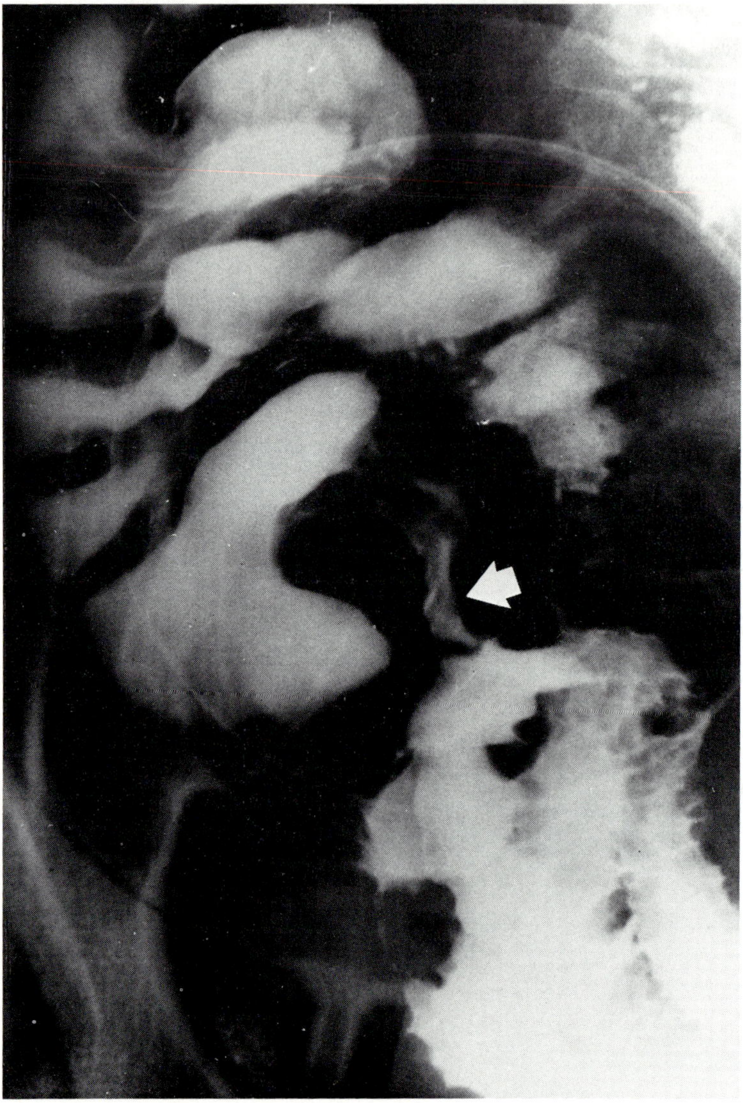

Fig. 9-8. Stenosis of the terminal ileum (arrow) following 6,000 rads of radiation therapy for cervical carcinoma.

The most marked changes are submucosal in location and produce the typical radiological appearance of submucosal disease processes. The small bowel folds become 1) thickened (greater than 2.0 mm.), 2) straightened, and 3) rigid (Figs. 9-4A, B, and 9-5). Frequently the margins are sharply spiculated and the small bowel has a picket fence or stack of coins appearance (Fig. 9-4B).[26,31,32] These findings, however, are

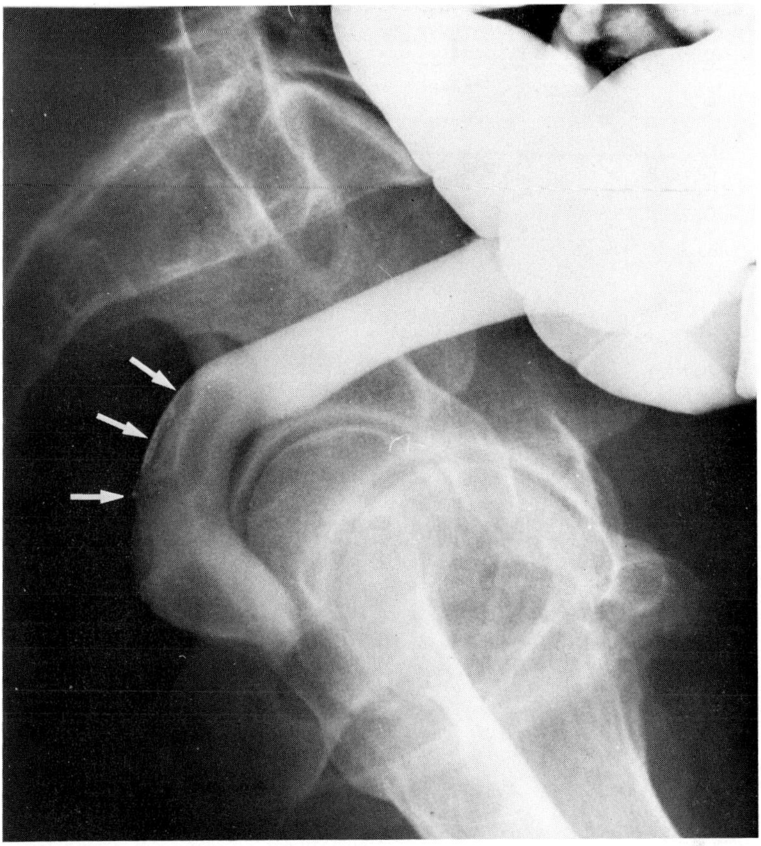

Fig. 9-9. Smooth rectal narrowing with widening of the presacral space and slight mucosal irregularity (arrows) is demonstrated on the lateral rectal film of a barium enema. The patient was two years post 4,800 rads to the pelvis for carcinoma of the cervix.

nonspecific and are produced by any disease process that causes the submucosa of the small intestine to be thickened. Hemorrhage, edema, lymphoma, carcinoma, and fibrous tissue all may simulate radiation enteritis, but small bowel ischemia and regional enteritis most closely simulate the changes seen in chronic radiation enteritis.

Thickening of the bowel wall is present in almost every instance of radiation injury to the small intestine. Radiographically the loops of bowel are separated and frequently have sharp angles, kinks, and bends, which are unchanging from film to film (Fig. 9-6). While small bowel thickening is usually diffuse in any one area of involvement, areas of focal fibrosis and thickening of the submucosal may produce nodular filling defects in the small bowel which simulate metastatic disease (Fig. 9-7).[26]

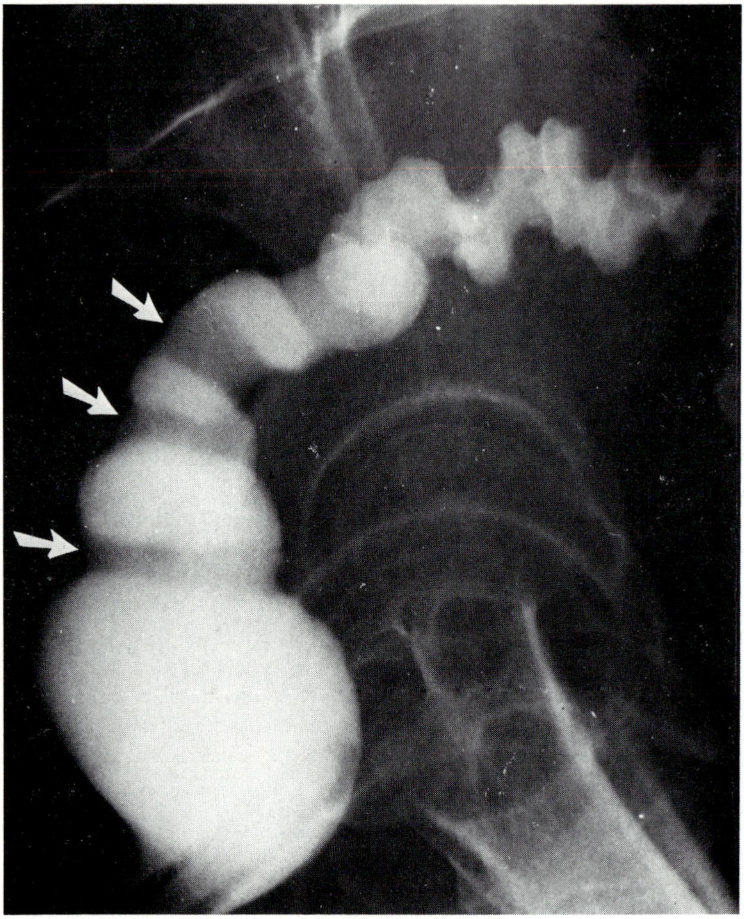

Fig. 9-10. Acute radiation induced proctitis in a patient receiving 6400 rads in 34 days followed by 3,500 rads of radium implants for cervical carcinoma. The lateral rectal radiograph reveals marked thickening of the rectal folds (arrows), narrowing and spasm. No ulceration is identified.

Mesenteric fibrosis, adhesions, and retraction often cause the bowel loops to become matted together and congealed into a mass of intestine such that it is impossible to separate any one loop of bowel from another. While this appearance may occur anywhere within the abdomen, it is most frequent in the pelvis, as the pelvic location does not permit palpation to be employed to study individual loops of intestine. It may be difficult to distinguish radiation-induced adhesions and fibrosis from post operative change, unless radiation enteritis is detected in other regions of the bowel.

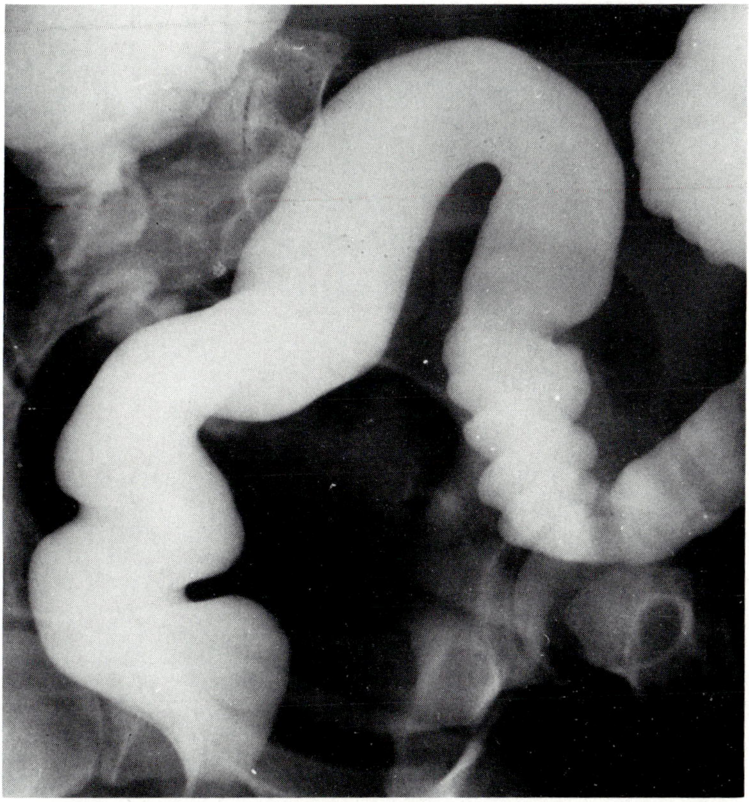

Fig. 9-11A. Acute radiation proctitis: A barium enema in 1972 prior to radiation therapy demonstrated the rectosigmoid colon to be normal.

As the mesentery becomes fibrotic, the mesenteric side of the small bowel is drawn toward the fibrotic area and the folds of the intestine become drawn toward one side of the bowel. This finding is found not only in radiation enteritis but in any process that produces adhesions or induces fibrosis. Metastatic tumors, carcinoid tumors, retractile mesenteritis and postoperative adhesions all appear radiographically similar.

Stenosis (Fig. 9-8) is the late result of progressive fibrosis, vasculitis and venous obliteration. Multiple strictures may be present at varying points along the small bowel, producing intestinal obstruction. The stenosis may be as short as 5 mm. and radiographic detection may be extremely difficult.

Fistulae between loops of small bowel and the colon and bladder are serious sequelae of radiation therapy. Careful monitoring of the passage

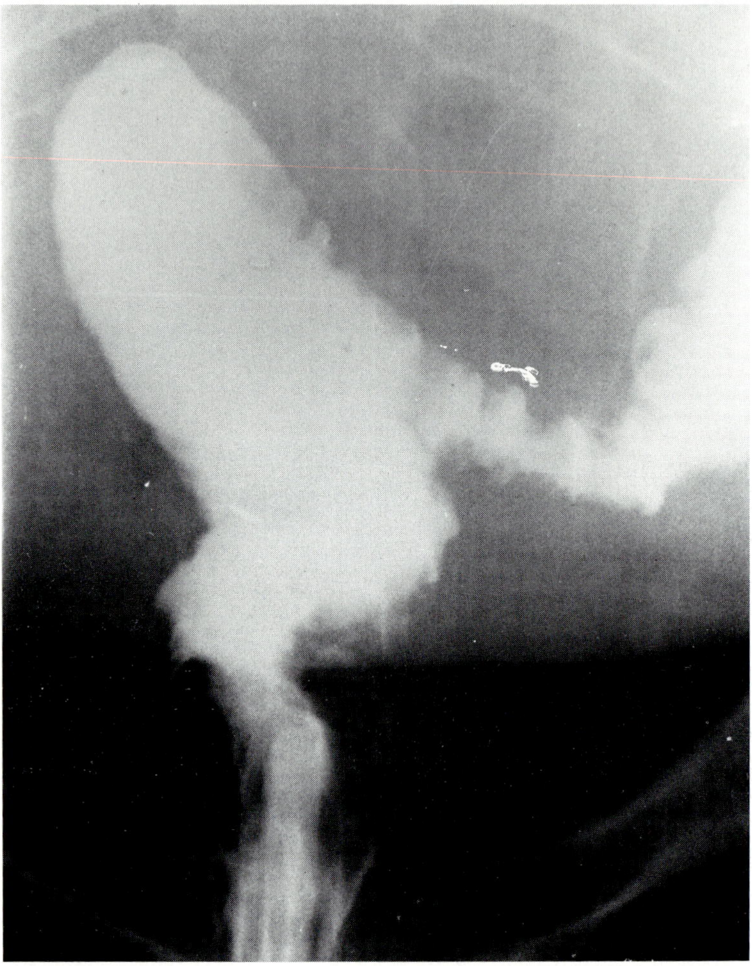

Fig. 9-11B. A barium enema in 1974, one month following pelvic radiation therapy with 5,800 rads reveals mucosal ulceration, spasm, and thickening of the folds producing a radiographic picture identical to acute ulcerative colitis.

of the barium as it proceeds through the intestine is necessary to confirm a diagnosis of these enteric fistulae.

Colon

The most frequently injured segments of the large bowel are the rectum and sigmoid colon. Radiographically, radiation injury to the rectum and sigmoid colon initially manifests itself as an area of smooth

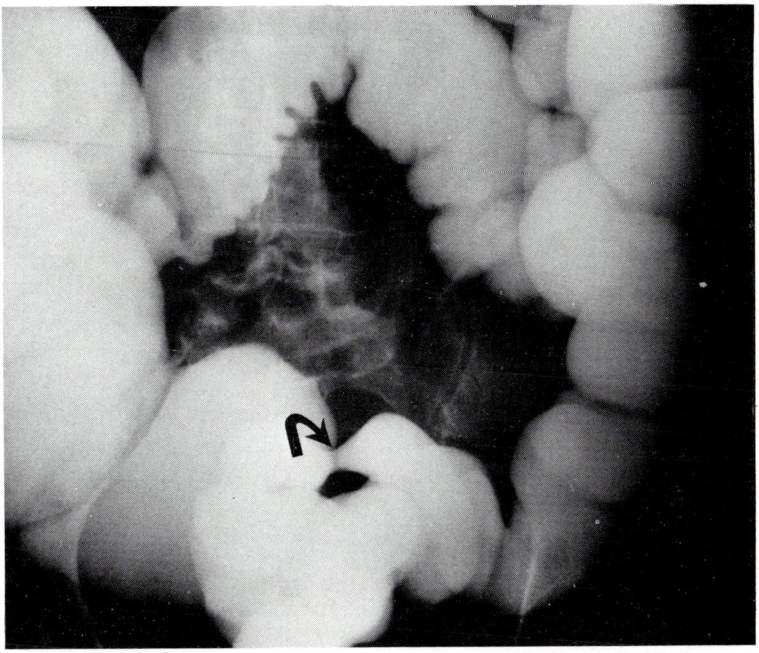

Fig. 9-12. Colonic stricture (arrow) twelve years after pelvic radiation therapy. Surgery revealed marked fibrosis of the colonic wall and vascular structures.

narrowing (Fig. 9-9) or as a spasm with a friable mucosa, demonstrable on double contrast radiography. There may be thickening of the mucosal folds secondary to edema (Fig. 9-10) or, rarely, a rectal ulcer. In the early stages a radiation-induced proctitis or sigmoiditis may be indistinguishable from acute ulcerative colitis or proctitis (Figs. 9-11 and 13).

Ongoing fibrosis and vascular damage may produce progressive focal rectal or sigmoid narrowing and stenosis. The stenotic segment is usually tapered and has a benign appearance (Fig. 9-12), but may be short, ulcered, and difficult to distinguish from recurrent tumor (Figs. 9-13 and 14). Todd[13] termed these rectal lesions "pseudocarcinoma" when they appeared following radiation treatment of cervical carcinoma.

As the injury becomes chronic the entire rectum and sigmoid colon may become diffusely narrowed with smooth or thickened mucosa (Fig. 9-15). The findings may be subtle at fluoroscopy, and mild degrees of rectal narrowing overlooked. A balloon catheter must not be inflated in the rectum of any patient having had pelvic irradiation, since the rectum is often rigid and forced balloon distention may result in a rectal perforation.

Rectal stenosis is most common six to 18 months after irradiation therapy and may be associated with symptoms of obstruction. Pain and bleeding may occur if an associated rectal ulceration is present (Fig. 9-16).

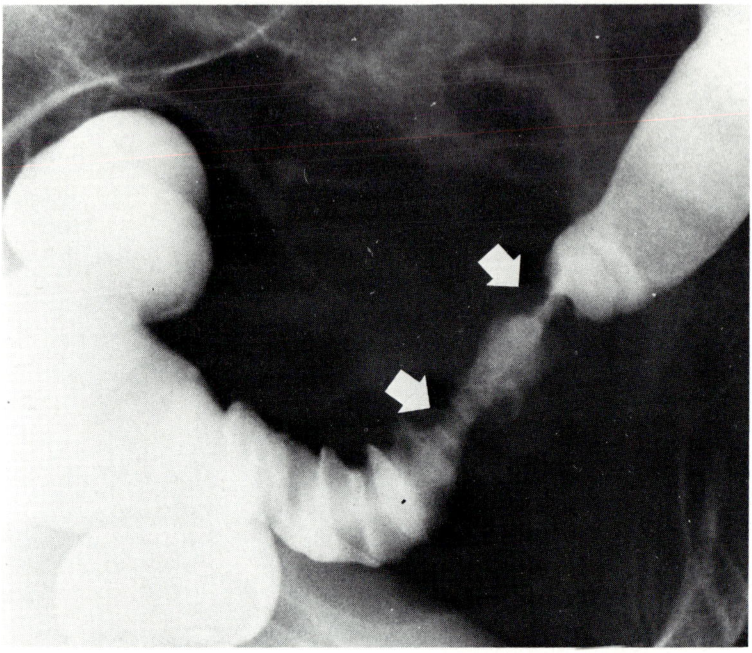

Fig. 9-13. A barium enema two years following radiation therapy for cervical carcinoma reveals a stricture in the sigmoid colon (arrows). Pathologic examination showed sigmoid ulceration, marked fibrosis of the muscularis and vascular fibrosis and obliteration.

Progression of vascular injury may result in a focal perforation and abscess, which simulate diverticulitis or lead to the development of a rectovaginal (Fig. 9-17), rectal-enteric, or rectal-vesical fistula. Demonstration of the fistula tract is best done with an enema using a water contrast media; however, the radiological examination is frequently difficult to perform because of the severe pain these patients suffer.

The transverse colon and other colonic segments are also susceptible to radiation injuries, but reports of injury are rare due to the infrequency with which these colonic segments are irradiated.

TREATMENT

New radiation therapeutic equipment allows for larger doses of radiation to be given to tumors without serious skin reaction. However, larger tumor doses potentially expose the intestinal tract to higher levels of radiation. To minimize intestinal damage the initial therapeutic step

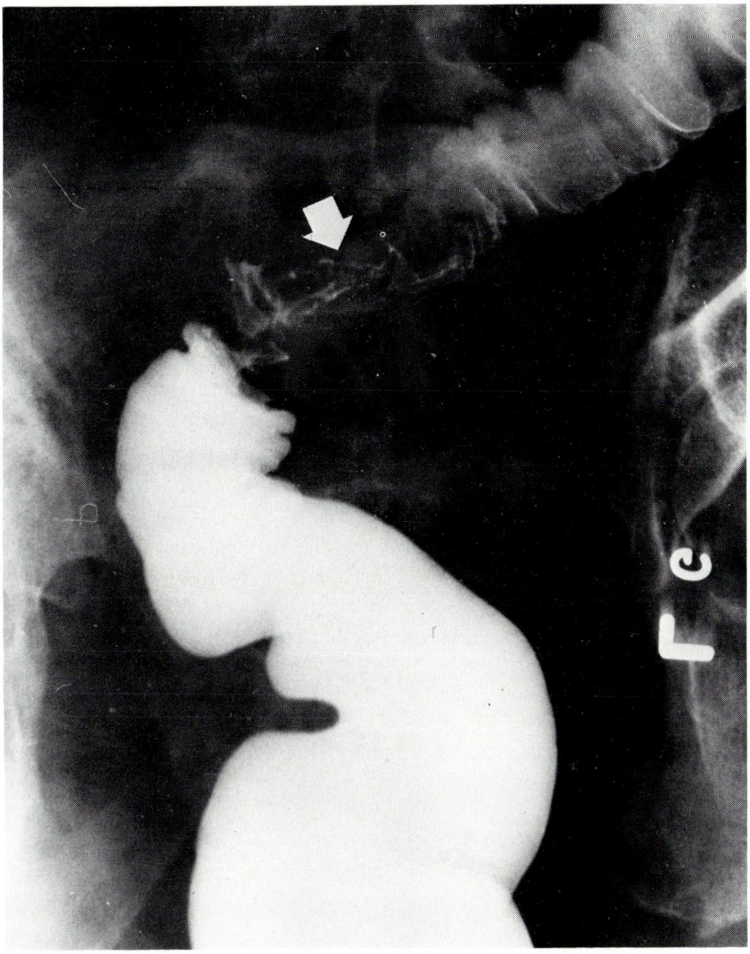

Fig. 9-14. Radiation damage to the sigmoid colon producing narrowing (arrow), spasm and fixation which simulates a colonic carcinoma.

should be careful treatment planning. This will avoid unnecessary intestinal exposure. An awareness of a history of prior surgery, vascular disease, inflammatory bowel disease, concomitant chemotherapy,[61] or other conditions which increase the risk of radiation damage to the bowel must be carefully elicited.

It is beyond the scope of this chapter to detail every medical and surgical modality used in treating radiation-induced intestinal injuries. As a general principle, it is wise to individualize therapy as much as possible and to avoid surgical intervention unless indicated.

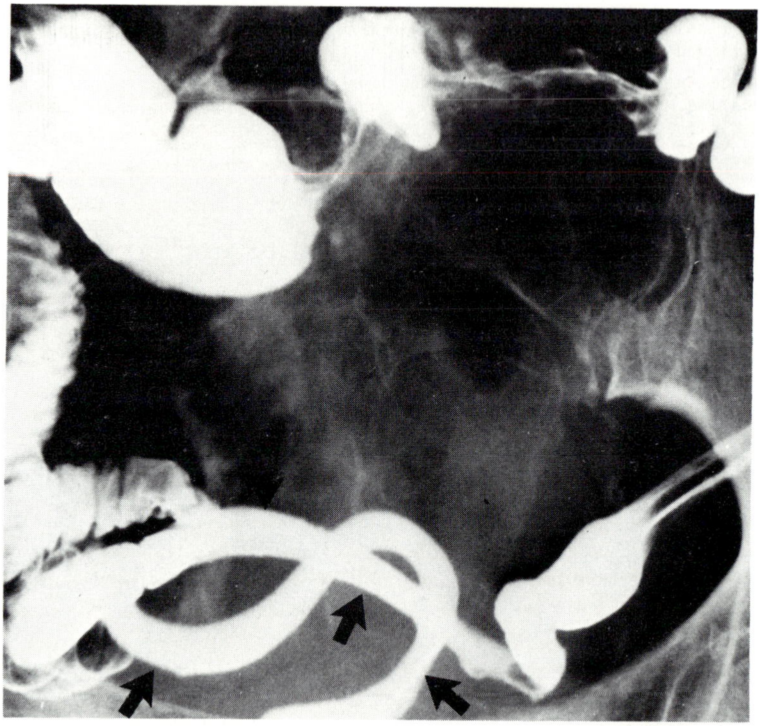

Fig. 9-15. Diffuse, severe rectal and sigmoid colon narrowing (arrows) eight years after radiation therapy for cervical carcinoma. The mucosa is smooth and has no ulceration.

Most symptoms of radiation intestinal injury may be managed by medical means. Radiation-induced gastric ulceration may be treated conservatively and, while the ulcer may not heal quickly, long-term medical management may control symptoms and result in healing in some instances.

Choleretic enteropathy may be treated with cholestyramine. Antibiotic therapy may be useful in eliminating bacterial overgrowth due to intestinal stasis and may decrease radiation-induced malabsorption. Narrowed areas in the rectum and esophagus have been treated with dilatation and steroid enemas are used to treat radiation proctosigmoiditis.

Surgery is usually reserved for complications of obstructions, massive hemorrhage, fistulae, intestinal necrosis, perforation and/or radiation-induced carcinoma. Surgery is always difficult in irradiated tissue, and most surgeons advocate wide resections and removal in block of all tissue in the irradiated field.[36] Dissection of adhesions is not advocated unless the bowel is to be removed. Despite advances in surgical tech-

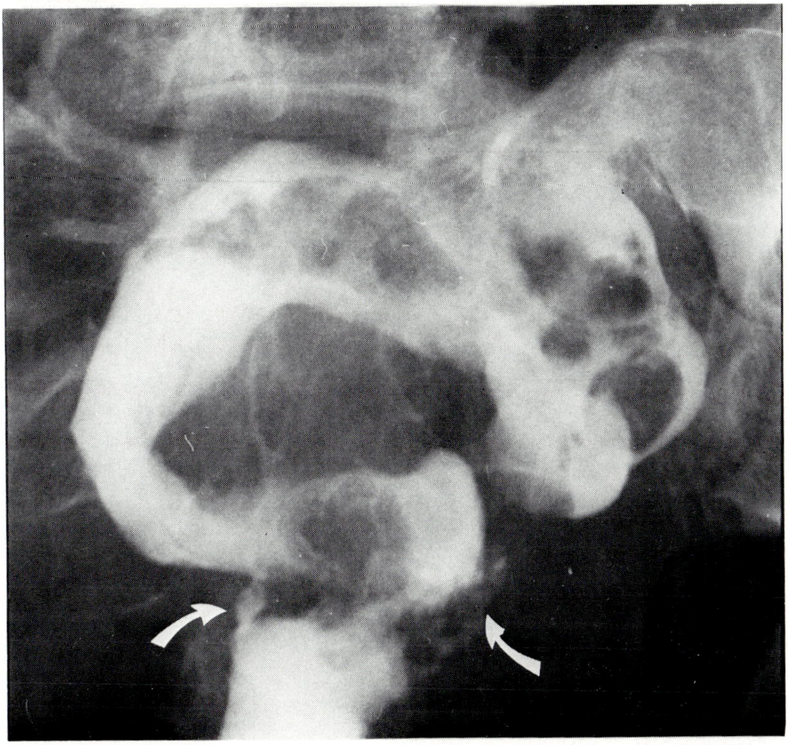

Fig. 9-16. Severe radiation proctitis following 8,000 rads to the pelvis. The barium enema reveals focal narrowing of the rectum and ulceration (arrows) which extends through the rectal wall producing a severe peritonitis. The rectum was found to be necrotic at surgery.

nique, an aggressive surgical approach does not appear to offer much except when severe radiation complications are present.

NEWER ASPECTS OF TREATMENT AND PREVENTION

In 1953 Gray et al. demonstrated that hypoxic tissue was less radiosensitive than normal tissue.[62] Various investigators have attempted to protect normal tissue by inducing local hypoxia.[63–65] Others attempted to increase tumor radiosensitivity by increasing oxygen tension within the tumors.[66]

Recently Steckel et al.[63] demonstrated that superior mesenteric artery infusion of vasopressin or propranolol-epinephrine reduced radiation injury to the dog's intestine. Rappleye et al.[67] showed a similar

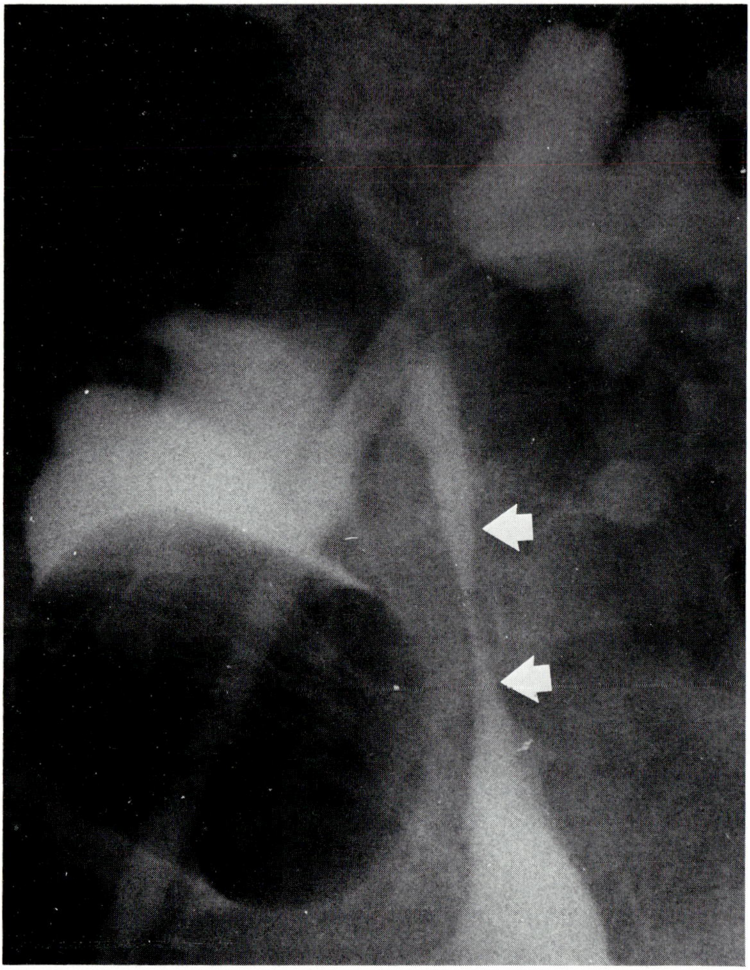

Fig. 9-17. A barium enema in a patient with a radiation induced recto-vaginal fistula (arrow). Distended by a balloon catheter of any patient having had pelvic radiation increases the chance of rectal perforation.

protective effect of vasopressin in irradiated mice. Presumably these agents act by decreasing mesenteric blood flow and inducing a degree of intestinal hypoxia. Bosniak et al.[68] demonstrated that radiation-induced vascular spasm could be prevented by intra-arterial papaverine while Stryker et al.[69] reported that oral prednisone, rather than having a protective effect following pelvic irradiation, actually had an adverse action.

Recently, antibiotic therapy has been shown to have some beneficial effect on the intestinal tract of patients with regional enteritis,[70] and Spratt et al.[55] in 1961 demonstrated that sulfasuxidine given prior to irradiation of isolated ileal loops reduced the inflammatory cell response and decreased lethality. Additional investigations are needed to further delineate the role bacteria play in radiation injury and in pharmacological methods of protecting the intestine during radiation exposure. However, despite the attractiveness of some of these research findings, to date, none of these experimental techniques has been proven to be of use in preventing radiation damage to the human gastrointestinal tract.

REFERENCES

1. Walsh D: Deep tissue traumatism from roentgen ray exposure. Br Med J 2:272–273, 1897
2. Edsall DL: The attitude of the clinician in regard to exposing patients to the x-ray. J Am Med Assoc 47:1425–1429, 1906
3. Franz K, Orth J: Fall einer rontgen schadigung. Berl Klin Wchnschr 54:622–664, 1917
4. Von Franqué O: Schwere Darm-und Hautschadigung bei Rontgentiefentherapie int Schwerfilter. Zentralbl F Gynak 42:1–4, 1918
5. Heck W, Schwere Darm: und Hautschadigung bei Rontgentie Fentherapie mit Schwerfilter. Strahlentherapie 11:796–802, 1920
6. Haendly P: Pathologisch-anatomische Ergebnisse der Strahlenbehandlung. Strahlentherapie 12:1–87, 1921
7. Mathias: Rontgenverbrennungen des Dickdarms. Centralbl F allg Path u Path Anat 33:65, 1922–1923
8. Fischer B: Uber Bestrahlungsnekrosin des Darmes. Strahlentherapie 13:333–358, 1922
9. Schwarz E: Uber Schadigungen bei der Rontgenbehandlung von Myomen und hamorrhagiochen Metropathien. Strahlentherapie 15:398–411, 1923
10. Sanders A: Zur Zenntnis der Rontgenschadigungen am Darm. Strahlentherapie 18:457–472, 1924
11. Elliott AR, Jenkinson EL: Ulcerations of the stomach and small intestine following roentgen therapy. Radiology 23:149–156, 1934
12. Newell QU, Crossen HS: Late complications in irradiation treatment of cancer of the cervix. Surg Gyn Obst 60:763–768, 1935
13. Todd TF: Rectal ulceration following irradiation treatment of carcinoma of the cervix uteri pseudocarcinoma of the rectum. Surg Gyn Obst 67:617–631, 1938
14. Warren S, Friedman NB: Pathology and pathologic diagnosis of radiation lesions in the gastrointestinal tract. Am J Path 18:499–507, 1942
15. Mulligan RM: The lesions produced in the gastrointestinal tract by irradiation. Am J Path 18:515–527, 1942
16. Aune EF, White BV: Gastrointestinal complications of irradiation for carcinoma of uterine cervix. J Am Med Assoc 147:831, 1951
17. ReQuarth W, Roberts S: Intestinal injuries following irradiation of pelvic viscera for malignancy. Arch Surg 73:682, 1956
18. Smith AN, Douglas M, McLean N, et al.: Intestinal complications of pelvic irradiation for gynecologic cancer surgery. Gyn Obst 127:721–728, 1968
19. Kottmeier HL: Complications following radiation therapy in carcinoma of the cervix and their treatment. Am J Obst Gynec 88:854–866, 1964

20. Maruyama Y, VanNagell JR, Uhey J, et al: Radiation and small bowel complications in cervical carcinoma therapy. Radiology 112:699–703, 1974
21. Joelsson I, Raf K, Soderberg G: Stenosis of the small bowel as a complication in radiation therapy of carcinoma of the uterine cervix. Acta Radiol (Ther) (Stockh) 10:593–604, 1971
22. Kottmeier HL, Gray MJ: Rectal and bladder injuries in relation to radiation dosage in carcinoma of the cervix. Am J Obstet Gynec 82:74, 1961
23. Fabrikant JI, Anlyan WG, Creadick RN: The management of radiation injuries to the intestines. South Med J 52:1186, 1959
24. Nance FC, Persson AV, Piker JF: Radiation injuries to the lower gastrointestinal tract. Am Surg 34:21–25, 1968
25. DeCosse JJ, Rhodes RS, Wentz WB, et al: The natural history and management of radiation induced of the gastrointestinal tract. Ann Surg 170:369–384, 1969
26. Mason GR, Dietrich P, Friedland GW, et al: The radiologic findings in radiation-induced enteritis and colitis. A review of 30 cases. Clin Radiol 21:232–247, 1970
27. Rogers LF, Goldstein HM: Roentgen manifestations of radiation injury to the gastrointestinal tract. Gastrointest Radiol 2:281–291, 1977
28. Wigby PE: Post-irradiation stricture of the rectum and sigmoid following treatment for cervical cancer. Am J Roentgenol 49:307–320, 1943
29. Seaman WB, Ackerman LV: The effect of radiation on the esophagus: A clinical and histologic study of the effects produced by the Beta tron. Radiology 68:534–541, 1957
30. Stryker JA, Hepner GW, Mortel R: The effect of pelvic irradiation on ileal function. Radiology 124:213–216, 1977
31. Goldstein HM, Rogers LF, Fletcher GH, et al: Radiological manifestations of radiation induced injury to the normal upper gastrointestinal tract. Radiology 117:135–140, 1975
32. Roswit B, Malsky SJ, Reid CB: Severe radiation injuries of the stomach, small intestine, colon and rectum. Am J Roentgenol 114:460–475, 1972
33. Chau PM, Fletcher GH, Rutledge FN, et al: Complications in high dose whole pelvis irradiation in female pelvic cancer. Am J Roentgenol 87:22–40, 1962
34. Strockbine MF, Hancock JE, Fletcher GH: Complications in 831 patients with squamous cell carcinoma of the intact uterine cervix treated with 3,000 rads of more whole pelvis irradiation. Am J Roentgenol 108:293–304, 1970
35. Powell-Smith C: Factors influencing the incidence of radiation injury in cancer of the cervix. J Can Assoc Radiol 16:132–137, 1965
36. Localio SA, Stone A, Friedman M: Surgical aspects of radiation enteritis. Surg Gyn Obst 129:1163–1172, 1969
37. LoIudice T, Baxter D, Balint J: Effects of abdominal surgery on the development of radiation enteropathy. Gastroenterology 73:1093–1097, 1977
38. Perkins DE, Spjut HJ: Intestinal stenosis following radiation therapy. A roentgenologic-pathologic study. Am J Roentgenol 88:953–966, 1962
39. Colcock BP, Hume A: Radiation injury to the sigmoid and rectum. Surg Gyn Obst 306–312, 1959
40. Radiation Enteropathy. Chapter VII, in RA Cooper, Jr (ed) Radiation Oncology: Radiation Biology and Radiation Pathology Syllabus. Chicago, American College of Radiology, 1975, pp 97–113
41. Withers HR: Regeneration of intestinal mucosa after irradiation. Cancer 28:75–81, 1971
42. Nielsen J: Clinical results with rotational therapy in carcinoma of the esophagus. A preliminary report based on 174 cases. Acta Radiol 26:361–391, 1945
43. Freid JR: Roentgen therapy of carcinoma of the esophagus. Am J Roentgenol 59:551–564, 1948

44. Phillips TL, Margolis L: Radiation pathology and the clinical response of the lung and esophagus, in Vaeth JM (ed): Radiation Effect and Tolerance, Normal Tissue. Basic Concepts in Radiation Pathology, Proceedings of the Sixth Annual San Francisco Cancer Symposium. Baltimore, Univ Park Press, 1972
45. Friedman M: Calculated risks of radiation injury of normal tissue in the treatment of cancer of the testis, in Amer Cancer Society (ed): Proceedings of the Second National Cancer Conference. New York, Amer Cancer Society, 1954
46. Reeves RJ, Sanders AP, Isley JK, et al: Fat absorption from the human gastrointestinal tract in patients undergoing radiation therapy. Radiology 73:398, 1959
47. Duncan W, Leonard JC: Malabsorption syndrome following radiotherapy. Quarterly J Med 34:319, 1965
48. Reeves RJ, Cavanaugh PJ, Sharpe KW, et al: Fat absorption studies in patients undergoing CO-60 teletherapy and/or radium application. Am J Roentgenol 94:848, 1965
49. Lipkin M, Quastler H, Muggia F: Protein synthesis in the irradiated intestine of the mouse. Radiation Res 19:277, 1963
50. Berk RN, Seay DG: Cholerheic enteropathy as a cause of diarrhea and death in radiation enteritis and its prevention with cholestyramine. Radiology 104:153–156, 1972
51. Hoffman AF: The syndrome of ileal disease and the broken enterohepatic circulation: Cholerheic enteropathy. Gastroenterology 52:752–757, 1967
52. Mennie AT, Dalley VM, Dinneen LC, et al: Treatment of radiation-induced gastrointestinal distress with acetylsalicylate. Lancet 2:942, 1975
53. Casserett GW, Eddy HA: Effects of radiation on vasculature of intestine. Conference on Time-Dose Relationships in Radiation Biology as Applied to Radiotherapy, Carmel, California, Sep 1969
54. McIntosh HC, Hutton JE: Clinical and roentgen aspects of irradiation stricture of the rectum and sigmoid. Am J Roentgenol 52:647–662, 1944
55. Spratt JS, Heinbecker P, Saltzstein SL: The influence of succinylsulfathiazole (sulfasuxidine) upon the response of canine small intestine to irradiation. Cancer 14:862–874, 1961
56. MacMahon CE, Rowe JW: Rectal reaction following radiation therapy of cervical carcinoma: Particular reference to subsequent occurrence of rectal carcinoma. Ann Surg 173:264–269, 1971
57. Slaughter DP, Southwick HW: Mucosal carcinoma as a result of irradiation. Arch Surg 74:420, 1957
58. Smith JC: Carcinoma of the rectum following irradiation of cancer of the cervix. Proc Roy Soc 55:701, 1962
59. Fletcher GH, Brown TC, Rutledge FN: Clinical significance of rectal and bladder dose measurements in radium therapy of cancer of uterine cervix. Am J Roentgenol 79:421–450, 1958
60. Feiring W, Jampol ML: Perforation of a gastric ulcer following intensive radiation therapy. N Engl J Med 242:751–753, 1950
61. Schenken LL, Burholt DR, Hagemann RF, et al: The modification of gastrointestinal tolerance and responses to abdominal irradiation by chemotherapeutic agents. Radiology 120:417–420, 1976
62. Gray LH, Conger AD, Ebert M, et al: The concentration of oxygen dissolved in tissue at the time of irradiation as a factor in radiotherapy. Br J Radiol 26:638–648, 1953
63. Steckel RJ, Snow HD, Collins JD, et al: Successful radiation protection of the normal intestinal tract in the dog. Radiology 111:451–455, 1974
64. Bacg ZM: Chemical Protection Against Ionizing Radiation. Springfield, Thomas, 1965, pp 328

65. Kligerman MM, Bond VP, Held BT, et al: Anoxic protection of small intestine of dogs by intra-arterial catheterization. Radiology 78:284, 1962
66. Tobin DA, Vermund H: A randomized study of hyperbaric oxygen as an adjunct to regular fractionated radiation therapy for clinical treatment of advanced neoplastic disease. Am J Roentgenol 111:613–621, 1971
67. Rappleye AT, Johnson GH, Olsen ID, et al: The radioprotective effects of vasopressin on the gastrointestinal tract of mice. Radiology 117:199–203, 1975
68. Bosniak MA, Hardy MA, Quint J, et al: Demonstration of the effect of irradiation on canine bowel using in vivo photographic magnification angiography. Radiology 93:1361–1368, 1969
69. Stryker JA, Abt AB, Allegra JC, et al: The effect of prednisone and irradiation on the rectum in dogs. Radiology 121:183–187, 1976
70. Moss AA, Carbone JV, Kressel HY: Radiologic and clinical assessment of broad-spectrum antibiotic therapy in Crohn's disease. Am J Roentgenol 131:787–790, 1978

William M. Wara
Gordon M. Gamsu
Jeffrey A. Golden*

10
Radiation Pneumonitis

Radiation pneumonitis, more recently termed radiation pneumonopathy or radiation pleuropneumonitis, has been known for some time. The first reports appeared in the 1920s, shortly after the advent of kilovoltage equipment capable of penetrating and delivering significant doses to the internal structures of the thoracic cavity.[1] An historical review with clinical and pathological descriptions is given by Rubin and Casarett.[2]

The occurrence of radiation pneumonitis varies widely among patients. The development and severity of the disease depends on the dose of irradiation delivered, the time over which the course of therapy is given, the volume of lung irradiated, and certain modifying factors such as concomitant chemotherapy. In patients who have been treated for carcinoma of the breast the incidence, depending on the series, varied from a few percent to over 70 percent.[3] Symptomatic radiation pneumonitis is seen most commonly in patients receiving whole lung irradiation for the palliation of pulmonary metastases.[4,5] In patients with bronchogenic carcinoma who are being treated with radiation therapy, the lung tissue immediately surrounding the tumor will be irradiated. Most of these patients will develop pneumonopathy which, in many cases, will be of a moderately symptomatic degree. Fatal radiation pneumonitis is rare in the treatment of localized bronchogenic carcinoma.

* The authors wish to thank Lee Rachel McLaughlin for editorial and secretarial assistance.

RADIOBIOLOGIC CONCEPTS

X-rays and gamma rays consist of photons and are used in treatment of lung tumors. Other types of irradiation—protons, alpha particles, neutrons and pi-mesons—are being investigated, but are not ready for routine clinical application. X-rays and gamma rays are absorbed by tissue exponentially and their biological effect is mediated through the production of charged ions and free radicals in the target material. The actual distribution of energy deposited in the target material, and therefore the volume affected, will vary with the energy of the radiation, the size of the radiation source, the dimensions and shape of treatment beam, the use of filters, the source to target distance, and the collimation system.

Modern radiation therapy, when given with curative intent, is largely limited to megavoltage (MeV) irradiation, i.e., it employs an energy source of greater than one million electron volts. Megavoltage, compared with kilovoltage irradiation has the advantages of greater penetration, less absorption by bone tissue, less side scatter, and reduced dosage to skin and subcutaneous tissues. A Cobalt-60 radiation source gives gamma rays of 1.17 and 1.33 MeV. Linear accelerators in common use produce x-rays ranging from 4 to 25 MeV.

In general, linear accelerators have more sharply defined radiation beams than do Cobalt-60 machines. In addition to the collimation system built into each machine, special radiation shielding blocks, wedge filters and tissue compensating filters are utilized to shape the high dose volume and to protect sensitive normal tissues.

The biological basis of radiation therapy is complex. The intent, of course, is to destroy the tumor with a radiation dose that can be tolerated by whatever normal tissue must be included in the irradiated volume. Even when the radiation equipment and treatment planning are optimum (we refer in particular to treatment fields, rotation, protective radiation blocks, and tissue compensating filters) some normal tissue is virtually always included. The success of treatment thus depends upon many interrelated factors, including: 1) careful treatment planning designed to limit the high dose treatment volume to noncritical structures; 2) the inherent sensitivity of the irradiated normal and tumor cells; 3) the total numbers of the various cell types present; 4) the ability of normal cells to migrate into the irradiated volume and the ability of tumor cells to metastasize out; 5) the repopulation capability of normal versus tumor cells; 6) rearrangement of cells in the cell cycle between radiation fractions; 7) the relative ability of tumor and normal cells to repair sublethal radiation damage between treatment fractions; and 8) the oxygen tension and time required for reoxygenation of hypoxic tumor cells. (Hypoxia may decrease radiosensitivity by threefold.) While each of these factors, when studied experimentally, has been shown to be important, the extent to which each influences a particular clinical situation is usually unknown. In practice, the radiation therapist, after selecting the approach that gives the best physical distribution of absorbed dose, tends to apply the maximum dose consistent with an acceptable risk for critical normal structures. Certain tumors known to be particularly radiosensitive may be treated with a lesser dose, but in general, it is the sensitivity of normal tissues that limits radiation therapy.

We have developed a formula for predicting pulmonary damage that relates dose, time, and number of fractions of irradiation based upon clinical and animal results.[6] With this formula we can reduce different treatment regimens to equivalent single doses using the concept of nominal standard dose (NSD) developed by Ellis.[7] Using a ret dose, we can predict the threshold for development of radiation peneumonitis. Since Ellis' formula $[D = (NSD) \cdot N^{0.24} \cdot T^{0.11}]$, wherein N equals the number of fractions and T the total time, is based on skin response, it is not appropriate for lung, nervous, or kidney damage. Our data suggest a steeper slope for pulmonary damage, and that more importance lies in daily dose than total time in the causation of pneumonitis. With this model we can also predict that the likelihood of developing pneumonitis increases with an increase in dosage (Table 10-1).

HISTOPATHOLOGIC CHANGES IN THE LUNG

Ionizing radiation damages cells capable of proliferation by inducing mitotic death. Cells that are not capable of mitosis will be injured as a secondary phenomenon. The primary mechanism of radiation injury con-

Table 10-1
Dose versus Risk of Pneumonitis*

Dose (rads)	Percent Risk of Pneumonitis *Number of Fractions (5 times per week)*		
	10	20	30
1500	6%	0%	0%
2000	53%	5%	0%
3000	100%	80%	60%
3500	100%	93%	70%

* Richards MJS and Wara WM: Radiation pneumonitis complicated by *pneumocystis carinii*. Int J Radiation Oncology Biol Phys 4:287–291, 1978

sists of direct and indirect radiochemical breakage of DNA molecules within the chromosomes. Mitosis must occur before cellular damage will manifest itself; the expression of damage in the lung will be a function of the kinetics of the cells composing the lung.[8]

The morphological changes in lung tissue following irradiation can be divided into three phases during the first six to nine months. An exudative phase is seen during the first 30 days; a pneumonic phase occurs throughout the second and third months; and a reparative phase occurs between the third and sixth to ninth months. In the exudative phase endothelial and epithelial damage appear with interstitial edema, alveolar proteinosis, and hyaline membranes.[9,10] In about 40 percent of the cases capillary congestion and platelet aggregation may be present. In the pneumonic phase, alveolar type II cells, as well as alveolar macrophages, proliferate and fill the air spaces.[11,12] Capillary damage is extensive and collagen deposition begins. In the reparative phase, there is proliferation of multiple cells including mast cells. Collagen is produced with subsequent fibrosis and profound distortion of lung architecture. At six to nine months and beyond, fibrosis of the alveolar walls predominates with a marked reduction in the number, size and volume of the alveoli. The number of patent capillaries and small vessels is markedly reduced. With high-dose irradiation, complete fibrotic replacement of the lung may occur[13] (Table 10-2).

Recent information has been presented on the immediate reaction of the alveolar epithelial cells, especially type II pneumocytes, within the first two months, as seen with electron microscopy. Cytoplasmic edema, congestion, and platelet aggregations have been described.[13] Type II pneumocytes showed a marked focal and perivascular hyperplasia with no changes in type I pneumocytes. In the reparative phase, type two pneumocytes are regenerated, appear larger than normal, and have thickened basement membranes.

Table 10-2
Histopathological Changes After Irradiation

Phase I	Phase 2	Phase 3
Exudative	Pneumonia	Reparative
0-30 days	2-3 months	3-9 months
Cellular damage and interstitial edema	Airway consoliation	Fibrosis
	Collagen formation	Reduced compliance
Reduced ventilation and perfusion	Reduced compliance	

ALTERATIONS IN PULMONARY FUNCTION

By the time clinical symptoms are evident, one to two months after irradiation, changes in pulmonary function will have occurred. During the exudative phase, decreased ventilation and perfusion to the irradiated area, as well as ventilation/perfusion mismatch, are observed. Pulmonary blood flow has begun to decline as early as 25 days postirradiation, reaching a maximum decrease by 100–150 days.[14] Many studies have demonstrated changes in pulmonary mechanics when large lung volumes have been irradiated. Total lung capacity, vital capacity, and forced expiratory volume in one second will all be reduced. Diffusing capacity and lung compliance may also be diminished.[15] Decreased pulmonary compliance occurs with the radiographic appearance of the pneumonic phase, and persists into the chronic fibrotic phase. Radioisotope studies of regional blood flow, which reveal abnormalities earlier than radiographs, appear to be the most sensitive indicators of functional damage.

CLINICAL FEATURES

The clinical syndrome related to radiation pneumonopathy varies with the volume of lung irradiated and the dose delivered. In general, doses below 2,000 rads to small lung volumes will not produce symptoms. With doses sufficient to cause acute pneumonopathy, or larger volumes, the initial findings may be clinical or radiographic. Symptoms usually occur six weeks to three months following irradiation. The initial symptom is usually cough, which may be mild or severe.[2,3] Dyspnea, low grade fever, and tachypnea may be prominent features. Following whole lung irradiation, severe dyspnea, cyanosis, marked tachypnea, and fever may progress to death within weeks. Patients whose irradiation comprised less than a volume equivalent to one lung show a gradual decrease in symptoms as the process evolves from the exudative to the fibrotic phase. Corticosteroid treatment may dramatically improve symptoms. Physical findings may include tachypnea, fine respiratory rales, a pleural friction rub, and, in severe cases, cyanosis.

Both the clinical presentation and radiographic changes of radiation pneumonitis may be mimicked by infection. Opportunistic organisms may cause pneumonias resembling radiation pneumonopathy.[6] The radiographic manifestations of lymphangitic carcinomatosis may also resemble radiation pneumonitis.

RADIOGRAPHIC FINDINGS

The first radiographic findings of radiation pleuropneumonitis generally coincide with the onset of symptoms 6 to 12 weeks following completion of treatment.[14,16,17] The first manifestation is an ill-defined, hazy increase in density in the irradiated field, obscuring the pulmonary vasculature (Fig. 10-1 A–C). This may progress to pulmonary consolida-

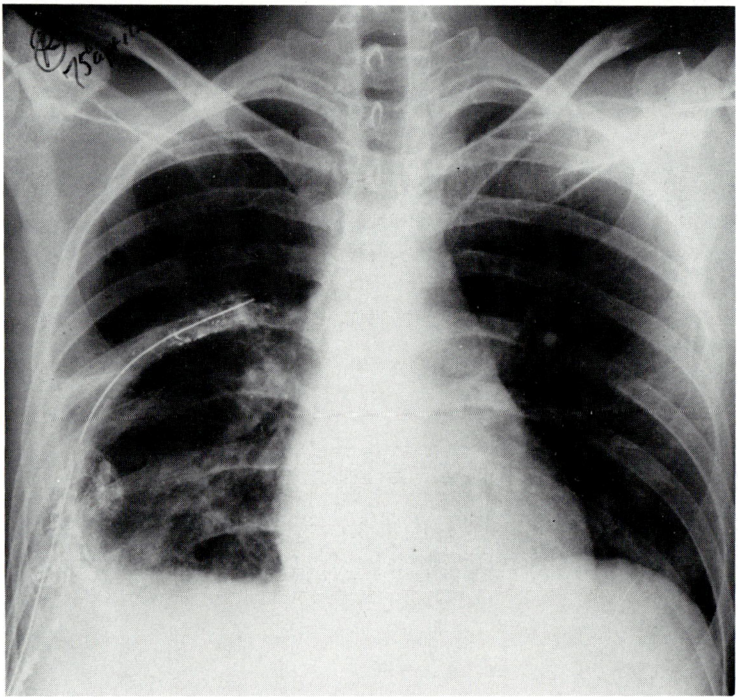

A

Fig. 10-1A. A frontal radiograph in a 24-year-old male five weeks following 800 rad in one fraction whole-body irradiation plus cytoxan in preparation for a bone marrow transplant, revealing a right chest tube with contrast in the right hemithorax outlining an empyema cavity. The right lung was shielded from irradiation.

Fig. 10-1B. One week later after the sudden onset of shortness of breath, the left lung reveals a diffuse opacification with air bronchograms. The right lung remains clear.

Fig. 10-1C. One week later the left lung is further consolidated with more distinct air bronchograms being visible. The left lung has lost volume as revealed by mediastinal shift to the left and elevation of the left hemidiaphragm. At postmortem examination the left lung revealed extensive radiation pneumonopathy.

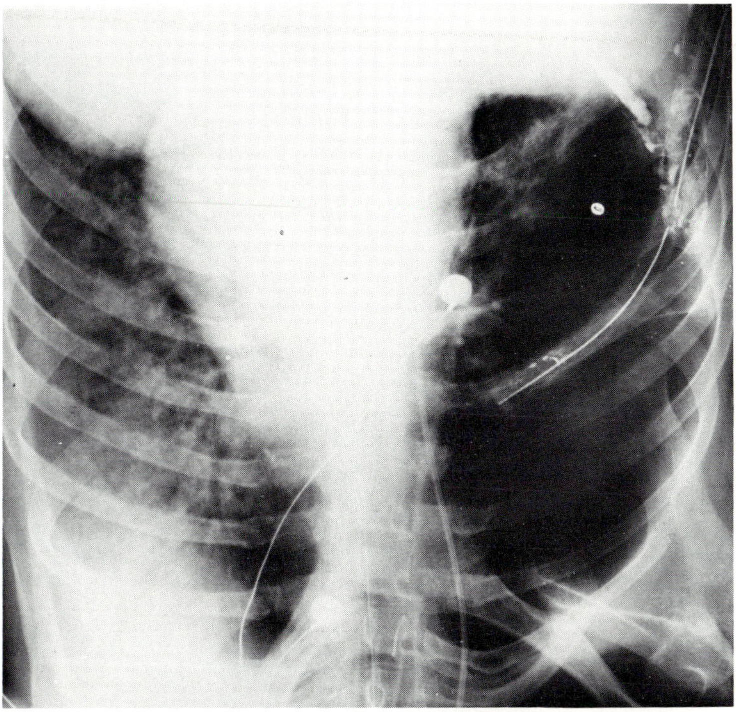

B

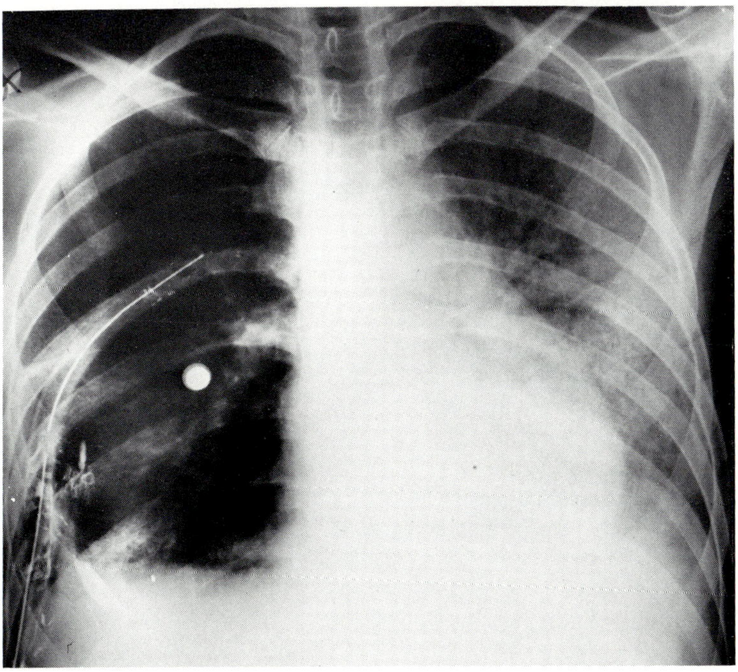

C

tion with air bronchograms, or to a nodular or acinar pattern. The radiographic changes have a relatively sharp edge and are limited to the field of irradiation (Fig. 10-2 A,B).

Patients receiving a dose just sufficient to cause pneumonitis may show complete radiographic resolution. In the majority, however, the pneumonic changes progress to a chronic and usually irreversible fibrosis. The appearance changes from consolidation to dense linear streaks which radiate from the area of involvement. Marked cicatricial volume loss will occur (Fig. 10-3 A–C). Retraction toward the area of scarring results. In the lower lobes the diaphragm will be elevated, while hilar retraction and elevation occur with upper lobe irradiation (Fig. 10-4). The mediastinum may shift toward the ipsilateral side. The permanent changes of fibrosis take six to 24 months to evolve. Radiation changes after two years are unusual and an alternative process should be considered.

Pleural or pericardial effusions are uncommon. Cavitation is usually from necrosis of the tumor, but rarely occurs without residual cancer

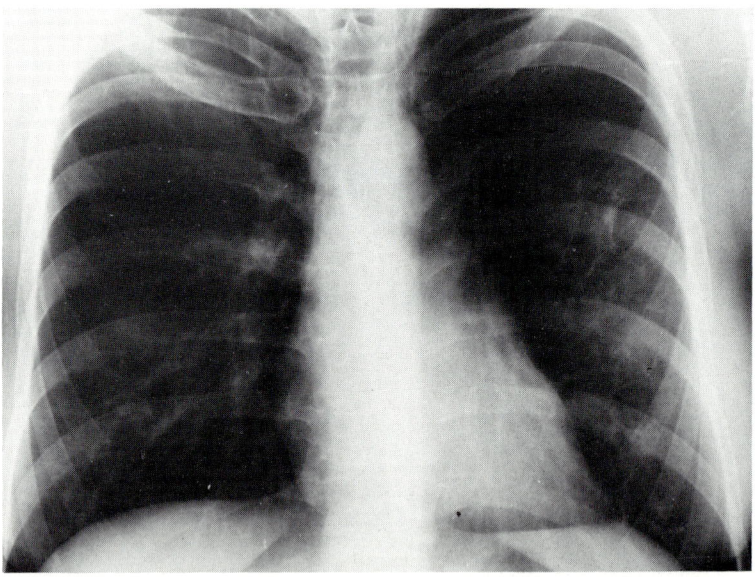

Fig. 10-2A. A frontal radiograph in a 22 year old female immediately prior to irradiation for a recurrent left midlung field metastasis from an undifferentiated carcinoma of unknown primary site. The patient received whole lung irradiation to 2,100 rads with a boost to 4,900 rads to the left midlung over a six week period. The residue of a previous left thoracotomy is visible together with a small nodule in the left midlung field. The remainder of the lungs is clear.

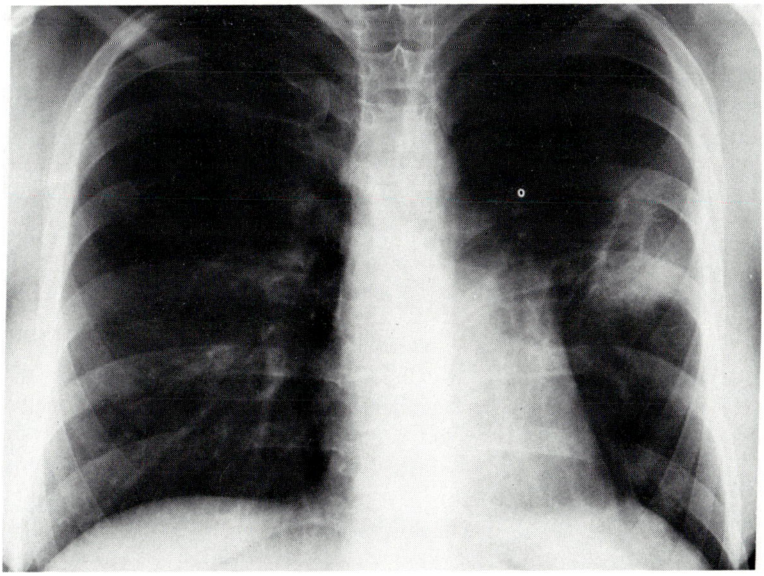

Fig. 10-2B. Ten weeks later a reasonably well-defined area of increasing density is present in the left midlung field. The density conforms to the area of irradiation. The remainder of the lungs is clear. The area of increased density represents the pneumonic phase of radiation pneumonitis.

evident in the wall of the cavity. Spontaneous pneumothorax is an unusual complication of radiation pneumonopathy. Other complications are usually associated with tumor destruction and include bronchial obstruction, rib fractures, and tracheo-esophageal fistula. Respiratory insufficiency due to radiation fibrosis of large volumes of lung is uncommon. Chronic pericarditis and pleurisy with chronic effusions do occur, but are also uncommon.

The possibility of radiation changes outside the treatment field has been extensively discussed. These changes can almost always be attributed to an alternative process such as infection.

MODIFYING FACTORS IN RADIATION PNEUMONITIS

The three interdependent primary factors to be considered in the development of clinical radiation pneumonopathy are the volume of lung irradiated, the radiation time and fractionation, and the total dose.[4] Irradiation of one third to one half of a lung will usually produce symptomatic disease. Whole lung irradiation can lead to severe symptoms and even death. The dose required for the treatment of bronchogenic carcinoma or pulmonary metastases will almost always produce regional changes in perfusion and regional radiographic changes, but may be asymptomatic. Although the total dose is important, even more important is the number of fractions into which the dose is divided: the greater the number of fractions, the less severe the damage from irradiation.

A number of chemotherapeutic drugs potentiate or add to the effect of lung irradiation, whether given before, during, or after irradiation. Enhancement of radiation effect is seen with actinomycin D, bleomycin, adriamycin, and cytoxan.[18] Actinomycin D has the greatest effect and appears to be a true potentiator, while the other drugs are additive.[17] Withdrawal from steroids may also precipitate radiation pneumonitis; these drugs must be used with caution when given with lung irradiation.

The above factors all contribute to the differential diagnosis in a suspected case of radiation pneumonitis. The internist, radiation oncologist, and radiodiagnostician must all consult and, based on the patient's history and appropriate diagnostic tests, exclude such possibilities

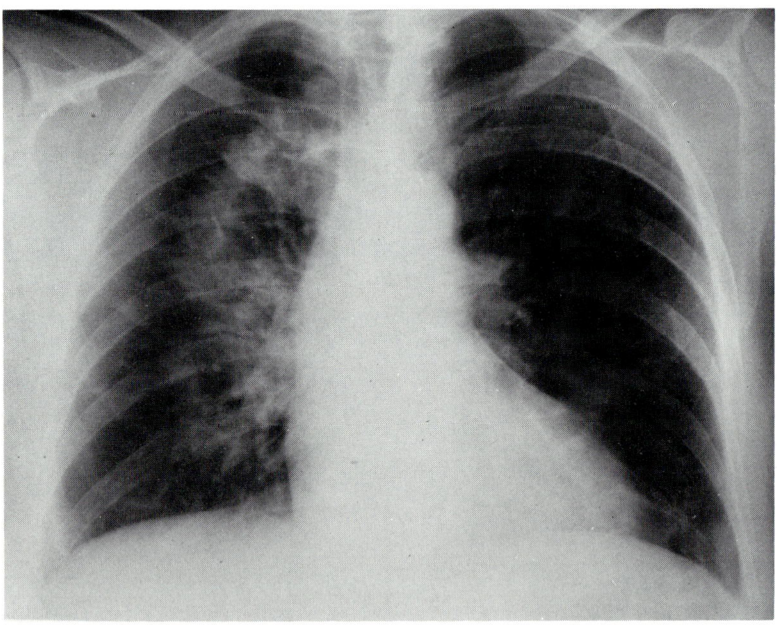

Fig. 10-3A. A frontal radiograph in a 59-year-old female with shortness of breath and fever. Film obtained seven weeks following 4,960 rads to a 9 × 8 cm. field over the right hilus. The left lung is hyperlucent from a prior left radical mastectomy. An ill-defined area of consolidation is present in the right perihilar midlung, conforming to the area of irradiation, representing the pneumonic phase of radiation pneumonitis.

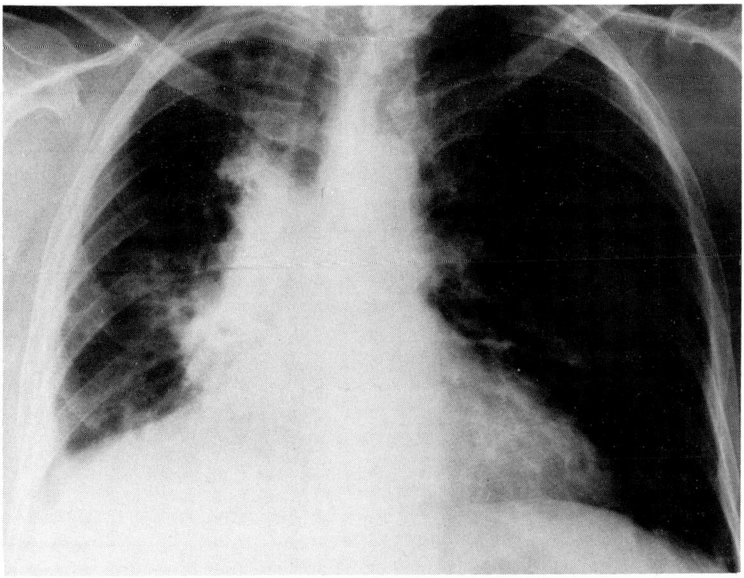

Fig. 10-3B. Four months later. The right lung has lost considerable volume. The prior area of consolidation shows patchy increasing density representing pulmonary fibrosis. Continued patchy consolidation is visible. The above features represent the reparative phase of radiation pneumonitis.

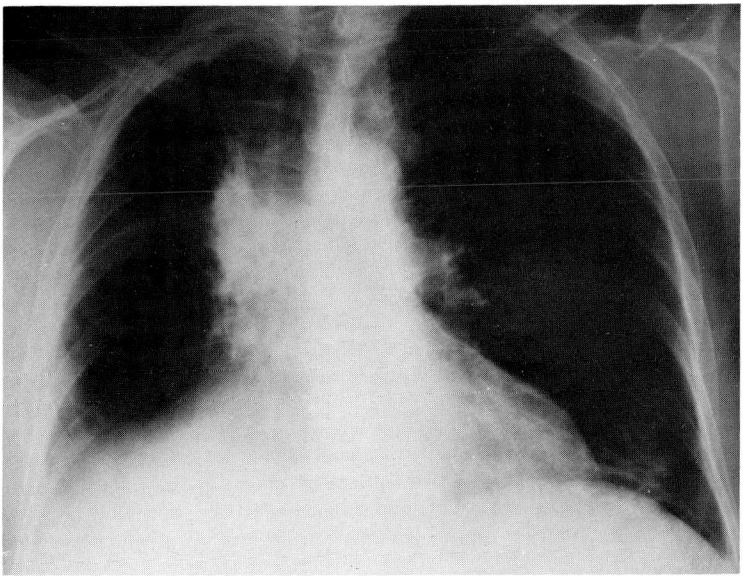

Fig. 10-3C. Fifteen months later. The right lung shows further volume loss. The area of radiation pneumonitis now demonstrates a marked increase in density with linear streaking into the surrounding lung parenchyma. Fibrosis from radiation pneumonitis has occurred. The radiographic features were unaltered over the ensuing year.

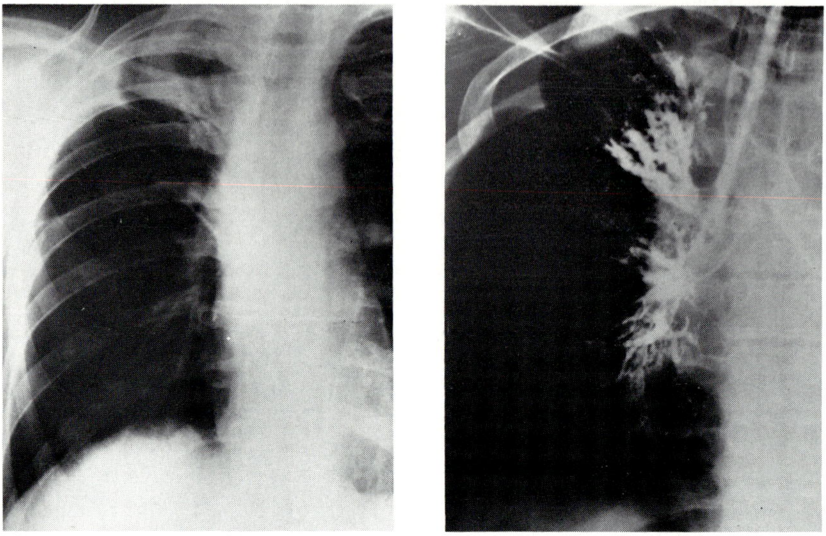

Fig. 10-4. A frontal radiograph (above left) in a young female following right radical mastectomy and right supraclavicular irradiation to 5000 rads in 25 treatments, revealing extensive volume loss and increased density in the right upper lobe. Pleural thickening over the right apex is evident. The patient was complaining of cough, sputum production and hemoptysis. A bronchogram (above right) reveals extensive bronchiectasis in the irradiated lobe. Lobectomy was required for control of hemoptysis.

as: recurrent neoplasm, lymphangitic spread of cancer, effect of radiomimetic chemotherapeutic drugs, and superinfection by opportunistic organisms. All causes of pneumonitis must be ruled out, and a consistent radiation history obtained before a clinician may diagnose radiation pneumonitis. We have made quite clear that this diagnosis is difficult to make; many of the above factors may mimic the radiation syndrome, leading to inappropriate therapy.[6] Therefore, great care and multidisciplinary cooperation must be obtained before this diagnosis is reached.

TREATMENT

Radiation pneumonitis can be avoided to some extent by minimizing the radiation dose to the lung through proper treatment, planning, and shielding of areas of the lung not considered critical to treatment of the patient's disease. When pneumonitis is mild, cough suppressants, aspirin, and activity restriction may be sufficient for relief of symptoms. Patients should be followed closely and given supplemental oxygen when necessary.

In human studies, summarized by Rubin and Casarett,[2] corticosteroids, given prophylactically, failed to prevent pneumonitis. However, steroids should be given as soon as symptoms develop (usually prednisone in doses of 60 to 100 mg. per day). The response rate depends on the radiation dose delivered. No evidence is available to indicate whether steroids can alter the pathological process once the pneumonic phase has progressed to a reparative or chronic fibrotic phase.

Antibiotics have been used both prophylactically and at the time pneumonitis develops. Again, there is no evidence of their efficacy. Antibiotics should be reserved for patients with specific infections. Specimens from the lung should be cultured for any specific organisms and their sensitivities should be determined.

Anticoagulants have been used in the treatment of radiation pneumonitis in an attempt to minimize vascular damage. The few clinical reports have not been optimistic. In occasional circumstances, symptoms may be so severe, with limited lung involvement, that surgical resection may be indicated for palliation. Caution should be exercised in the selection of these patients, since surgery performed in areas that have been subjected to high doses of irradiation is characterized by a high incidence of postoperative complications and morbidity.

A rational approach to the management of patients with radiation pneumonopathy is as follows: patients with mild asymptomatic disease should be followed both clinically and with radiographs. If a significant volume of lung is involved, corticosteroid therapy may be beneficial. The dose of the drug can be gradually tapered after resolution of symptoms. Secondary infections should be excluded. Oxygen should be administered to maintain arterial oxygen tensions at acceptable levels. The increasing use of multi-modality treatments, which combine irradiation and chemotherapy, will probably result in more patients developing radiation pneumonitis in the future.

REFERENCES

1. Groover TA, Christie AC, Merritt EA: Observations on the use of the copper filter in the Roentgen treatment of deep seated malignancies. Southern Med J 15:440–444, 1922
2. Rubin P, Casarett GW: Clinical Radiation Pathology, Philadelphia, WB Saunders, 1968, pp 423–470
3. Gross NJ: Pulmonary effects of radiation therapy. Ann Int Med 86:81–92, 1977
4. Wara WM, Phillips TL, Margolis LW, Smith V: Radiation pneumonitis: a new approach to the derivation of time-dose factors. Cancer 32:547–552, 1973
5. Margolis LW, Phillips TL: Whole-lung irradiation for metastatic tumor. Radiology 93:1173–1179, 1969
6. Richards MJS, Wara WM: Radiation pneumonitis complicated by pneumocystis carinii. Int J Radiation Oncology Biol Phys 4:287–291, 1978

7. Ellis F: Relationship of biological effect to dose-time fractionation factors in radiotherapy, in M Ebert, A Howard (eds): Current Topics in Radiation Research vol 4. Amsterdam, North Holland Publishing Co, 1968, pp 357–397
8. Hall EJ: Radiobiology for the Radiologist, Hagerstown, Harper & Row, 1973
9. Bennett DE, Million RR, Ackerman LV: Bilateral radiation pneumonitis, a complication of the radiotherapy of bronchogenic carcinoma. Cancer 23:1001–1018, 1969
10. Jennings FL, Arden A: Development of radiation pneumonitis—time and dose factors. Arch Pathol 74:351–360, 1962
11. Moosavi H, McDonald S, Rubin P, et al: Early radiation dose-response in lung: an ultrastructural study. Int J Radiation Oncology Biol Phys 2:921–931, 1977
12. Phillips TL, Benak S, Ross G: Frontiers of Radiation Therapy and Oncology. Baltimore, Karger, Basel and University Park Press, 1972, pp 21–45
13. Phillips TL, Wyatt JP: Radiation fibrosis, in Fishman AP (ed): Pulmonary Diseases. New York, McGraw-Hill (in press)
14. Prato FS, Kurdyak R, Saibil EA, et al: Physiological and radiographic assessment during the development of pulmonary radiation fibrosis. Radiology 122:389–397, 1977
15. Emergil C, Heinemann HO: Effects of irradiation of chest on pulmonary function in man. J Applied Physiology 16:331–338, 1961
16. Fried JR, Goldberg H: Post-irradiation changes in lungs and thorax: a clinical, roentgenological and pathological study, with emphasis on late and terminal stages. Amer J Roentgenol 43:877–895, 1940
17. Phillips TL, Fu KK: Quantification of combined radiation therapy and chemotherapy effects on critical normal tissues. Cancer 37:1186–1200, 1976
18. Soble AR, Perry, H: Fatal radiation pneumonia following subclinical Busulfan injury. Amer J Roentgenol 128:15–18, 1977

PART 3

Occupationally Induced Disease

Ronald G. Grainger
Anne E. Walker
A. Milford Ward*

11

Vinyl Chloride Monomer-Induced Disease: Clinical, Radiological and Immunological Aspects

The story of vinyl chloride-induced disease has been described as a watershed in the history of occupational medicine.[1] The understanding of this disease has precipitated new attitudes toward occupational hazards and has made obligatory an immediate response to the first evidence of damage due to industrial processes.

Within the last decade, the complicated multi-system symptomatology, the signs, and the radiological and pathological features have been defined. The toxic chemical, vinyl chloride monomer (VCM), and the specific industrial processes with which it is associated have been identified. The pathogenesis of vinyl chloride disease (VCD) has been intensively studied and there is now strong evidence that immunological processes are involved. Since 1974, the levels of permissible exposure to VCM have been lowered substantially by industrial legislation; there is a good possibility that current exposure levels will not be high enough to induce disease in the future.

Our own involvement with vinyl chloride came about when workers at a local polyvinyl chloride (PVC) manufacturing plant developed symptoms of the disease. We present here our clinical, radiological, and immunological studies of workers from this factory.

MANUFACTURE OF POLYVINYL CHLORIDE

The process of converting vinyl chloride monomer (VCM) to polyvinyl chloride (PVC) by polymerization was discovered in Germany

* The authors wish to thank Mrs V. Morris for her assistance in preparing the manuscript.

in the mid 1930s. Production is now world-wide, resulting in an annual output of approximately eight million tons. The uses of PVC are many and varied as it is used extensively both in the home and in industry.

PVC is manufactured by the polymerization of VCM; 500 to 1,500 molecules of the monomer produce one molecule of PVC, depending on particle size.[2] VCM (monochloro ethylene, or C_2H_3Cl) is a liquid gas at normal temperature and pressure. It has a pleasant odor, which can be detected at a concentration of 400 parts per million.

The polymerization process takes place in a large reactor or autoclave approximately 6 ft. 6 in. in diameter and 11 ft. 3 in. high with a capacity of approximately 290 cu. ft. (Fig. 11-1). Liquid VCM is dispersed in water with a suspending agent and a catalyst. During polymerization, the mixture is constantly agitated by a central paddle, and carefully controlled pressure is applied within the reactor. As the process is exothermic, the autoclave is continuously water-cooled. Polymerization takes approximately eight hours, and at the end of this time, 92–95 percent of the monomer has been converted to polymer. Excess monomer is then drawn off and the thick slurry of PVC in water is run out of the bottom of the reactor, centrifuged, dried, bagged, and sent for processing. The PVC slurry contains a considerable quantity of VCM: up to 500 parts per million.

Despite constant stirring during polymerization, some of the thick slurry of PVC settles on the inner lining of the autoclave and on the central paddle. To ensure the purity of the next batch of PVC, this residual scale has to be removed before the vessel is recharged. Descaling used to be performed manually; an operator would climb into the autoclave

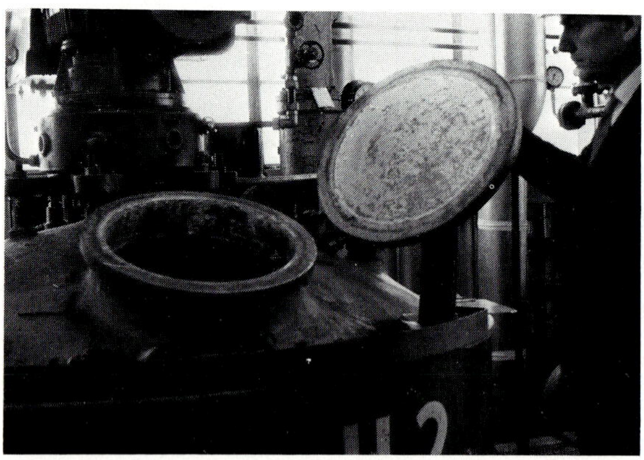

Fig. 11-1. The reactor or autoclave is a cylinder with a domed top and bottom. The illustration shows a worker opening the upper hatch door through which the cleaners climbed to descale the inner walls. The total height of the reactor is 11′3″ and the internal diameter is 6′6″. The capacity is approximately 290 cu.ft.

through the hatch in the dome (Fig. 11-1) and mechanically descale the vessel wall with hammer and chisel.

The health hazards of PVC manufacture appear to be entirely related to exposure to VCM. VCM gas is readily absorbed by the lungs. Workmen have most often been exposed to VCM when the reactors are first opened after polymerization, during manual descaling of the reactor, and during maintenance work on pipes carrying the liquid VCM. However, the drying of the PVC slurry and bagging of the final PVC powder are not without hazard.

The PVC slurry contains approximately 500 parts per million of VCM, whereas the dry powder contains less than five parts per million. Microscopic examination reveals that PVC particles have a markedly pitted surface in which unpolymerized VCM may be retained. The smallest particles of PVC (0.5 μm in diameter) are easily inhaled and may carry unpolymerized VCM into the lungs.

CLINICAL EFFECTS OF EXPOSURE TO VINYL CHLORIDE MONOMER

Acute

Exposure to high concentrations of VCM gives rise to temporary narcosis, dizziness, weakness of the legs, impaired coordination, and sudden loss of consciousness. (At one time, VCM was considered for use as an anesthetic; it is chemically related to chloroform.) Only in the last four years have environmental levels of VCM been adequately and accurately monitored in PVC manufacturing plants. Current levels are probably as low as five parts per million, but it is possible that twenty years ago, levels were as high as 1,000 parts per million, and in 1973 around 500 parts per million. VCM has a pleasant smell and an agreeable taste. The initial symptoms of narcosis are not unpleasant, and it is probable that some workers have deliberately "sniffed" the VCM.

Chronic Exposure

In 1966,[6] acro-osteolysis (AOL), and in 1973 angiosarcoma of the liver were identified as complications of chronic exposure to VCM (Chapter 15). Suciu[4] described Raynaud's phenomenon, sclerodermatous skin changes, and liver dysfunction in PVC production workers. Experiments with rats exposed to high levels of VCM indicated a high incidence of liver, bone, and ceruminous gland tumors. An American epidemiological study of PVC production workers revealed an association between angiosarcoma of the liver and prolonged exposure to VCM.

Lange[5] introduced the name vinyl chloride-induced disease for the systemic disorder that included dysfunction of the liver and lungs, splenomegaly, osteolysis, sclerodermatous skin changes and thrombocytopenia in PVC production workers. Specifically, the disorder was characterized by the following.

LIVER

Angiosacroma of the liver. In 1974, the B. F. Goodrich PVC production plant in Louisville, Kentucky, voluntarily and admirably revealed that six of its employees who had been exposed to VCM had recently died of angiosarcoma of the liver (ASL).[30] All six employees had worked as reactor cleaners and had been exposed to high concentrations of VCM. Confirmatory experimental evidence that VCM could induce ASL in animals was soon produced.[31]

ASL is a rare histological variety of malignant liver tumor and is variously described as Kupffer cell sarcoma, hemangio-endothelioma, and hemangioblastoma. The essential histological feature is that the liver vascular sinusoids are lined by proliferating tumor cells of endothelial or Kupffer cell origin. There is a dense intra-sinusoidal network of reticulin fibers.

ASL is almost always the result of exposure to toxic substances such as thorium dioxide (after angiography and other radiodiagnostic procedures), prolonged arsenic intoxication (therapeutic, vineyard workers) as well as vinyl chloride monomer (VCM reactor cleaners).

Within months of the initial Goodrich announcement, several other patients with VCM-induced ASL were reported in the United States, the United Kingdom, Sweden and Germany. By 1976, as many as 47 cases of ASL secondary to VCM exposure had been reported; two of these patients were from United Kingdom.[32] Almost all of these patients had worked as reactor cleaners in PVC production plants and had therefore been exposed to the high concentrations of VCM which were prevalent before the danger was appreciated. It is calculated that the mean period from initial exposure to VCM to the development of ASL is about 17 years.

Clinically, the patients present with features of abdominal tumor, liver failure, ascites, and hemorrhage. Radiology reveals a large liver, often with splenomegaly and ascites. Angiography demonstrates stretching of the intrahepatic arteries around tumor masses, abnormal tortuous distorted arteries with rapid filling of hepatic veins (Fig. 11.11). Ultrasound and isotope studies provide confirmatory evidence of multiple intrahepatic masses.

The diagnosis of ASL is made by histological examination on tissue, preferably obtained by laparotomy rather than percutaneous needle biopsy, which may cause severe hemorrhage. The outcome is inevitable fatal.

In VCM-induced ASL there is often a diffuse fibrosis of the portal, perivascular and periductal tracts, of a type rather different to the much more frequent alcoholic cirrhosis. Grey scale ultrasonography of the liver

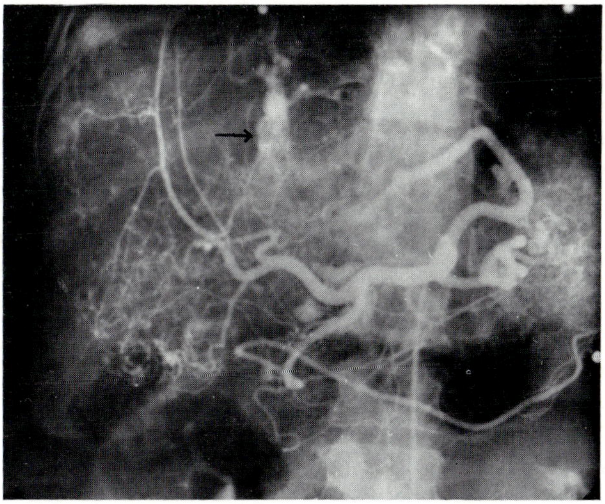

Fig. 11-2. Selective coeliac arteriogram showing stretching of intrahepatic arteries by masses, some of which are hypovascular and others which are hypervascular. Abnormal tumor vessels with premature filling of intrahepatic veins (arrow). This angiosarcoma is not the result of vinyl chloride exposure but is due to an injection of thorotrast for venography twenty years earlier.

may reveal evidence of this with a distorted liver pattern, an enlarged portal vein and splenomegaly.[33]

It is surprising that as far as is known, no person who has developed ASL has also had skin or bone changes of the type described above as being caused by VCM exposure. It seems that two different mechanisms are involved in VCM-induced liver tumor and in the cutaneous and acroosteolytic manifestations.

BONES

Acro-osteolysis (AOL) due to exposure to VCM was first described by Cordier[6] in 1966. Industrial AOL has a triad of signs—lytic bone changes, Raynaud's phenomenon and sclerodermatous skin change. The incidence in PVC production workers was approximately 3 percent, and was almost exclusively confined to men who had worked as manual cleaners of autoclaves or reactors.[3,7]

SKIN CHANGES

Sclerodermatous skin changes affect mainly the hands, and vary from minute ivory-colored papules on the dorsal aspect of the hands and fingers to complete tethering of the skin of both hands, thereby interfering with manual dexterity. In severe cases with AOL, the fingers are clubbed and the nails become shortened and curved into a typical watch-glass appearance (Fig. 11-3). In one severely affected man, the skin changes involved the hands, arms, face, trunk and proximal thighs. Histologically, the skin changes differ from idiopathic scleroderma only in that the skin appendages are preserved in the VCM-induced disorder. Direct microscopy of the nail folds shows capillary abnormalities similar to those observed in patients with idiopathic scleroderma.[11] Blood flow studies confirm that both capillary and finger blood flow are impaired. Sympathectomy has proved helpful in relieving the Raynaud's phenomenon in some patients.[7,10]

LUNG FUNCTION

Dyspnea is a common symptom in PVC production workers. Miller[8] reported that 80 percent of PVC production workers had restrictive airways disease after 20 years of exposure. Reduction in lung volume and vital capacity have also been reported. Chest radiographs usually show little abnormality, but reticular and nodular opacities have been reported, and will be further discussed below. Marked defects in lung perfusion were found in production workers at the local factory examined in our study.[9] In one case, histology of the lung revealed focal thickening of the alveolar wall, and macrophages in the alveolar spaces. The affected individual had worked on the production of a particularly fine PVC powder with a particle size of 0.5 μm. One other case of PVC-induced pneumoconiosis has been described.

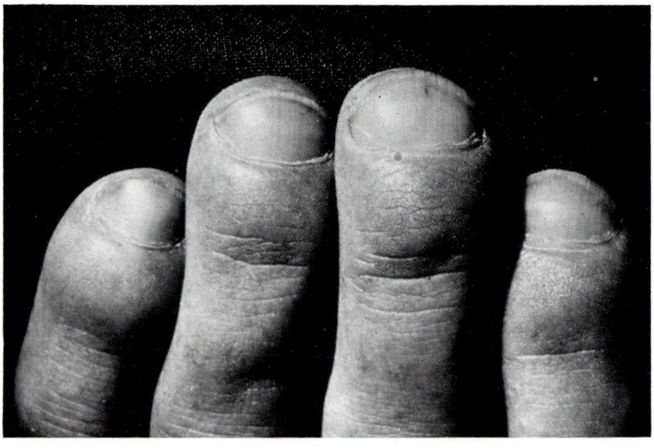

Fig. 11-3. Fingers of reactor cleaner with vinyl chloride disease. Note short terminal segments of fingers and marked convexity of the shortened nails to produce clubbing of the watch glass type.

Table 11-1
Symptoms in 37 PVC Production Workers—British Study by Present Authors (A.E.W.)

Symptoms	Number Affected	Percentage
1. Excessive fatigue, weariness	22	59.4
2. Coldness of hands	20	54.0
3. Aches in bones or joints	20	54.0
4. Tingling or discomfort of feet	17	45.9
5. Dyspnoea	17	45.9
6. Tingling or discomfort of hands	16	43.2
7. Coldness of feet	16	43.2
8. Muscles aches or pains in limbs	15	40.5
9. Impaired power of hand-grip	15	40.5
10. Loss of libido	13	35.1
11. Pain behind the eyes	3	8.1

THROMBOCYTOPENIA

This is a well-documented finding in VCD. Veitman[12] found that 80 percent of VCD patients had platelet counts between $17,000 \times 10^6$ and $14,300 \times 10^6$ per liter, and Wegman[12] states that 35 percent of PVC workers had abnormal platelet counts. Bone marrow studies reveal no abnormality.

ENDOCRINE ABNORMALITIES

Hypothyroidism has been reported in VCM-exposed workers. Suciu[4] found six cases in 168 workers. Sexual impotence is a common complaint in VCM-exposed workers. Low levels of 17 ketosteroids have been reported.[4,12]

MISCELLANEOUS SYMPTOMS

Although direct symptomatic enquiries may be suspected of maximizing symptoms, exposed workers continue to suffer many unexplained and persistent symptoms. These are well documented and it is interesting to compare the presenting symptoms in 37 British workers seen personally in 1974 (Table 11-1) with those from a German study published in 1975 (Table 11-2).[12]

RADIOLOGICAL ASPECTS

Acro-osteolysis induced by VCM is associated with radiological changes which are fascinating, unexpected, probably unique, and pathognomonic. AOL consists of localized zones of bone necrosis and absorption in the hands (and feet), associated with marked coldness and ischaemia of the fingers, which is induced by exposure to cold (Raynaud's syndrome). The condition was recognized in PVC manufacturing workers

Table 11-2
Initial Symptoms in 70 Patients from PVC Factory—German Study[12]

Symptoms	Number of Patients	Percentage
1. Upper abdominal complaints	42	60.0
2. Tiredness	27	38.6
3. Frequent dizziness	26	37.1
4. Paraesthesiae (numbness and tingling) in fingers and/or toes	22	31.4
5. Increased perspiration	19	27.1
6. Sensation of cold in individual fingers or hands	18	25.7
7. Arthralgia	17	24.3
8. Sexual potency difficulties	13	18.6
9. Pain in the head	9	12.9
10. Pain in the calves	9	12.9

in several different countries in the 1960s.[13] Presumably earlier cases had occurred, but were not at the time recognized as being related to VCM or PVC.

The bone absorption is always remarkably well defined, often consisting of multiple, clear-cut, deep erosions, as though a bit of bone had been removed by a bone punch. The erosions usually are not outlined by compact bone, but a thin white margin may be seen (Fig. 11-9). The erosions always involve bone surfaces—usually bony prominences, but occasionally articular surfaces. Fragments of bone may be detached, particularly at the tufts of the terminal phalanges, and these detached fragments may undergo further fragmentation and absorption. There is now firm evidence that the healing of bone lesions by new bone formation may occur in the months or years after exposure to VCM has been terminated (Fig. 11-5).

There is no periosteal reaction, nor do any localized changes in the overlying skin and subcutaneous tissues appear. The fingers may be clubbed and the nails shortened when the terminal phalanx is affected (Fig. 11-3). The bone lesions are not usually tender or painful.

The distribution of the bone lesions is a highly characteristic feature. The extremities, especially the hands and fingers, are most severely involved (hence the name acro-osteolysis). The tufts of the terminal phalanges of the fingers are the most severely affected bone areas. The VCM-induced bone changes of AOL tend to show a remarkable right–left symmetry (Figs. 11-4 through 11-9).

Articular bone erosions occur most frequently in the interphalangeal and metacarpo-phalangeal joints of the fingers (and toes), but other joints, especially those of the sacroiliac, may also be affected by these characteristic clear-cut bone erosions.

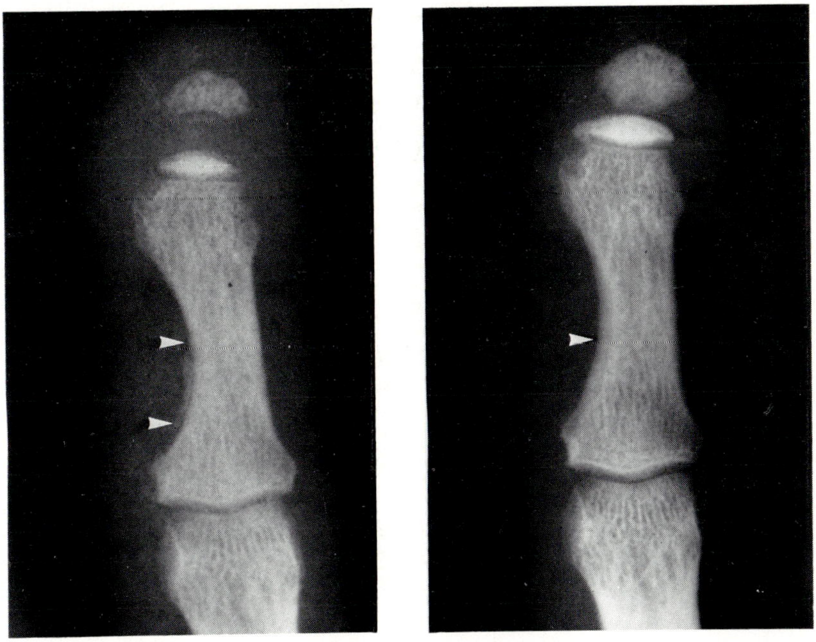

Fig. 11-4. Above left: A.D., 20/11/74. Left middle finger showing transverse band of bone absorption across the mid shaft of the terminal phalanx. Some fragmentation at the base of the separated tuft. Marked shortening of the terminal phalanx with clubbing of the soft tissues. Note periosteal cortical absorption on the radial side of middle phalanx (arrow). Erosions at the corner of this bone. Above right: A.D., 11/7/77. Left middle finger showing considerable healing. The separated distal fragment has consolidated and now has a triangular proximal end approaching the base of the phalanx. The terminal phalanx remains very short. Note healing of the previously eroded cortex on radial side of the middle phalanx (arrow). Cortication and healing of the previous erosions at the corners of this bone.

THE PHALANGES

It is probable that Raynaud's ischemic skin changes always precede radiological evidence of bone lesions in the fingers.

Radiological changes are always more marked and frequent in the distal parts of the terminal phalanges of the fingers. The earliest changes are small, angular, marginal defects in the terminal phalangeal tufts; these lesions may be simulated by congenital variations in ossification and by previous trauma. There may be small detached fragments of bone related to the defects; these fragments may later be absorbed. As the tuft changes are very liable to observer error, they are not to be relied on unless the sign is unequivocal and there is no history of trauma.

Transverse defects in the terminal phalanges are due to circumferential erosions. The erosions link up to traverse the phalanx, and in doing

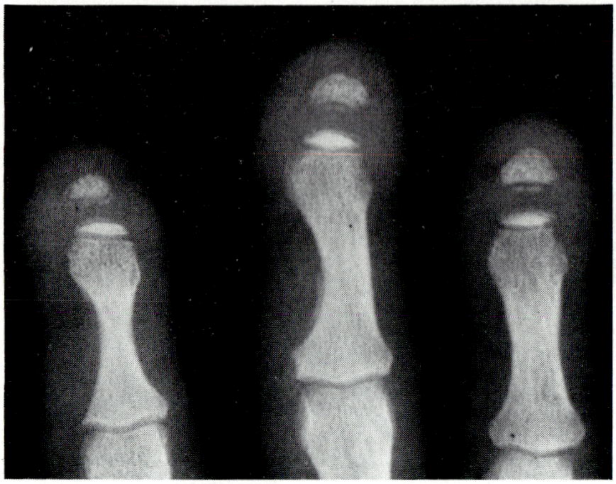

Fig. 11-5A. A.D., 20/11/74. Left index, middle and ring fingers showing identical changes with absorption of the middle third of each of the terminal phalanges. (The right fingers showed identical changes.)

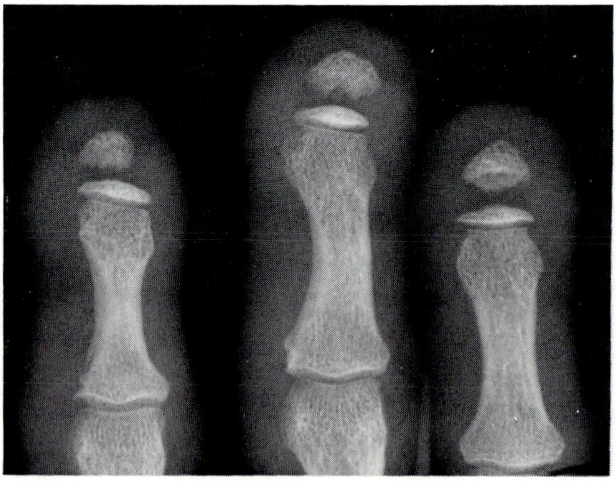

Fig. 11-5B. A.D., 20/9/76. Same fingers showing considerable healing with the proximal surface of the detached tuft becoming consolidated and growing towards the bases. (The right fingers showed identical healing changes.)

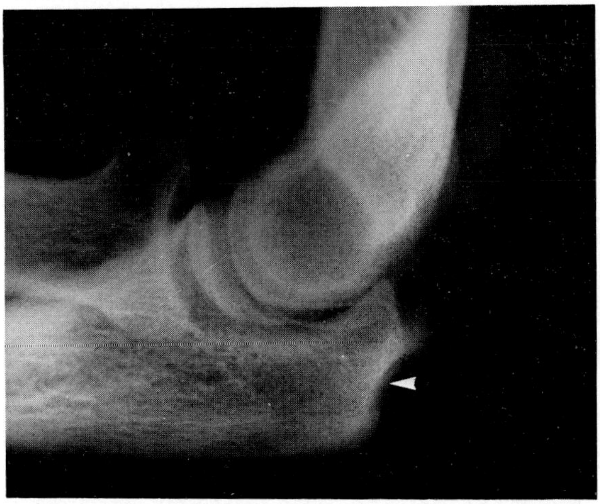

Fig. 11-6. A.D., 20/11/74. Left elbow showing erosion of the cortex of the olecranon process (arrow). (A similar lesion affected the right olecranon.)

so, detach the phalanx's distal portion, which may fragment and/or undergo sclerosis (Figs. 11-4 and 5). These transverse defects were seen by Dinman et al.[14] in 1.2 percent of 5,011 PVC workers (Table 11-3).

The loss of a substantial portion of the mid-shaft of the terminal phalanx results in approximation of the detached distal fragment to the base, thereby shortening the distal segment of the finger (Figs. 11-4 and 5) and accentuating the finger clubbing, which is often a prominent feature (Fig. 11-3).

The combined effect of tuft marginal erosions and transverse defects across the shaft may result in complete absorption of the distal portion of the terminal phalanx; this was found in 0.18 percent of Dinman's series (Table 11-3).

Table 11-3
Prevalence of Radiological Changes in Terminal Phalanges*

Characteristic	Controls 2,407 (percent)	PVC workers 5,011 (percent)
Marginal defects	2.04	7.11
Transverse defects	0.25	1.22
Total resorption of distal portion phalanx	0.08	0.18
Shortening	0.46	1.26
Clubbing	0.08	0.80

* From Dinman et al. 1971.[14]

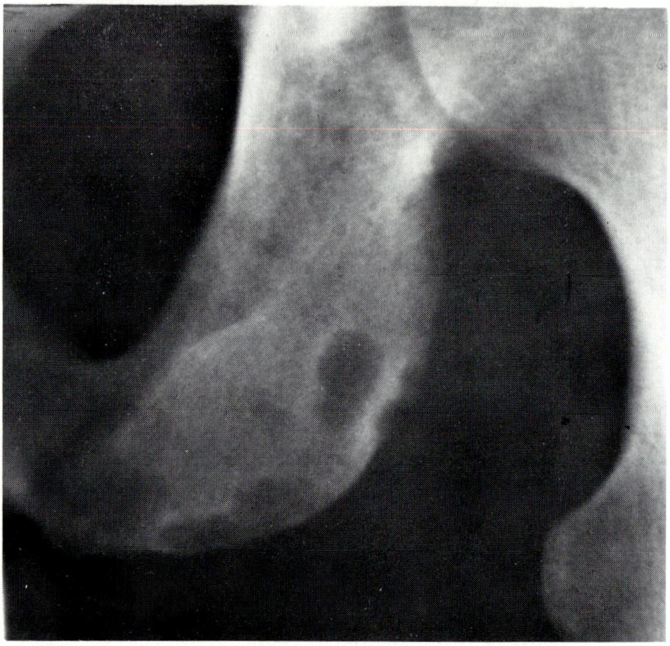

Fig. 11-7. A.D., 20/11/74. Multiple bone erosions of the left ischial tuberosity. All of these lesions involve cortical bone and the bone surface. (Similar lesions affected the right ischium.)

The changes of AOL are much less marked in the middle and proximal phalanges. The subperiosteal compact cortical bone along the shaft may be absorbed, exposing the underlying trabeculae (Fig. 11-4). This change is more marked on the radial aspect of the intermediate phalanges, producing an appearance similar to the subperiosteal bone resorption of hyperparathyroidism, but the delicate, lace-like trabeculation seen in that disease has not been observed in AOL.

The fingers are always more severely affected than the toes with regard to both Raynaud ischemic skin changes and bone-destructive lesions.

Following cessation of exposure to VCM, the bone defects may begin to heal.[15] Small detached fragments become incorporated into larger fragments (Figs. 11-4 and 5); the detached end of the terminal phalanx grows toward its base, often with an arrowhead front (Fig. 11-5) until contact is made. The two ends of the bone may then completely fuse, so reconstructing a "new" terminal phalanx. The contours of the new struc-

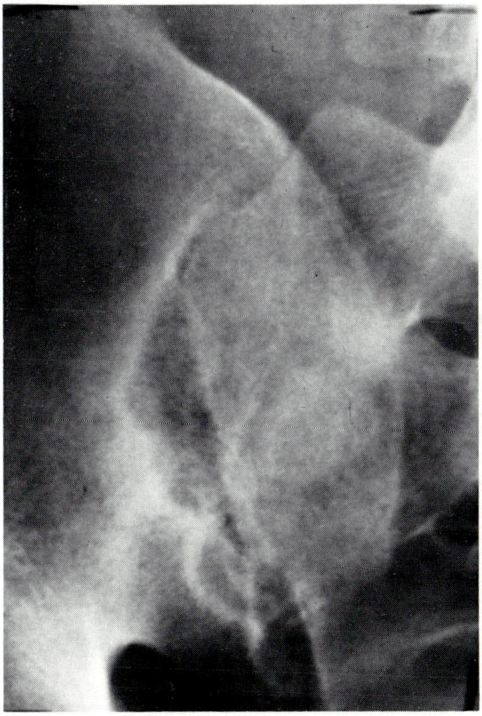

Fig. 11-8. A.D., 20/11/74. Right sacroiliac joint showing deep erosions into the iliac bone. (Similar lesions were present in the left sacro-iliac joint.)

ture are, however, quite different from those of the original phalanx. The new structure is shorter, broader, and stumpier, resulting in a permanently short terminal segment of the finger (with an excess of pulp and soft tissue) and accentuating the finger clubbing (Figs. 11-3 through 11-5).

DIFFERENTIAL DIAGNOSIS OF THE BONE CHANGES IN THE FINGERS

Scleroderma, whose radiological appearance is most similar to that of VCM-induced disease, is more common in women. Its skin changes differ from those of VCM disease in that ulceration of the tips of the fingers, loss of appendages and soft tissue calcification frequently occur. Esophageal and bowel involvement, with characteristic radiological appearances, are seen in idiopathic scleroderma but have not been reported in the industrially induced disorder.

Hyperparathyroidism may cause radiological phalangeal changes

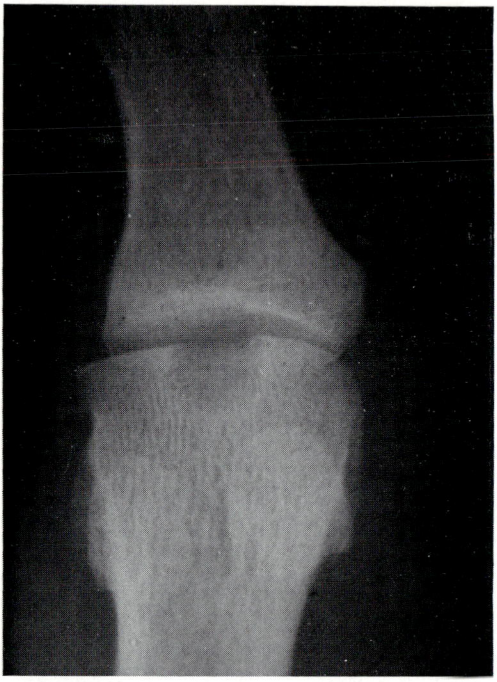

Fig. 11-9. A.D., 20/11/74. Deep erosion of central portion of articular surface of the head of the first left metatarsal. (The head of the first right metatarsal had a similar but smaller articular erosion.)

very similar to those caused by VCD, but the large osteoclastoma lesions, vascular calcifications and biochemical changes that occur in hyperparathyroidism are absent in VCD.

Ischemic atrophy of the phalanges as seen in diabetes, frost-bite, and ergotism may closely simulate VCM-induced changes; the history and clinical features are decisive.

Neuropathic lesions caused by syringomyelia, tabes (usually toes), leprosy, and congenital insensitivity to pain may resemble VCM-induced changes; furthermore, peripheral nerve lesions may produce similar erosive and destructive changes in the extremities. But the associated clinical features and the history will decide.

Rare conditions such as familial acro-osteolysis[16] (sometimes associated with osteo-sclerosis of the Albers-Schonberg type) and idiopathic acro-osteolysis may produce changes in the phalanges very similar to those of VCM-induced AOL; however, there may be a family history, whereas there is no history of VCM exposure in the other conditions.

Severe psoriatic arthropathy and sarcoidosis may produce bone lesions having a slight resemblance to AOL, but the clinical features are quite different.

It cannot be too strongly emphasized that exposure to VCM is the key factor in confirming a diagnosis of VCD. Almost every patient diagnosed to have AOL due to VCM exposure has worked as a reactor or autoclave cleaner; it is the manual scraping and cleaning of the reactor's inner walls that subjects the workers to levels of exposure sufficient to induce bone necrosis.

OTHER BONE LESIONS

Phalangeal lesions have been emphasized here because of their invariable predominance, but bone lesions may occur in other locations. They are always present on corticated bone surfaces—either articular or nonarticular—and appear as punched-out, clear-cut, small areas of bone destruction, sometimes bordered by a thin white margin. The lesions occur predominantly on bony prominences or pressure points, such as the olecranon process (Fig. 11-6), os-calcis ischial tuberosities (Fig. 11-7), or the angle of the mandible. Neither periosteal reactions nor overlying local skin changes (other than the scleroderma of VCD) are present, and the lesions are painless, requiring a skeletal radiological survey for their detection and enumeration. The bone erosions have a very strong predilection to be symmetrical both in site and in size on the two sides of the body (Figs. 11-4 through 11-9).

One of our own patients[17] was a 35-year-old male who had worked in PVC production (including reactor cleaning) for five-and-a-half years. He continued cleaning and scraping reactors for several months after AOL symptoms had developed. He appears to have the most severe and extensive bone and skin changes ever recorded in AOL due to VCD, with severe destructive changes in the phalanges (Figs. 11-4 and 11-5), ulnar styloids, olecranon processes (Fig. 11-6), medial and lateral humeral epicondyles, outer ends of the clavicles, upper ends of the humeri, halluces, cuneiforms, malleoli, os calces, lower poles of the patellae, greater trochanters, ischial tuberosities (Fig. 11-7), sacroiliac joints (Fig. 11-8),[7] and angles and vertical rami of the mandibles. Most of the radiographs in this chapter are of this patient. It should be added that considerable healing of the phalangeal lesions occurred a few years after exposure to VCM was terminated (Figs. 11-4 and 5).

ARTICULAR LESIONS

The sacroiliac joints appear to be particularly prone to the bone changes of VCD. Dodson et al.[18] reported four sacroiliac cases; several others have also been recorded. The lesions are the usual clean-cut erosions, sometimes corticated, usually multiple, extending deeply from the articular surface into the adjacent bone, particularly of the ilium, but also of the sacrum (Fig. 11-8). The appearances are quite different from those of ankylosing spondylitis in which the erosive changes are much less well defined, shallower, and accompanied by changes in the surrounding bone; ankylosing spondylitis eventually heals with bone ankylosis. It will be interesting to follow up patients with VCD changes in the sacroiliac joints in order to determine the end stage.

Articular erosions may also occur in several other joints, particularly those of the hands, arms, feet and legs (Fig. 11-9). The bone lesions consist of well-defined articular erosions; there is no surrounding osteoporosis, no joint effusion and no para-articular swelling (Fig. 11-9).

VASCULAR CHANGES IN THE HAND

Four of our more severely affected VCD patients had retrograde radial arterial catheterization and hand arteriography (RGG). Each showed occlusion of some of the digital arteries (Figs. 11-10 and 11); the occluded segments were both long and short.

Digital arterial occlusions were by no means invariable in fingers severely affected by Raynaud's phenomenon or AOL. There was an increase in the number of small vessels in the vascular tufts of the pulps at the fingertips. The cause of this change is not known; while it could represent an attempt to produce collateral circulation, it may alternatively result from stasis of blood flow in the fingertips—an effect of shortening and bone destruction. Similar hyperemia of the terminal pulp's vascular rete has been reported in hypertrophic pulmonary osteoarthropathy.[19] (Clubbing of the fingers is a feature of both AOL due to VCM and hypertrophic pulmonary osteo-arthropathy.)

PULMONARY RADIOLOGICAL CHANGES

Dyspnea was a frequent presenting symptom in our series (Table 11-1). Radiology of the chest was normal in this group, but Selikoff et al.[20, 21] reported that the chest radiographs of 13.3 percent of 985 PVC polymerization workers showed linear, nodular or reticular changes. Ventilation and perfusion isotope scans have shown occasional lung perfusion defects in our group.[9] Lung function tests have been difficult to interpret partly because of the high incidence of tobacco smoking, but six of our patients showed impaired carbon monoxide diffusion defects.

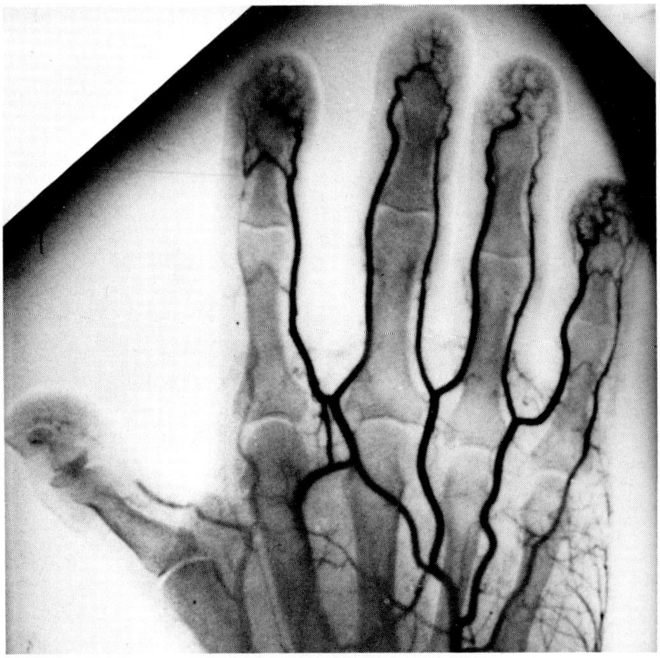

Fig. 11-10. A.D., 1975. Arteriography of left hand showing occlusion of the ulnar digital artery of the thumb, and the radial digital artery of the index finger.

THE PATHOGENESIS AND IMMUNOLOGY OF VINYL CHLORIDE DISEASE

The multisystem clinical features of VCD strongly suggest that a circulatory factor is involved in its pathogenesis. The histological finding of perivascular inflammatory infiltrate and the end-stage narrowing of dermal vessels with subintimal fibrosis are also suggestive of a circulating, complex disorder.[22] The accumulated clinical, histological and immunological evidence suggest that VCD is a complex-mediated disease, with thrombocytopenia and splenomegaly being secondary features that follow complement activation and a persisting immune response.

Evidence is presented here to suggest that a metabolite of VCM (probably chlorethylene epoxide) binds to IgG, promoting aggregation of IgG molecules. Exposure to cold precipitates these complexes; the complexes in turn stimulate complement activation, causing platelet aggregation and fibrinogen conversion to fibrin. Both of these processes occlude capillaries and other small vessels. Raynaud's phenomenon, as well as the

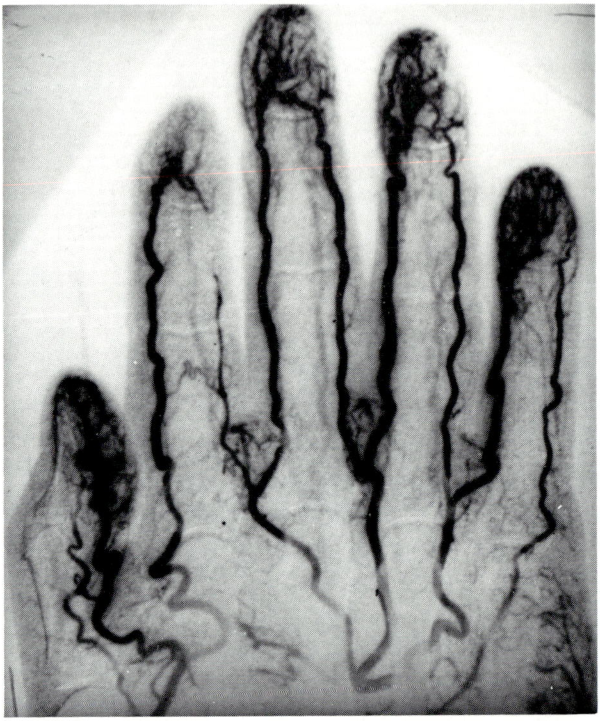

Fig. 11-11. V., 1975. Arteriography of right hand showing patchy occlusion of the ulnar digital artery of the index finger. Note dense arterial rete in the pulp of the terminal segments of all the fingers except the index.

dermal osseous and other clinical manifestations, are explainable with this small vessel occlusion hypothesis.

Metabolism of Vinyl Chloride Monomer

Animal studies in the metabolism and excretion of VCM have shown that VCM may be eliminated in three principal ways: (1) expiration by the lungs of unchanged VCM, (2) expiration of CO_2 derived as a metabolite of VCM, and (3) urinary excretion of the metabolites of VCM.

The major urinary metabolites are thio-diglycolic acid, S (2–chlorethyl) cysteine, N–acetyl S (2–chlorethyl) cysteine, and urea. Intermediate or alternative metabolites of VCM include monochloracetic acid, 2–chloroethanol, 2–chloroacetaldehyde, and chlorethylene epoxide.[23]

It appears that the proportion of VCM that is metabolized is greater when the animal is exposed to a small dose. Saturation of the major or primary metabolic pathway results in redirection through alternative and potentially toxic metabolic pathways.[24] The cyclic chlorethylene epoxide is a highly unstable alkylating agent with a very short biological half-life but a high potential biological activity. It has a marked affinity for free sulphydril pool in rats. This affinity for sulphydril radicals allows the chlorethylene epoxide to cross-link between and to aggregate molecules of IgG and other plasma proteins in vivo. The metabolite–IgG complexes and aggregates are readily precipitated on cooling.

Immunological Abnormalities

The major immunological abnormalities in VCD include hyperimmunoglobulinemia with a polyclonal increase in IgG, cryoglobulinemia, cryofibrinogenemia, and in vivo activation of complement via the classic activation pathway.[22] There is also evidence to suggest mild T-cell depression with a reduction in the circulating T-cell population and a reactive increase in the circulating B-cell population. Immunofluorescent examinations of skin and lung biopsies have demonstrated the deposition of IgG with associated complements C3 and fibrin in relation to the histological lesions described in small blood vessels.

Hypothetical Mechanisms in the Immunological Pathogenesis of Vinyl Chloride Disease

The association of known immunological abnormalities and metabolic data relating to VCD permits the formulation of a hypothetical model for the pathogenesis that will explain the diverse features of this multi-system illness.

An alternative metabolite of VCM—probably chlorethylene epoxide—binds to IgG, producing a structural conformational change that promotes aggregation of the IgG molecule. (The aggregated molecules or structurally anomalous monomers may also become antigenic, but this is probably of minor significance.) The IgG aggregates remain soluble, but they are cryoprecipitable and may initiate complement activation. Precipitation of the IgG aggregate by cold causes complement activation that results in platelet aggregation (with consequent apparent thrombocytopenia), and conversion of fibrinogen to fibrin with polymerization. Occlusion of small vessels results from both of these mechanisms. Occlusions of the skin capillaries may cause the anomalies observed by Maricq;[25] the resulting ischemia will stimulate new collagen biosynthesis.[26] Occlusion of small "end" vessels in cortical bone may result in the characteristic lytic lesions, while occlusion of dermal vessels may result in sclerodermatous changes.

The final phase in this hypothetical mechanism is self-perpetuating, which explains why the disease appears to progress for many months after removal from VCM exposure.

EXPERIMENTAL EVIDENCE

Eighty-eight workers from a local VCM polymerization plant were studied by one of us (A.E.W.). They were divided into three groups on clinical evaluation (Table 11-4): 9 patients with definite VCD, 44 patients with possible VCD, and 35 asymptomatic patients.

Immunochemical and immunological investigations showed a gradation of abnormalities throughout the three groups: polyclonal increases in IgG, cryoglobulinemia, in vivo complement conversion, and a cell-mediated immune defect (Table 11-4).

The cryoglobulin was a mixed cryoglobulin comprising IgG, C_3, and fibrinogen.

The rheumatoid factor as assessed by latex agglutination was universally negative, but hemagglutination showed low titer positive results in eight of the nine persons in Group I, and ten of the 44 in Group II, indicating the presence of aggregated IgG in the serum of the more severely affected individuals.

Direct immunofluorescent examination of skin and muscle biopsies from Group I individuals showed close correlation between the presence of cryoglobulin and that of IgG, C_3, and fibrin both within the lumen of small vessels and adherent to the vascular endothelium.

Ultracentrifugal analysis. IgG preparations from Group I patients appeared visually less stable than those from Group III and from healthy volunteers. Sedimentation velocity analysis indicates the presence of high molecular complexes exceeding 19S, but these complexes are produced in vitro due to the instability of IgG prepared from VCD patients (Group I). Some preparations give lower than normal values for IgG; for these, the normal S°20W concentration dependence of the sedimentation coefficient

Table 11-4
Immunological Abnormalities in Vinyl Chloride-Induced Disease (VCD) and VCM-Exposed Workers

Clinical Group	Number	Cryoglobulin	In vivo C_3 conversion	PACIA assay positive (MAG or RF)
I VCD	9	8 (90%)	6 (66%)	5 (55%)
II possible VCD	44	15 (33%)	19 (44%)	12 (27%)
III VCM exposed	35	0	0	0

is reversed. The molecular disintegration after initial dimerization[27] and the reversed concentration dependence of the S value constitute further evidence of the structural anomaly within the IgG molecule.

Interaction with Protein A indicates a chemically induced IgG structural anomaly. Addition of Protein A to purified IgG from VCD patients resulted in immediate precipitation of a heavy complex. This feature was not observed with normal IgG or IgG from asymptomatic VCM-exposed workers (Group III). In a gel-phase technique, stable Protein A:IgG complexes have only been seen in either (definite or possible) VCD patients, or in rheumatoid arthritis. The structural anomaly of IgG in rheumatoid patients is well documented[28] and the finding of similar results in VCD patients is further evidence of a chemically induced IgG structural anomaly.

The PACIA assay for circulating complexes[29] depends on the presence of immune complexes or immunoglobulin aggregates in the test sample that inhibit agglutination of IgG-coated latex particles by an agglutinator substance. The agglutinators currently employed are murine agglutinator (MAG) and rheumatoid factor (RF). The presence of significant quantities of circulating complexes in 50 percent of Group I and Group II workers with MAG suggests that the majority of complexes in VCD are greater than 20–22 S, although positive results with the RF agglutinator show that 11–55 S complexes are also present.

Conclusions of Experimental Evidence

Ultracentrifugal analysis and PACIA assay give direct evidence of the presence of circulating complexes in VCD. This confirms the indirect evidence obtained from cryoprecipitation and in vivo complement activation. Further direct evidence is provided by immunofluorescent microscopy. Evidence for the molecular anomaly in IgG is provided by the Protein A interaction and by sedimentation velocity analysis. It has not yet been proven that the metabolite:IgG complex is antigenic, but the presence of aggregated IgG is sufficient to activate complement by the classic activation pathway, thereby triggering the final recycling stage in the pathogenesis of vinyl chloride-induced disease.

Summary of Immunological Studies

It is postulated by us that the pathogenesis of vinyl chloride-induced disease is the occlusion of small blood vessels in skin, bone and other tissues by aggregation of platelets, and the conversion of fibrinogen to fibrin (which encourages thrombosis). It is suggested that these vessel-occluding processes are initiated by the precipitation (particularly by cold) of immunoglobin (IgG) aggregates that have resulted from structural changes induced in the IgG molecule by a metabolite of vinyl chloride monomer. This metabolite may well be chlorethylene epoxide.

ETIOLOGY OF VINYL CHLORIDE-INDUCED DISEASE

At the present time, it is not known how VCM produces such a wide range of abnormalities in so many body systems—both in humans and in animals. One possibility is that of a direct toxic effect on the tissues by VCM or one of its metabolites. Another possibility is that the tissue damage is secondary to vascular and/or immunological change. Most probably a combination of these (and possibly other unknown) factors is responsible for the many and varied pathological changes.

The immunological changes described above strongly favor the hypothesis that an immunological chain of reactions may be the cause of small vessel damage and occlusion, ultimately resulting in ischemic tissue changes.

VCM enters the body by direct inhalation of gas and when small particles of PVC (carrying VCM) are inhaled. Inhaled particles of PVC may, themselves, exert a toxic reaction.

It is very interesting that no PVC polymerization worker has been reported to be suffering from both AOL and angiosarcoma of liver. This suggests that VCM may initiate more than one type of toxic reaction, or that there is considerable individual variation in organ susceptibility to toxic levels of VCM. As angiosarcoma of the liver usually develops after a long latent period (15–20 years), some workers with AOL due to VCM may subsequently develop liver tumors.

CONCLUSION

Since 1974, the levels of exposure to VCM in PVC production plants have been reduced to five parts per million. No further cases of VCM-induced disease should appear if these new standards are maintained. It is, however, quite possible that highly exposed workers employed in the industry before 1974 will develop angiosarcoma of the liver at a later date.

The safety of workers handling finely particulate PVC polymer is not yet established; this aspect requires further study and careful monitoring of both the industrial processes and the exposed workers.

REFERENCES

1. Gauvain S: Vinyl chloride. introduction to the problem. Proc Roy Soc Med 69:275–277, 1976
2. Barnes AW: Vinyl chloride & the production of PVC. Proc Roy Soc Med 69:277–280, 1976
3. Lilis R, Anderson H, Nicholson WJ, et al: Prevalence of disease among vinyl chloride & polyvinyl chloride workers. Ann NY Acad Sci 246:22–41, 1975
4. Suciu I, Drejman I, Valaski M: Investigation of diseases due to vinyl chloride. Medicina Interna (Bucharest) 15:967–978, 1963
5. Lange CE, Jühe S, Stein G, et al: Vinyl chloride disease—an occupational systemic sclerosis. Int Arch Occ Health 32:1–32, 1974
6. Cordier, JM, Fievez C, Lefevre MJ, et al: Acro-osteolysis combined with skin lesions in 2 workers exposed in cleaning autoclaves. Cahiers Med Travail 4:14–19, 1966
7. Wilson RH, McCormick, WE, Tatum CF, et al: Occupational acro-osteolysis. Report of 31 cases. JAMA 201:577–581, 1967
8. Miller A, Teirstein AS, Warshaw R, et al: Changes in pulmonary function in workers exposed to vinyl chloride and polyvinyl chloride. Ann NY Acad Sci 246:42–51, 1975
9. Darke CS: Vinyl chloride & the production of PVC. Proc Roy Soc Med 69:277–281, 1976
10. Takouchi Y, Mabuchi C: A case of occupational acro-osteolysis presumably caused by vinyl chloride. Japan J Industrial Health 15:385–394, 1973
11. Maricq HR, Johnson MN, Whetstone CL, et al: Capillary abnormalities in polyvinyl chloride production workers. JAMA 236:1368–1371, 1976
12. Veltman G, Lange CE, Jühe S, et al: Clinical manifestations & course of vinyl chloride disease. Ann NY Acad Sci 246:6–17, 1975
13. Harris DK, Adams WGF: Acro-osteolysis occurring in men engaged in the polymerisation of vinyl chloride. Brit Med J 3:712–714, 1967
14. Dinman BD, Cook WA, Whitehouse WM, et al: Occupational acro-osteolysis. 1. An epidemiological study. Arch Environ Health 22:61–73, 1971
15. Williams DMJ, McLachlan MSF: Healing of phalangeal defects in acro-osteolysis. J Soc Occ Med 26:98–99, 1976
16. Cheney WD: Acro-osteolysis. Am J Roentgenology 94:595–617, 1965
17. Preston BJ, Lloyd Jones K, Grainger RG: Clinical aspects of vinyl chloride disease. Proc Roy Soc Med 69:284–286, 1976
18. Dodson VN, Dinman BD, Whitehouse WM, et al: Occupational acro-osteolysis III. A clinical study. Arch Environ Health 22:83–91, 1971
19. Laws JW, El Sallab RA, Scott JT: An arteriographic & histological study of digital arteries. Brit J Radiology 40:740–747, 1967
20. Lilis R, Anderson H, Miller A, et al: Pulmonary changes among vinyl chloride polymerisation workers. Chest (Supplement) 69:299–303, Feb 1976
21. Selikoff IJ: Discussion. Proc Roy Soc Med 22:281, 1976
22. Ward AM, Udnoon S, Watkins J, et al: Immunological mechanisms in the pathogenesis of vinyl chloride disease. Brit Med J 1:936–938, 1976
23. Green T, Hathway DE: The biological fate in rats of vinyl chloride in relation to its oncogenicity. Chem Biol Interac II: 545–562, 1975
24. Williamson KS: Review of animal studies. Proc Roy Soc Med 69:281–283, 1976
25. Maricq HR, Darke CS, Archibald R McL, et al: In vivo observations of skin capillaries in workers exposed to vinyl chloride. An English-American comparison. Brit J Ind Med 35:1–7, 1978

26. Jayson MIV, Bailey AJ, Black C, et al: Collagen studies in acro-osteolysis. Proc Roy Soc Med 69:295–297, 1976
27. James K, Henney CS, Stanworth DR, Structural changes occurring in 7S globulins. Nature: 202, 563–566, 1964
28. Johnson PM, Watkins J, Scopes PM, et al: Differences in serum IgG structure in health and rheumatoid disease. Circular dichroism studies. Ann Rheumatic Diseases 33:366–370, 1974
29. Cambiaso CL, Riccomi H, Masson PL, Automated determination of immune complexes by their inhibitory effect on the agglutination of IgG coated latex particles by rheumatoid factor or Clq. Ann Rheumatic Diseases, Supplement 1:36, 40–44, 1977
30. Block JB: Angiosarcoma of the liver following vinyl chloride exposure. JAMA 229:53–54, 1974
31. Maltoni C, Le Femine G: Carcinogenicity bio-assays of vinyl chloride: Current results. Ann NY Acad Sci 246:195–218, 1975
32. Lee FI, Harry DS: Angiosarcoma of the liver in a vinyl chloride worker. Lancet 1:1316–1318, 1974
33. Taylor KJW, Barrett JJ, Williams DMJ et al: Preliminary results of Grey scale ultrasonography in the detection of vinyl chloride related liver and spleen disease. Proc Roy Soc Med 69:292–295, 1976

John K. Davidson

12
Dysbaric Osteonecrosis

Aseptic necrosis of bone is a late complication resulting from exposure to a hyperbaric environment such as the compressed air of a tunnel under construction or the high pressures of deep-sea diving. The condition does not appear until at least six months or a year after the first exposure to increased atmospheric pressure. Symptoms of pain and limitation of movement in the affected shoulder or hip joint may be the presenting feature but, more often, the condition is first recognized radiologically, when evidence of osteonecrosis is demonstrated at an annual radiographic survey in a symptomless person.

Various terms have been applied to this condition: caisson disease of bone, caisson arthrosis, aseptic necrosis of bone of caisson workers, barotraumatic arthropathy, aseptic barotraumatic osteonecrosis, etc. That forty-nine different terms have been used, however, is understandable when the etiology and natural history have only recently been more clearly understood. Dysbaric osteonecrosis is now the accepted term and applies to the skeletal lesions that develop in divers and tunnel or caisson workers who have been exposed to increased atmospheric pressure. Osteonecrosis may also, though rarely, develop in aviators who are exposed to low pressure or a hypobaric environment, and lesions in this group are included in the term dysbaric osteonecrosis.

Men working in a caisson, or in tunnels being built through water–bearing ground are rarely exposed to pressures exceeding four atmospheres absolute (ATA) or 44 lbs. per square inch gauge (psig). In the UK the standard shift is of eight hours duration. Compressed air is required in tunnel construction to prevent water from seeping through the bed of the river, and thereby flooding the work. The air pressure varies with both the height of the water immediately above and the porosity of the ground. When men are about to work in compressed air either in a tunnel or caisson, they enter a man lock where, within a few minutes, the pressure is raised to that of the working chamber. The men then enter the working chamber where they remain for periods of time that vary according to the particular job. The majority remain for an eight hour shift. Upon completion of their work they re-enter the man lock and are decompressed to atmospheric pressure. The decompression procedure depends upon the pressures to which they have been exposed and the length of exposure. The procedure is specified by legislation: the Work in Compressed Air Special Regulations, 1958[1] with subsequent modifications in the Blackpool Trial Decompression Table, 1966.[2] For a six-hour exposure at 3 ATA the decompression time would be approximately 115 minutes, according to the modified Blackpool Tables. Following each shift the men remain at the working site for an hour, for it is within this first hour that symptoms of Type I or the more serious Type II decompression sickness are most likely to develop. Should these symptoms arise, the men are immediately recompressed in a separate medical recompression chamber.

Divers are also exposed to a hyperbaric environment. For approximately every 11 meters of descent into sea water the pressure increases by one atmosphere (1 ATA). Although divers may go to a depth of 150–200 meters and are, therefore, exposed to higher pressures than tunnel workers, their period of exposure is usually considerably shorter. Over 1,000 divers are currently employed at any one time in oil exploration in the North Sea. Divers may work from a diving bell or be connected to the surface by continuous air lines. Currently, commercial dives are regularly made to depths of 130–170 meters and dives as deep as 340 meters are planned. As in the case of tunnel workers, the decompression period depends on the depth and length of time to which divers have been exposed. For example, for a dive of 15 minutes at 13 meters the decompression time would be 12 minutes; for a dive of 30 minutes at 200 meters the decompression time would be approximately 36 hours. Currently, the change from air to oxyhelium mixtures is made at about 20 meters.

Saturation dives are carried out quite commonly. In the saturation dive, the diver remains under pressure for periods of from four to ten days. Following this, a single lengthy decompression is required. Experimental simulated dives have been made to depths of 650 meters. More commonly, especially for recreation, use is made of the self-contained underwater breathing apparatus (Scuba). Scuba divers rarely go to depths beyond 60 meters, and dysbaric osteonecrosis is virtually unknown at depths of less than 60 meters.

Following decompression, both the compressed air worker and the diver may develop either Type I or Type II decompression sickness. Type I, consisting of pain in one or more of the limbs with the joint characteristically held in a semi-flexed position, is often referred to as the "bends." The pain is relieved by recompression, whereby the causative bubble is made smaller and goes back into solution. Type II, potentially more serious, is always accompanied by a constitutional upset. Common neurological symptoms are limb weakness, paraesthesia, etc., which are thought to result from a bubble entering the circulation of the CNS. Cardiovascular symptoms may arise as a result of involvement of the coronary circulation.

DYSBARIC OSTEONECROSIS

Although dysbaric osteonecrosis was first described in compressed air workers by Bornstein and Plate in 1911[3] and in divers by Seifert in 1936,[4] only in recent years has much attention been paid to the insidious danger of a hyperbaric environment. For many years reports were confined to those patients presenting with a painful hip or shoulder joint, and who had a history of decompression sickness. More recently, large radiographic surveys have demonstrated that a significant percentage of symptomless compressed air workers have bone lesions. Similar surveys in divers have revealed a low presence of bone lesions which, however, is increasing now that dives are being made to greater depths.

Prevalence

In 1964 the Decompression Sickness Panel of the Medical Research Council set up a Central Bone Registry in Newcastle upon Tyne which maintains a file of skeletal radiographic surveys of 2,390 compressed air workers; of those surveyed, an overall prevalence of 18.2 percent had lesions. In addition, since 1969 the Registry has maintained records of divers and now holds radiographs of skeletal surveys of 3,728 divers. Of these, 3.2 percent reveal definite bone lesions.

Similar skeletal surveys have been carried out elsewhere. Elliott and Harrison[5] reported a 4.0 percent prevalence of osteonecrosis in 350 symptomless divers in the Royal Navy. In a group of 934 US Navy divers, Hunter et al. found 1.7 percent to have osteonecrosis.[6] The report by Ohta and Matsunaga,[7] however, is particularly interesting and underlines how prevalent dysbaric osteonecrosis may be where supervision is poor and there is little understanding of the physiological problems involved. Ohta and Matsunaga studied Japanese shell fish divers who spent their professional lives (from the ages of fifteen to fifty years) diving to 70 meters throughout the year without any timed decompression. Each year three to five divers died from accidents or from decompression sickness. Positive osteonecrosis was found in 15 percent of those between 16 and 19 years, and in 76 percent of those over age 40. The overall incidence was 50.5 percent. Hauteville et al.,[8] reporting a survey of 105 French navy divers, indicated that the prevalence of bone lesions may be as high as 46.7 percent. However, they found a high incidence of bone islands and cystic areas and considered that these might represent positive evidence of osteonecrosis.

Few comparable skeletal surveys concern themselves with compressed air workers. An analysis of data from the MRC Bone Registry shows that among workers with no previous experience the prevalence of bone lesions varies from nine percent to 17 percent.[9,10,14] These figures should be interpreted with caution, however, for an important factor is the length of time between first exposure to compressed air and radiological survey. Lesions require time to become radiologically evident and their incidence increases in later radiological surveys.

Radiological and Pathological Correlation

Occlusion of the blood supply to bone tissue causes necrosis, recognized histologically by an absence of osteocytes in the bone lacunae. An attempt at repair starts by revascularization. Granulation tissue grows in from the living bone to the necrotic segment and new bone is laid on the scaffold of dead trabeculae. For a reason that is not clearly understood, the process of repair becomes arrested before it is complete. Formation of new bone continues. The new tissue accumulates, forming a zone of thickened trabeculae, and so causes an increase in bone bulk. At this stage, at least six months after the ischemic episode, areas of increased density become radiologically apparent. Prior to this, necrotic bone is radiographically indistinguishable from living bone. Weight bearing or excess physical activity may cause structural failure of the articular surface with depression or sequestration of the cortex. These changes are readily recognized radiologically. Once structural failure has occurred, secondary osteoarthritis begins to develop.

The radiological changes within the bone shaft are identifiable as areas of increased density which progress to calcification. It is believed that this increased density is the result of revascularization of necrotic bone and that the calcification results from calcium deposition in the fibrous capsule surrounding the necrotic area.

Radiological Investigations

The radiographic skeletal survey consists of AP projections of each proximal humerus and each proximal femur, and AP and lateral projections of each knee including the distal two-thirds of the shaft of the femur and the proximal third of the shaft of the tibia. Additional projections might include an AP projection of the proximal humerus with the arm in internal rotation and a projection of the hip joint with the leg in the lateral position. The MRC Bone Registry has prepared helpful notes on the radiographic examinations that are readily available.

The radiographic examination of bones is now part of the statutory medical examination of compressed air workers and divers. The number of surveys of divers recorded in the Registry annually now exceeds 2,000—a measure of current diving activity in the North Sea.

The radiological demonstration of the earliest changes of dysbaric osteonecrosis demands high quality radiographs that clearly demonstrate the bone trabeculae. Probably the most common radiological flaw is underpenetration of the radiograph. Consequently, early absolute increases in radiographic density will not be detected (Fig. 12-4A). As already indicated, during revascularisation, new bone is laid on the dead trabeculae causing an overall increase in bone bulk. It is often necessary, therefore, for the kilo voltage to be increased in order that the trabeculae be clearly apparent. Other difficulties in interpretation result from poor positioning, particularly of the shoulder joint. The gonad must always be protected from ionising radiation; if this is done, dosage estimations indicate that the basic radiographic survey can be repeated at intervals of six months. Repeat examinations are usually carried out at intervals of one year unless clinical indications of damage to a joint are present.

Radiographic Classification

Following the first radiographic skeletal survey at the Clyde Tunnel in Glasgow and the study of radiographs in the Bone Registry, the following radiographic classification was drawn up which has been accepted internationally. The classification is summarized below. Detailed descriptions with sample radiographs are available elsewhere.[12,13]

Lesions are classified into two broad groups:

Juxta–articular lesions. These involve or are adjacent to an articular cortex and occur in the head of the humerus or femur. They may already be giving rise to disabling symptoms when first seen; if not, they may do so in the future and, therefore, have to be considered as potentially disabling. Characteristics: (A1) areas of density with an intact articular cortex (Fig. 12-1A); (A2) spherical segmental opacities; (A3) dense layer (Figs. 12-2 and 3); (A4) structural failure: *a*. translucent subcortical band, *b*. collapse of the articular surface, *c*. sequestration (Figs. 12-1B, 12-4B, and 12-6); (A5) osteoarthritis.

Head, neck and shaft lesions. These are situated at some distance from the joint surface and rarely, if ever, give rise to symptoms. Characteristics: (B1) dense areas; (B2) irregular calcified areas (Fig. 12-5); (B3) translucent areas.

Over the past 20 years the MRC Bone Registry has built up an incomparable bank of skeletal radiographs of compressed air workers and divers. From these it has been possible to observe osteonecrosis developing in serial radiographs. Some dense areas, or dense layers adjacent to an intact articular cortex may remain static for several years and, as long as the articular surface is intact, the patient remains symptom-free (Fig. 12-3, 12-4). Others may progress from dense areas adjacent to the articular cortex through the dense layer to a structural surface and then develop secondary osteoarthritis (Figs. 12-4A, B, and C). Symptoms commence when structural failure occurs. Similarly, it has been possible to observe shaft lesions that develop first as areas of increased density and then become more obvious areas of irregular calcification.

By far the most common radiological abnormalities are irregularly calcified areas in the bone shaft, which form 68 percent of all lesions in divers and 44 percent in compressed air workers. The next most common lesions are the dense areas in the shaft. These account for about 20 percent of lesions in compressed air workers, and 12 percent of those in divers. Juxta-articular dense areas and spherical segmental opacities with an intact cortex comprise about 20 percent of lesions in compressed air workers and 11 percent in divers.

Distribution of Lesions

In both compressed air workers and divers the femoral shaft is the most common site of bone lesions. Analysis showed that 383 of 2,200 compressed air workers had 977 lesions (Fig. 12-8) and that of the 3,728 divers, 118 had 206 positive lesions (Fig. 12-9). Lesions were frequently multiple and bilateral. The most common sites in both compressed air workers and divers were the femoral shaft, the head of the humerus, the tibial shaft, and the head of the femur, in that order.

Bone Necrosis in Relation to Occupational History

Data from an analysis of compressed air workers[14] indicate that the frequency of bone lesions increases with age and length of experience. In a group of 2,063 compressed air workers, the incidence of lesions increased from 6.0 percent in those under 24 years of age to 29.0 percent in those over age 40. Similarly, in a group of 1,831 men, an incidence of 13.0 percent in those with under five years of experience rose to 61.0 percent in those with over 20 years of experience. Significantly more compressed air workers have been treated for Type I decompression sickness than for Type II.

Histories of diving experience accompany the skeletal radiographic examinations of each diver. As in the case of compressed air workers, evidence of osteonecrosis markedly increases with age and experience. In a group of 2,516 divers the incidence increased from 0.4 percent in those under 24 years of age to 6.4 percent in those over 40 years. Similarly, an incidence of 1.5 percent in those divers with under five years of experience increased to 3.4 percent in those who had been diving for over 20 years. In those diving beyond 170 meters the incidence of bone lesions increased to 7.6%.[11] There is also a strong positive correlation between susceptibility to decompression sickness and subsequent development of a definite lesion.

Differential Diagnosis

The most common type of aseptic bone necrosis is that which develops in the femoral head following a fracture of the femoral neck or, more rarely, a dislocation of the hip. While its radiological appearance is identical to that of dysbaric osteonecrosis, the diagnosis is not likely to be confused because of the presence of the fracture.

Patients receiving high-dose steroid therapy may also develop osteonecrosis after several months to (more often) a year. The distribution of lesions is different, being more common in the weight-bearing joints such as the femoral head. One major differentiating feature in steroid-induced osteonecrosis is the presence of a structural failure in the medial femoral condyle or the talus. Such lesions are never found in dysbaric osteonecrosis. Hemoglobinopathies may cause lesions in the head of the humerus or in the femoral shaft that are identical to those in dysbaric osteonecrosis. Here, hematological tests are of value in the differential diagnosis. Other causes of osteonecrosis include Gaucher's disease, chronic alcoholism, pancreatitis, radiotherapy and radium therapy.

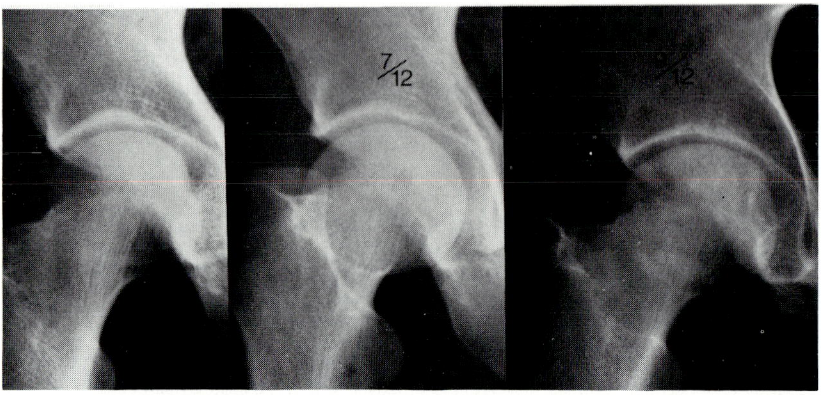

Fig. 12-1. The right femoral head shows no abnormality; at seven months there is possible increased density of the femoral head with an intact articular cortex (A1). At nine months there is slight depression of the superior articular surface.

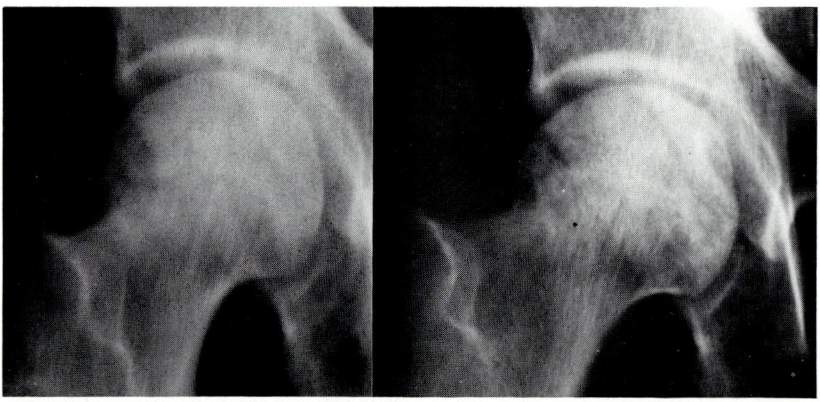

Fig. 12-2. Same case as Fig. 12-1; tomographs of the right femoral head at nine months show sequestration of a large segment of the superior articular surface, which is slightly depressed (A4c).
Compressed air worker aged 27 years; worked regularly in CA at pressures of up to 3½ ATA. Type 1 'bends' on three occasions. Eleven months after first exposure to CA began to experience pain in the right hip; radiograph at that time showed possible increase in density (Fig. 12-2, center). Two months later (Fig. 12-1, right) had more severe pain; structural failure of the articular surface is now evident. (Figs. 12-1 and 2 reproduced with permission of Dr. Yau Kim Pong).

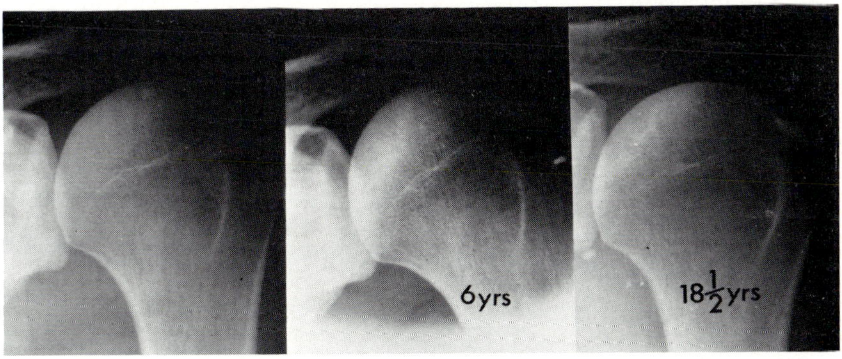

Fig. 12-3. On the left, the head of the left humerus shows no abnormality. At six years there is a dense curvilinear layer of increased bone density enclosing approximately half of the articular surface which is intact (A3). Eighteen-and-a-half years after the original radiograph (on the left), the dense layer is unchanged in appearance and the articular surface remains intact.
Experienced compressed air worker working for over 25 years at pressures of up to 3.5 ATA. The left shoulder is symptom-free because the articular surface has remained intact.

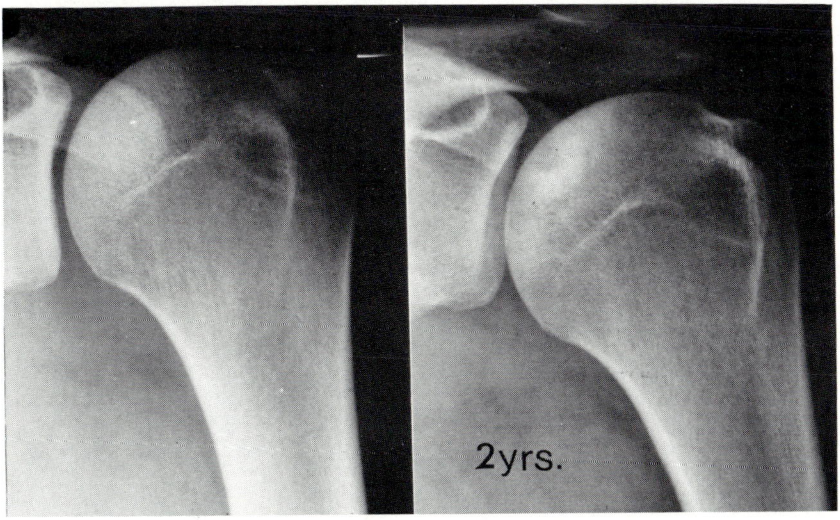

Fig. 12-4. On the left, the head of the left humerus shows no abnormality. Two years later there is a dense layer with an intact articular cortex (A3).
Diver aged 33 years with six years of experience. Dived to a maximum depth of 190 meters for 25 days. The left shoulder remains symptom-free.

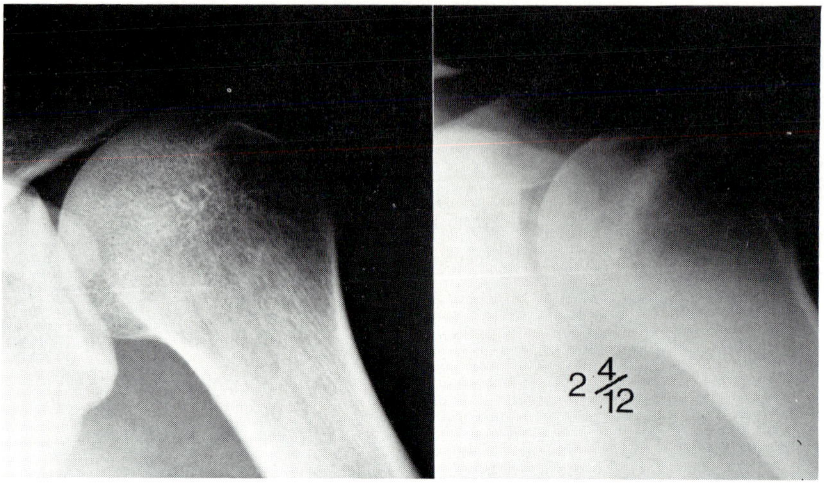

Fig. 12-5. On the left, the head of the left humerus shows no abnormality. At two years and four months there is possible increased density of the head of the humerus. The radiograph is of poor diagnostic quality.

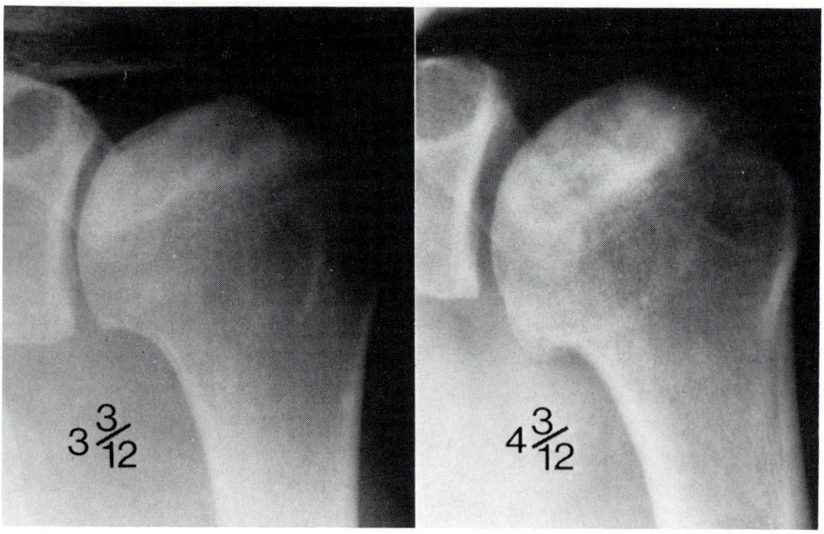

Fig. 12-6. At three years and three months there is sequestration of a small portion of the articular surface with increased density of the head of the humerus. At four years and three months the changes are more marked (A4c).
Diver aged 31 years with 12 years of experience dived to a maximum depth of 147 meters for one hour and ten minutes; also, a longest dive of 14 days at 77 meters. At the time the radiograph showed sequestration of the articular surface, symptoms of pain and disability were present in the left shoulder.

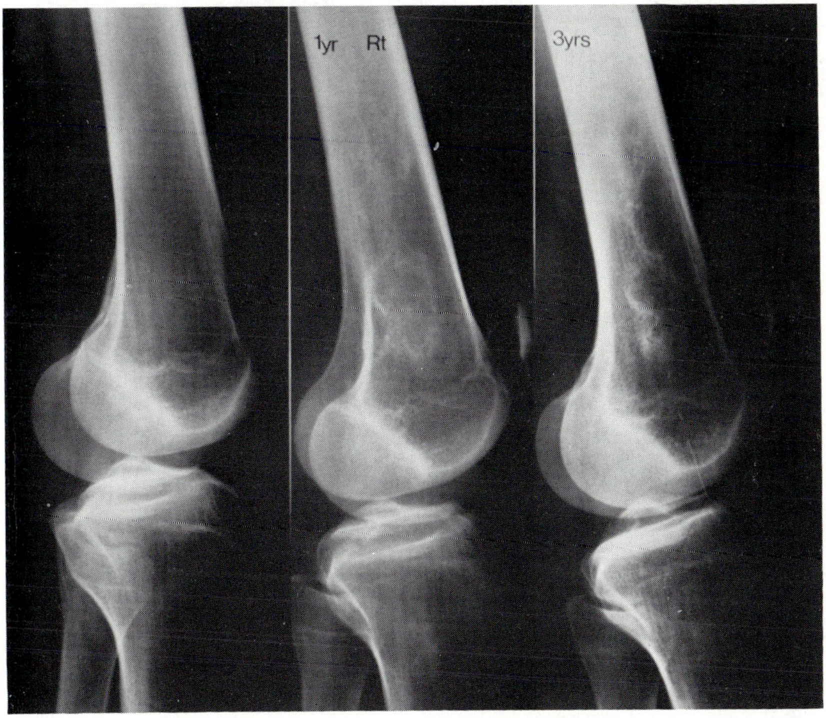

Fig. 12-7. Calcification developing in the shaft of the right femur over a period of three years. The calcification is now extensive and irregular, occupying almost the entire width of the medulla (B2). The knee joint is not involved and no symptoms are present.
Diver aged 34 years with four years of experience. Dived to a maximum depth of 148 meters for one hour.

Calcification in the shaft of the bone must be differentiated from an enchondroma. The ability to make this distinction, however, can be difficult in the early stages. Usually a medullary enchondroma shows circular foci of calcification that are in close apposition. These foci cover a much smaller area than that normally covered by a medullary infarct, which, when fully developed, may occupy an area of up to 45 cm^2.

Differentiation of early osteonecrosis from bone islands or small translucent cystic areas may be difficult. Each of these has mistakenly been interpreted as positive evidence of osteonecrosis.[8,15] In an investigation by Hauteville et al.[8] bone islands were found to be twice as common in divers than among controls, while cystic areas (*géodes bordées*) were almost eight times as prevalent in the divers. Amako et al.[15] found bone islands in 21.6 percent of 450 divers and in 0.5 percent of 1,979 controlled

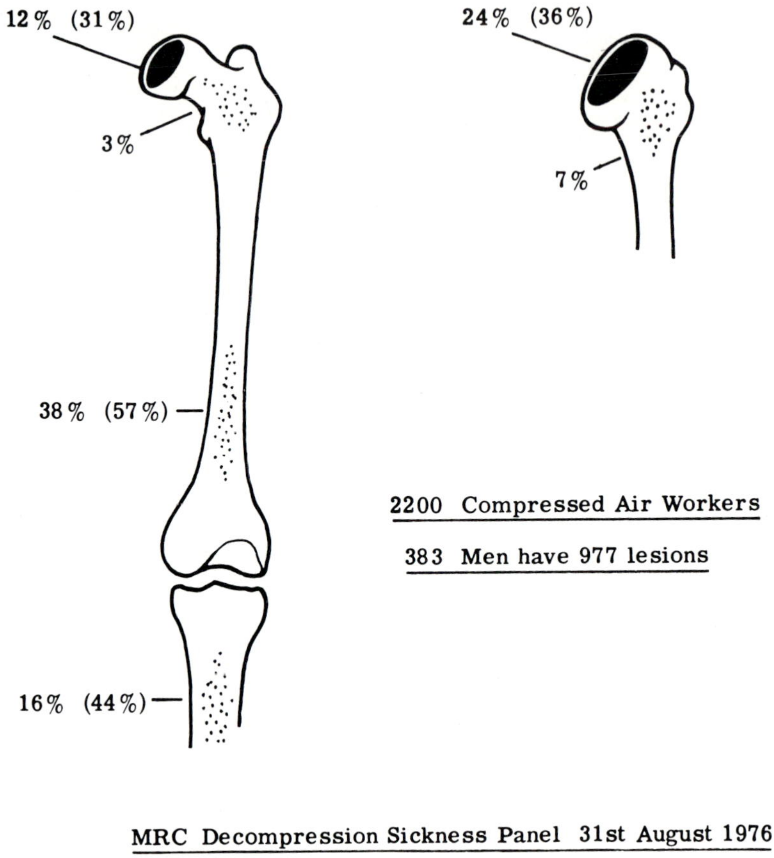

Fig. 12-8. Distribution of bone lesions in compressed air workers.

patients. He, too, interpreted bone islands to represent positive evidence of osteonecrosis, and this interpretation may partially explain why 268, or 59.5 percent of the divers were reported to have osteonecrosis. Subsequently, Davidson et al.[16] compared the skeletal radiographs of 100 Royal Navy divers to 100 controls and found no significant difference in the incidence of bone islands or cystic areas. The Davidson report included the autopsy and radiographic and histological studies of six diving fatalities. The clinical radiographs of five of these showed bone lesions; one showed a cystic area. Bone islands are usually compact and ovoid or oblong in shape with well-defined margins. Small translucent cystic areas with a fine sclerotic margin are usually seen in the femoral neck and may result from damage at the insertion of the joint capsule.

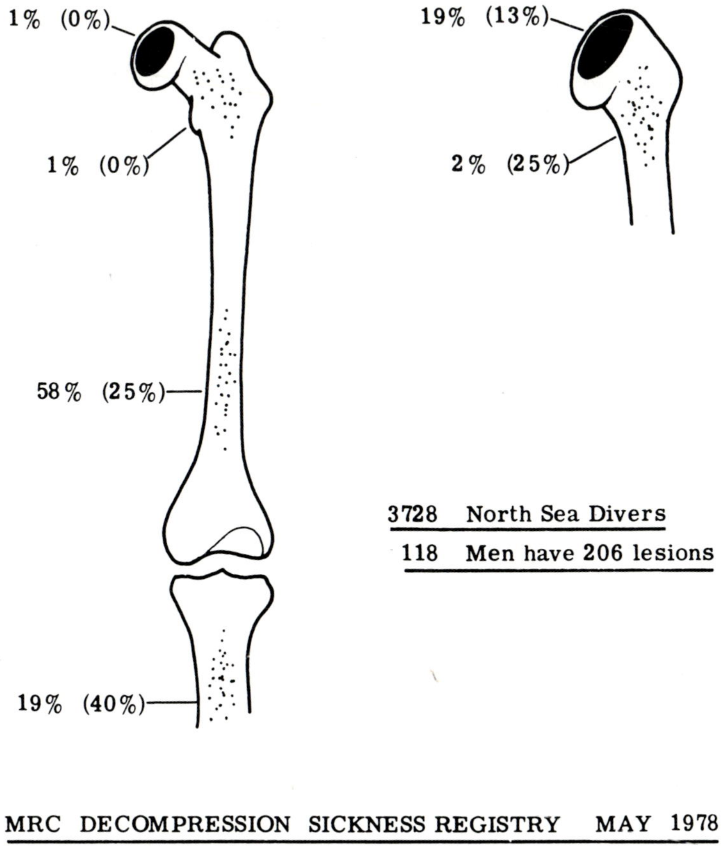

Fig. 12-9. Distribution of bone lesions in divers.

Research

The causative mechanism by which bone necrosis comes about is still not clear, but it seems likely that bubble emboli will cause occlusion of the multiple end arteries at vulnerable sites and thereby cause necrosis. The actual ischaemic episode is painless; it is impossible, then, to identify precisely when this occurs. Furthermore, the optimum management and treatment of symptomatic lesions is often unsatisfactory: attempts to repair necrotic bone and damaged articular surfaces have not been particularly successful. The results for excision of the hip joint and replacement with a prosthesis, on the other hand, are much more encouraging. The main disadvantage as applied to a young man, however, is that the life of a prosthesis is probably limited to 20 years.

For these reasons much research and effort have been directed toward the development of a suitable animal model by which bone necrosis may be studied in a laboratory environment with control of both compression and decompression. The experiments would be designed especially to reproduce bone necrosis and devise other ways of detecting dysbaric osteonecrosis at a much earlier stage.

The condition has been reproduced in rabbits following injection of glass microspheres into the right or left external iliac arteries.[17] More importantly, very encouraging results have been obtained from investigations using radio–isotopes. These experiments have indicated that bone lesions may be detected as early as three weeks after the ischaemic episode and several months before the lesions could be identified by radiology.[18] A safe and inexpensive method of detecting bone damage earlier would be of considerable advantage. Gregg et al.[19] in a study in rabbits found that marrow death is followed by a significant rise in serum ferritin levels. The authors indicate that this finding may be of value in the early diagnosis of dysbaric osteonecrosis.

Management and Treatment

Attempts at repairing the articular surface of the humeral or femoral head following structural failure have not been successful. Excision of the hip and replacement by a prosthesis have given good results, particularly in elderly arthritic patients. However, the life span of a prosthesis is likely to be limited to approximately 20 years; unfortunately, this would be a major disadvantage in young divers or compressed air workers with symptomatic bone lesions.

Symptom-free compressed air workers, or divers with positive radiological evidence of osteonecrosis should be informed that they do have a lesion and that exposure to great depths or high pressure, especially for those with a joint lesion, should be avoided. Some researchers express the view that, once it has been determined that an individual has a bone lesion, there should be no further exposure to a hyperbaric environment. Giving up this type of work and avoiding further exposure to a hyperbaric environment, however, does not necessarily signify that there will be no further deterioration in the progress of the lesion. Currently, there is no way of determining whether a symptomless juxta-articular lesion will advance to structural failure with subsequent osteoarthritis. The patient should be advised to have serial radiographic surveys at annual intervals for at least three years after last exposure to a hyperbaric environment.

Head, neck and shaft lesions will almost certainly remain symptomless. An increasing number of reports suggest that malignant fibrous histiocytoma is associated with osteonecrosis.[20] Sixteen cases of bone sarcoma have now been reported in association with osteonecrosis. Four of these were detected in compressed air workers, one in a patient with sickle–cell disease and six in patients of undetermined etiology. In all cases there was a long interval between bone infarction and the onset of sarcoma. Among the compressed air workers the interval varied from 17 to 28 years; lesions occurred on the femoral shaft in two, on the tibial shaft in one, and on the femoral head in one.

Dysbaric osteonecrosis is a major hazard to compressed air workers and an increasing hazard to divers now that dives are being made to greater depths. Early detection depends on reliable interpretation of good quality radiographs by at least two radiologists experienced in this type of work.

REFERENCES

1. HMSO: Work in Compressed Air Special Regulations. London, 1958
2. Medical Research Council Decompression Sickness Central Registry: Blackpool Trial Decompression Tables. Newcastle upon Tyne, University printing, 1966
3. Bornstein and Plate: Chronic joint changes due to compressed air sickness. Fortschritte auf dem Gebiete der Röntgenstrahlen und der Nuklearmedizin 18:197–206, 1911/1912
4. Seifert E: A rare disorder of the hip joint. Zentralblatt Chirurgie 63:2318–2321, 1936
5. Elliott DH, Harrison JAB: Bone necrosis—an occupational hazard of diving. J Royal Naval Medical Service 56:140–161, 1970
6. Hunter WL, Biersner RJ, Sphar RL, et al: Aseptic bone necrosis among US Navy divers: survey of 934 nonrandomly selected personnel. Undersea Biomedical Journal 5:25–36, 1978
7. Ohta Y, Matsunaga H: Bone lesions in divers. J Bone and Joint Surgery 56b:3–16, 1974
8. Hauteville D, Esquirol E, Hyacinthe R, et al: Les lésions osseuses latentes des plongeurs. Résultats comparés d'une enquête portant sur 105 plongeurs et sujets témoins. Revue du Rhumatisme 43:635–643, 1976
9. MRC Decompression Sickness Panel: Bone lesions in compressed air workers. With special reference to men who worked in the Clyde Tunnel (1958–1963). J Bone and Joint Surgery 48b:207–235, 1966
10. MRC Decompression Sickness Panel: Decompression sickness and aseptic necrosis of bone. Investigation carried out during and after the construction of the Tyne Road Tunnel (1962–1966). British J Industrial Medicine 28:1–21, 1971
11. Thickett VB, Evans A: Bone necrosis in British commercial divers, in Evans A, Walder DN (eds): Aseptic Bone Necrosis, Proceedings of Symposium of European Undersea Biomedical Society. London, CIRIA Underwater Engineering Group, 1977, pp 31–40
12. Davidson JK: Dysbaric osteonecrosis, in Davidson JK (ed): Aseptic Necrosis of Bone. Amsterdam/Oxford, Excerpta Medica, 1976, pp 147–212
13. Davidson JK: Dysbaric osteonecrosis and pulmonary changes in divers, in Steiner R

and Lodge Sir Thomas (eds): Recent Advances in Radiology No. 6. Edinburgh, Churchill Livingstone, 1979, pp 145–162

14. Trowbridge WP: Bone necrosis in British compressed air workers, in Evans A and Walder DN (eds): Aseptic Bone Necrosis. Proceedings of Symposium of European Undersea Biomedical Society, London, CIRIA Underwater Engineering Group, 1977, pp 41–49
15. Amako T, Kawashima N, Torisu T, et al: Bone and joint lesions in decompression sickness. Seminars in Arthritis and Rheumatism 4:151–190, 1974
16. Davidson JK, Harrison JAB, Jacobs P, et al: The significance of bone islands, cystic areas and sclerotic areas in dysbaric osteonecrosis. Clin Radiology 28:381–393, 1977
17. Cox PT: Simulated caisson disease of bone. Försvarsmedicin 9:520–524, 1973
18. Gregg PJ: The use of radio–isotopes in aseptic necrosis, in Evans A, Walder DN (eds): Aseptic Bone Necrosis. London, CIRIA Underwater Engineering Group, 1977, pp 77–83
19. Gregg PJ, Eastham EJ, Bell JI, et al: Serum ferritin and dysbaric osteonecrosis. Undersea Biomedical Research 4:75–79, 1977
20. Galli SJ, Weintraub HB, Proppe KH: Malignant fibrous histiocytoma and pleomorphic sarcoma in association with medullary bone infarcts. Cancer 41:607–619, 1978

Louis Kreel

13

Asbestosis and Mesothelioma on Computed Tomography

. . . this most excellent canopy, the air, look you, this brave o'erhanging firmament, this majestical roof fitted with golden fire, why it appears no other thing to me but a foul and pestilent congregation of vapours.

Hamlet II, ii, 320

Work in a well-ventilated space, if possible outdoors, when sawing, drilling, filing or sanding.

The Asbestos Safety Code

The fire- and heat-resisting properties of asbestos were not generally known to late nineteenth-century industry, but as an awareness of these properties spread in the early twentieth century, silicate minerals began to find their way into all phases of industrial production. Asbestos fibers were spun into cloth, mixed with cement to make pipes, used in brake linings, pipe lagging, electrical insulation, batteries, and even in the filter pads of certain types of respirators. It was, indeed, difficult to challenge the momentum of such an increasingly ubiquitous and desirable material, and considerable time was needed before the pathological effects of asbestos were investigated. The report of Seier (1928) was rapidly followed by those of Merewether and Price (1930), Krüger et al. (1931) and

Grateful acknowledgement is made to the Department of Health and Social Security of the United Kingdom, whose farsighted and generous help has assisted greatly in the development of this project. The assistance and considerable help of Stephen Henman and Malcolm Brooker, who have been managing the machine, is also gratefully acknowledged.

Gerbis and Ucko (1932). Each of these investigations implicated asbestos as a cause of pulmonary fibrosis.

We note with hindsight Pliny's mention of the difficulties in weaving asbestos and the use of respirators,[10] but the paper of Hurwitz[11] is more relevant. Although asbestos has been mined in Kuruman and Lydenburg since 1893, its pathological effects were only recognized radiologically some 70 years later. Equally interesting are the observations of Kiviluoto, who found an "epidemic" of asbestosis among inhabitants of a farming community in Northern Finland who were living near asbestos-producing mines.[13]

Once the long latent period was recognized, reports on the ties between asbestos exposure and pulmonary fibrosis, pleural plaques with calcification and mesothelioma proliferated. The clinical and radiological features became well established with reviews by Leathart,[20] Lawson,[19] Wagner et al.[30] and Hourihane.[9]

Another factor responsible for the delayed radiological detection of asbestos-related disease is that radiological changes are relatively minor when compared with the manifest disability of pulmonary fibrosis; expressed in another way, the radiological changes in other types of silicoses and pneumocomioses are much more obvious at equivalent stages of progression than are those of asbestosis. Equally significant, the effects of asbestos may eventually appear even when periods of industrial exposure are extremely short.[22]

RADIOLOGICAL SIGNS IN ASBESTOSIS

Abnormal signs can be related to both pleural and parenchymal disease. Abnormal shadowing resulting from parenchymal disease has been analyzed by Leathart,[20] Hurwitz,[11] Simon,[29] and Solomon.[28] These parenchymal appearances differ in their overall effect from other pneumocomioses, but they are by no means pathognomonic, and often resemble idiopathic interstitial fibrosis. Hurwitz drew attention to the 'honey comb' pattern and its similarity to the patterns characteristic of idiopathic fibrosis and scleroderma.[11]

The "clouding," "haze" or "ground-glass" appearance is a less definite sign, but there is general agreement that its presence is not merely technical and artefactual, or due to soft tissue shadowing. The clouding probably results from a superimposition of a very fine and uniform shadowing that is both alveolar and interstitial. On chest radiographs these parenchymal changes are more common in the lower and middle zones and are almost invariably bilateral.

In overt and late cases of the disease, the most common abnormalities were small, scattered opacities, that were 2–4 mm. in size, irregular, and ill-defined[29]; round opacities less than 2 mm. in diameter were less frequently seen. According to Soutar et al., the honeycomb pattern consists of several hairline ring shadows within areas of additional shadowing. The ring shadows range from less than 5 mm. to 10 mm. in diameter. Kerley "B", or septal, lines—short horizontal lines above the costo–phrenic angle that extend to the lung edge—were also relatively common to the honeycomb pattern.

Leathart stressed a "shagginess" that produced irregular outlines at the hilar regions and around the heart border. He also mentions hyper-transradiancy of one or both upper zones, presumably due to emphysema.[20]

Thickening of the fissures is certainly a feature of asbestosis.[28] All fissures may be affected, though in varying degrees; displacement of fissures is also common.

Large parenchymal shadows occur, but are almost invariably due to pulmonary tuberculosis or bronchial carcinoma. Occasionally a large static intrapulmonary shadow may be present which cannot be ascribed to either tuberculosis or carcinoma.[29]

Pleural Shadowing

The pleural calcifications of asbestosis are now so well recognized that, even in retrospect, the reason for Smith's inability to find any in his review is most surprising, especially since he found a number of cases resulting from exposure to talc. However, after the initial case of Jacob and Bohlig[12] and those reported for mixed dusts, including asbestos, by Frost et al. (1956) and Hurwitz (1961), there was no doubt that asbestosis characteristically showed calcified pleural plaques; such plaques could not be demonstrated in South African gold mine workers with silicosis. Radiological credence was thus given to Gloyne's pathological description of "stiff, horn–like plaques".[7] Furthermore, Hurwitz's assertion that "pleural changes are found more frequently than the classic diffuse pulmonary fibrosis" was subsequently confirmed.[1,9,13,29] Perhaps the most interesting reports are those of Kiviluoto[13] and Sargent et al.[22] Kiviluoto showed that an urban community living in the neighborhood of asbestos mines, but not actually engaged in mining itself, had developed asbestotic plaque, and Sargent et al. demonstrated that these changes can occur even after very short periods of industrial exposure (of the order of only eight to eleven months) and draws attention to the cases of Selikoff[25] and Hourihane et al.,[8] which discuss exposures of less than one week and six weeks, respectively.

Calcified pleural plaques are most easily recognized when they appear in profile as short, dense white lines 2–5 cm. in length on the diaphragmatic margin and adjacent to the rib cage. However, these calcifications may also form along the mediastinal margin and on the pericardium and can be up to 20 cm. in length. They are characteristically basal, bilateral and discontinuous.

En face these plaques are recognized with more difficulty, appearing more as "candle grease" shadowing. Thus, calcified plaques will be seen with greater clarity if lateral and oblique chest radiographs that are sufficiently exposed to distinguish calcification from adjacent soft tissue are also taken.

Anton conclusively demonstrated non-calcified pleural plaques on chest radiographs.[1] Faint shadows *en face* can be confirmed as pleural plaques by their flat profile at the periphery of the lung field, but because an area of normal pleura separates adjacent pleural plaques, a band of normal radiolucent lung can be seen between plaques in the *en face* view. Anton also points out that tomography is of no help in showing non-calcified pleural plaques, but he adds that on theoretical grounds, *axial* tomography would be most helpful.

A vertical band shadow behind the sternum and another in front of the posterior ribs was also considered a manifestation of pleural thickening in asbestosis.[29]

In asbestosis characterized by marked pleural thickening, the uncalcified pleural shadowing can be up to one cm. thick, raising the possibility of mesothelioma. Marked thickening of the fissures and fibrous parenchymal band shadows are usually associated with such cases. By observing oblique radiological views it is possible to see that, in some cases, circumferential pleural thickening is present and is most marked at or confined to the bases (Fig. 13-1).

"Pleural plaques" can be overdiagnosed. Companion shadows to ribs and occasional inward-protruding intercostal muscles may simulate uncalcified pleural plaques.

Hourihane emphasized not only that plaques are more prominent in the lower halves of the pleurae, but also that, in their earlier phases, they tend to follow the lines of the ribs, that is, they are on the inner margin of the rib and not in the intercostal spaces.[9]

The Position of the Diaphragm

According to George Simon, a raising or flattening of the diaphragm was an extremely common abnormality in the later stages of asbestosis. Simon characterized a raised diaphragm as being higher than the midpoint between the fifth and sixth ribs, anteriorly, and a depressed diaphragm as being below the seventh anterior rib.[26]

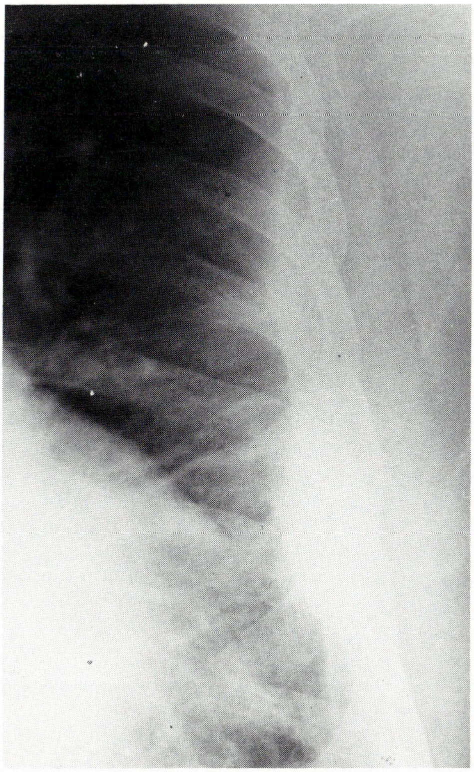

Fig. 13-1. Marked pleural thickening in asbestosis shown to be "circumferential" on CT and associated with restrictive abnormalities on lung function tests.

MESOTHELIOMA

Present in the majority of patients are intractable and frequently hemorrhagic massive pleural effusions; marked irregular pleural thickening usually develops in such patients before long.[3]

Pleural plaques can be demonstrated in the opposite lung in about half such cases; not infrequently, metastases and visibly enlarged hilar lymph nodes are present in the opposite lung as well.

It is, however, of interest to note that pleural plaques were not found at necropsy in 20 percent of the cases, and were not commented on in another 20 percent. Thus, in a large number of cases, pleural plaques will not be radiologically visible in the opposite lung.

Comment

The radiological signs of asbestosis are well known and have been described in great detail in the literature. There remain, nevertheless, a number of problems for the radiologist. Clearly, not all pleural plaques are visible on chest films, even using postero-anterior, lateral and oblique views; furthermore, "companion shadows" can be mistaken for plaques. As compared with other pneumocomioses, parenchymal lung involvement appears on the chest radiograph relatively late, and may show only minor changes even when there is obvious impairment of lung function.

In cases of mesothelioma the tumor is frequently hidden by the effusion. At later stages the chest radiograph shows superimposed shadowing, making assessment of the progress of the disease and of response to treatment difficult if not impossible.

Computed tomography, therefore, offers an additional modality for visualizing changes in asbestosis and mesothelioma in difficult cases.

GENERAL PRINCIPLES OF COMPUTED TOMOGRAPHY

Both conventional radiography and computed tomography (CT) use x-radiation. The transmitted photons are used to produce an image on film in the former, while in the latter, photon detectors are used. In CT, after sufficient readings have been taken (usually on the order of 300,000), a picture of an axial section of the body is reconstructed from tissue attenuation values, which are calculated by deducting the radiation on the photon detectors from the radiation of the x-ray tube. The system is concerned essentially with recording attenuation values; only subsequently is a picture reconstructed.

Each axial section is approximately 1 cm. thick and contains the attenuation values for all tissues within the section, which are arbitrarily subdivided into 1,000 EMI units or 2,000 Hounsfield units around water which is set at zero. Air is –500 EMI (or –1,000 Hounsfield units). The images created from the recorded attenuation values for each axial section can be shown in many different ways by using various window widths and window levels.

Window width refers to the total number of units covered in the picture. It may be as high as 400 or as low as one. With the widest window spread over a large range of EMI units, all tissues can be visualized, but the visual contrast between adjacent tissues is very low. With narrower windows a smaller range of tissues are visible, but visual contrast is increased. In a very real sense, then, the presentation of a single picture is an arbitrary editing of tissue attenuation values to illustrate particular features.

Window level settings, on the other hand, are directly related to particular attenuation values. Lung fields between −400 and −300 EMI units, adipose tissue between −50 and −5 EMI units, soft tissues between +5 and +40 EMI units, and bone between +100 and +300 EMI units are shown.

Thus, by varying both window width and window level settings, a large number of different appearances, representing the tissue attenuation values in a single axial section, can be created.

The information obtained from CT and conventional radiology, therefore, differs fundamentally in a number of ways. With conventional radiographs the radiation passes through all the tissues being examined, but once the picture is taken, the information cannot be manipulated. In CT the radiation passes through only one section at a time. The pictures, though, lend themselves to manipulation; furthermore, tissue attenuation values can be analyzed independently.

There are several disadvantages in using CT. Only one or two sections may be taken at a time, and the procedure is much more expensive and time-consuming than conventional chest radiography, although CT is probably on par with full conventional bilateral lung tomography.

To obtain pictures that are reasonably free of artefact, CT equipment must produce each section in an exposure time of less than 18–20 seconds, i.e., less than breath holding. Nevertheless, image quality will be downgraded by movement streaks in the lungs adjacent to the heart at the level of the ventricles. Because the lungs are examined in a series of 1 cm. sections, either a large number of these sections must be made to cover the whole lung, or, sections must be taken at preselected intervals ranging from 1.5–2.5 cm., depending on the clinical problem. In subsequent examinations of the same patient, difficulties in matching axial sections arise. Since each section is taken separately it is possible to have pictures of the same subject at varying degrees of inspiration or expiration; unless this inspiration/expiration information is available, comparisons will be invalid.

Positional and Gravity Effects

Because of its greater sensitivity, changes are seen in CT that cannot be visualized with conventional radiographs. CT sections of normal lungs taken while the patient is in the supine position (CT examinations are invariably performed with the patient horizontal) in suspended respiration are darker or less dense anteriorly and whiter or more dense posteriorly. This effect is more marked with breath holding in a neutral position than in deep inspiration. In fact, with breath holding in a neutral position the lungs in some patients appear so dense as to suggest "hypostatic" changes or early pulmonary edema, which in normal subjects can be immediately reversed on deep inspiration.[15]

If the subject is turned into the lateral decubitus position, the lowermost lung becomes denser and, in the prone position, the fronts of the lungs become denser. Again, the difference is considerably diminished in deep inspiration. Furthermore, in normal lungs bronchi and bronchioles can be seen.[16]

Another very important feature in normal subjects is the absence of any visible soft tissue along the inner margins of ribs that are adjacent to the lungs. Similarly, virtually no soft tissue is visible along the right vertebral body margins, but posterior to the descending aorta on the left side, a minimal amount of soft tissue is visible between the aortic margin and the head of the rib. The diaphragm has a regular, smooth margin in normal subjects apart from the streak artefact caused by cardiac movement. The costo–phrenic sulci are clear.

INDICATIONS OF ASBESTOSIS FROM CT

Pleural Plaques

The earliest evidence of the presence of pleural plaques is the appearance of additional soft tissue on the inner margin of a rib. The tissue growth is approximately 1–2 mm. thick and 2–3 cm. long. The tissue attenuation cannot be measured accurately because of the adjacent rib on one side and lung on the other. There is, however, no evidence to suggest calcification in this early phase (Fig. 13-2). Judging from their positions along rib margins and previous pathological descriptions, these early plaques would appear to be thickenings of parietal pleura only.

As pleural plaques become more extensive they can be seen in all areas of the lower two thirds of the thorax, but are most numerous posteriorly, around the vertebral bodies, and basally. An important feature of asbestosis plaques is their discontinuous appearance. Separate, apparently unrelated plaques, are found on different sections and in different positions along the inner rib margin (Fig. 13-3).

Asbestos pleural plaques usually have a thin white line along the innermost margin, suggesting early calcification; by the time calcification is visible on chest radiographs, the plaques appear as gross calcifications on CT sections (Figs. 13-4 and 5).

By the time pleural plaques have become continuous, their circumfer-

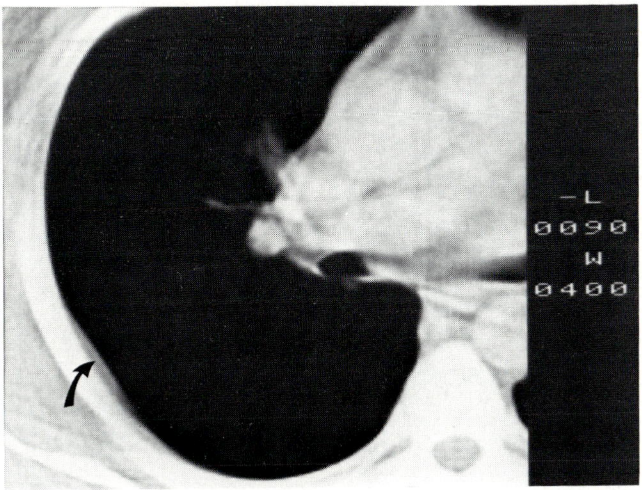

Fig. 13-2. Minimal pleural plaque formation not seen on a conventional chest radiograph.

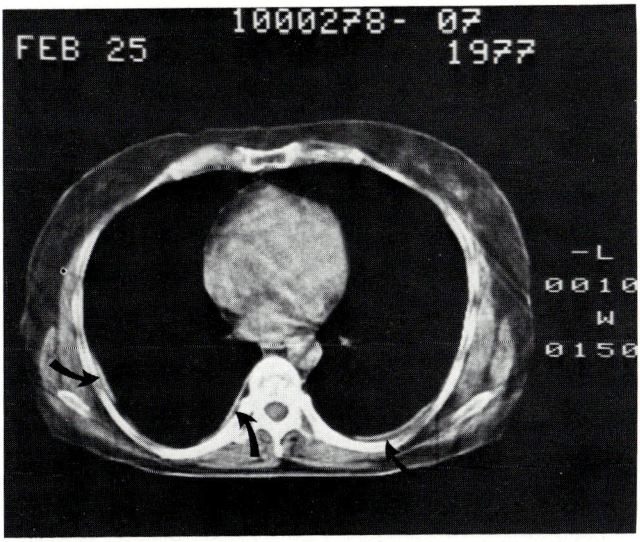

Fig. 13-3. Typical, multiple, bilateral discontinuous pleural plaques of asbestosis.

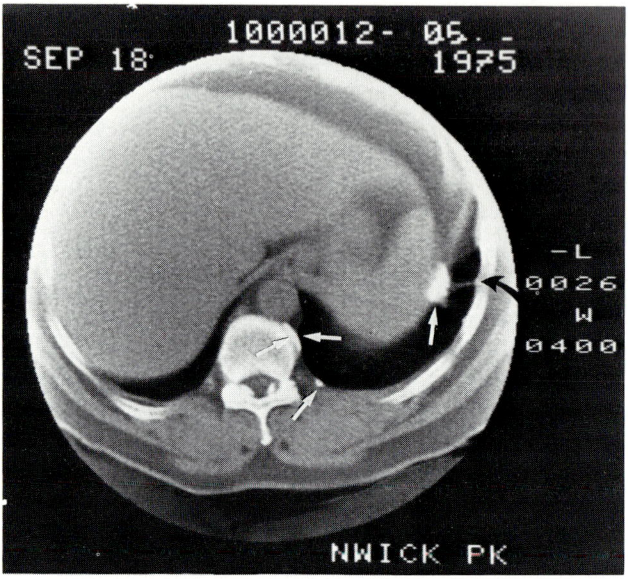

Fig. 13-4. Pleural plaques with calcification (white arrows) and a small adhesion intersecting the costo–phrenic angle (black arrow). Only one plaque was visible on the chest radiograph.

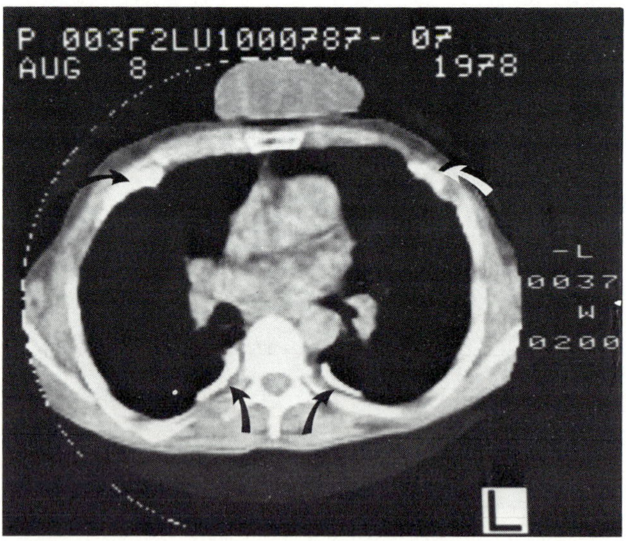

Fig. 13-5. Multiple calcified pleural plaques (arrows) quite easily visible on the chest radiograph.

ential nature is immediately obvious on axial sections (Fig. 13-6). Thick, white inner lines indicating calcification are also often present (Fig. 13-7).

Soft tissue bands that suggest pleural tags and are associated with plaques sometimes become clearly visible in the costo–phrenic angles (Fig. 13-4). Diaphragmatic thickening can also be seen along the rib attachments and may even be apparent immediately below the diaphragm. Irregularity of the diaphragmatic (Fig. 13-8) and cardiac margins, as well as attached calcified pleural plaques are common.

In outpatients, pleural effusions have neither been found in association with asbestosis in the early phase of minimal, or simple, soft tissue thickening, nor later, when there is obvious calcification. However, a pleural effusion is usually the first indication of mesothelioma.

Typically, in cases with circumferential pleural thickening, the posterior and lateral margins are most markedly involved towards the base and on the diaphragm with variable internal calcification; the mediastinal margin is usually affected only slightly, if at all (Figs. 13-6 and 7).

Thickening of the Fissures

Axial sections either tend to be in the same plane as the thickened fissures or to cut obliquely across the line of the fissure. Thickening of a fissure will therefore show as a white patch superimposed on the lung

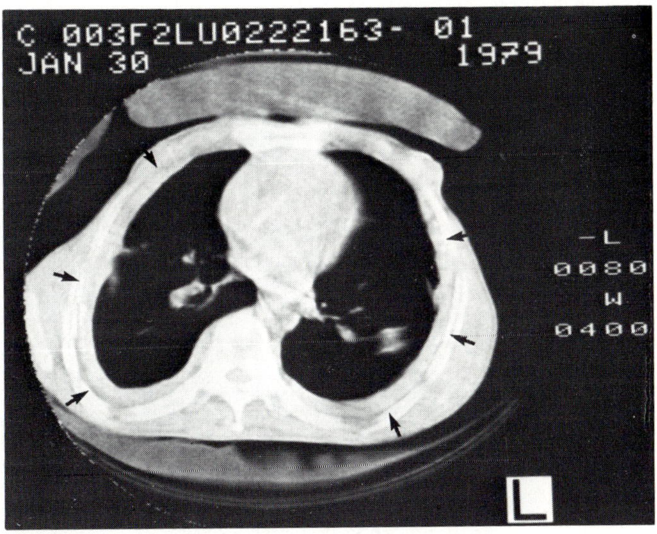

Fig. 13-6. Gross bilateral circumferential pleural thickening, more marked on the right, associated with restrictive abnormalities on lung function tests.

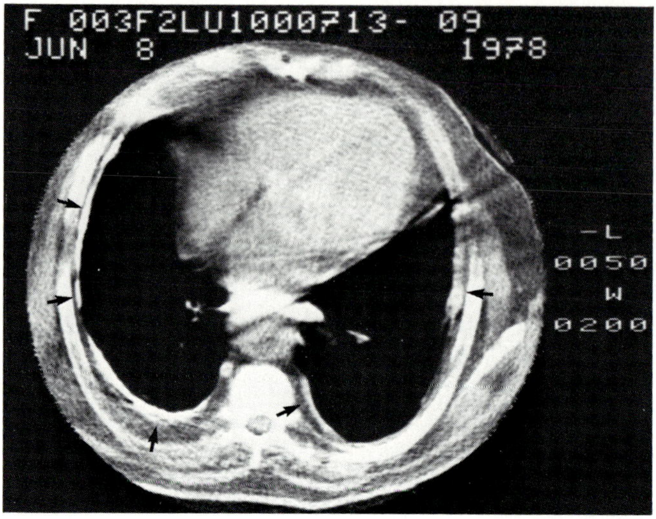

Fig. 13-7. Gross bilateral circumferential pleural thickening with obvious calcification and abnormalities of restrictive lung function.

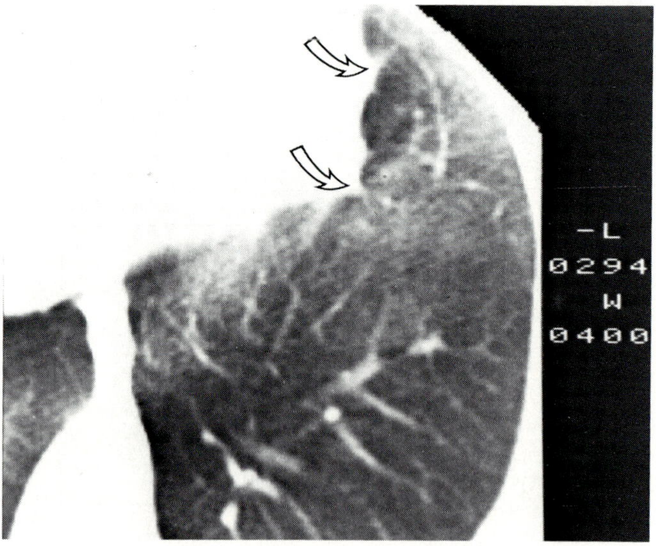

Fig. 13-8. Marked irregularity of the left hemidiaphragm in asbestosis.

field. Only at the thoracic wall or mediastinal margin does beaking and linear thickening appear. The thickened fissure appears as a linear thickening only when it is at right angles to the section. Normally, fissures are not visible, or only barely discernible as thin white lines.

Pulmonary Parenchymal Changes

The typical changes of interstitial fibrosis are seen on sections taken from the base of the lung and appear as a coarse network or "honeycomb" pattern which is superimposed on or replaces the normal branching pulmonary vascular pattern. It may best be observed at narrower window settings (Fig. 13-9). Patchy areas of increased density also occur particularly in juxtaposition to large pleural plaques (Fig. 13-10).

When interstitial fibrosis is present, the lung loses its normal "gravity perfusion" effect, its posterior aspects in the supine position no longer appear denser than the more anterior parts, and its appearance on inspiration differs little or not at all from that on expiration.

Thick white bands intersecting the parenchyma in the basal regions—especially near the diaphragm—are frequently seen in cases of severe, circumferential pleural thickening (Figs. 13-11 and 12).

Bullous formations are easily recognized, showing as low density or black areas devoid of normal lung structure. Bullae were found in a few

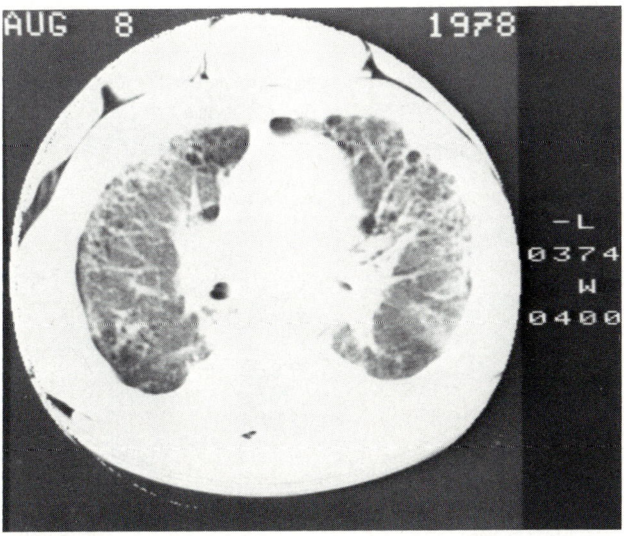

Fig. 13-9. Typical appearances of interstitial fibrosis which appear gross on CT but only slight on conventional chest radiographs.

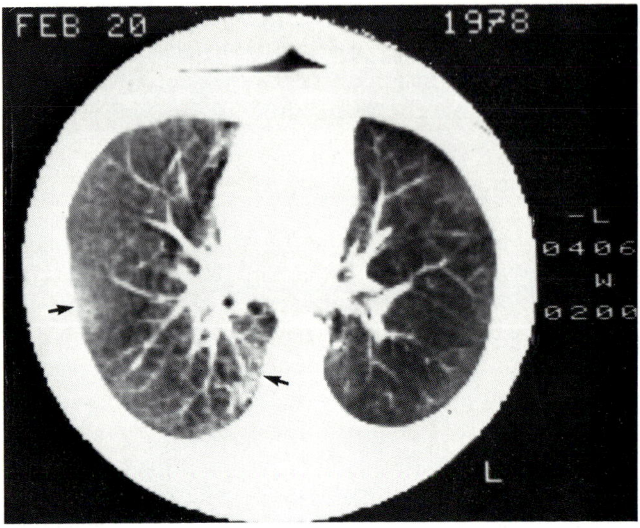

Fig. 13-10. Minimal interstitial fibrosis in two separate areas of the right lung.

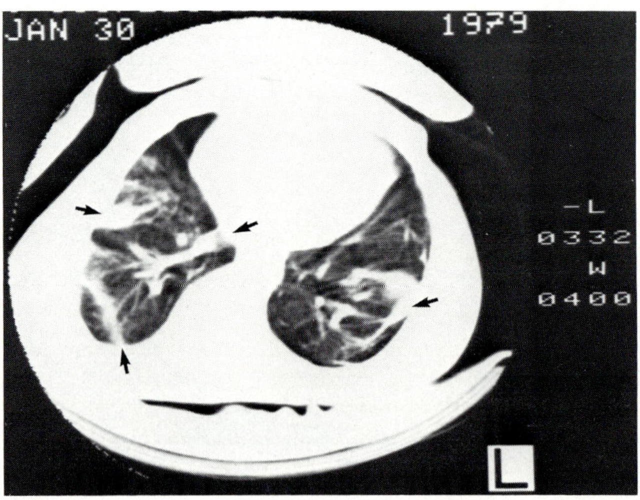

Fig. 13-11. Thick intersecting bands associated with marked pleural thickening in asbestosis.

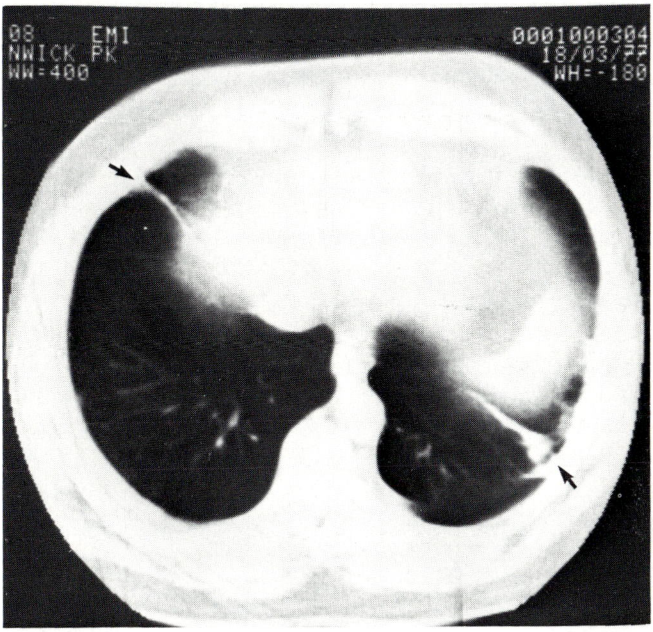

Fig. 13-12. Thick bands at the diaphragmatic level associated with asbestosis.

cases of asbestosis, but unlike the fibrosis occurring with silicosis, they were not a special feature.

Except in the case of tuberculous pleurisy, whose effects may stimulate the formation of asbestotic plaques, traces of old, unrelated diseases such as healed pulmonary tuberculosis, particularly at the apices, are easily recognized. However, adjacent localized pulmonary fibrosis is invariably present with tuberculous pleural thickening and is continuous and more marked at the upper lobes and apices. No plaques are strictly confined to the inner margin of a rib.

CT Signs of Mesothelioma

Unilateral pleural effusions are usually the earliest sign of mesothelioma, but there is nothing specific about their appearance. At the first signs of pleural effusion, careful examination may reveal the presence of asbestotic pleural plaques.

The characteristic feature of mesothelioma is the marked thickening and irregularity of the pleura. This thickening also extends onto the mediastinum and is associated with the contraction or diminished size of the hemithorax on the affected side. Unlike a pleural effusion, it does not change in shape or position with the patient lying decubitus (Fig. 13-13).

The pleural effusion and the irregular pleural thickening can occur together, either on opposite sides or on the same side (Fig. 13-14). By suitable positioning, the irregular tumorous pleural thickening can be distinguished from the effusion. This fact is particularly important in assessing the effects of treatment.

At the base of the pleural thickening, adjacent to the thoracic wall margin, a thick white line is often barely visible, suggesting residual basal calcification. Asbestotic pleural plaques may be seen in the ipsilateral hemithorax.

Local thoracic wall enlargement due to tumour infiltration at the site of pleural fluid aspiration has been noted in association with both local rib destruction and expansion and large, localized nodular calcifications within mesothelioma tissue (Fig. 13-15).

Tumor infiltration of a fissure shows as a marked irregular thickening. Peripheral (Fig. 13-16) as well as more central pulmonary nodules, which

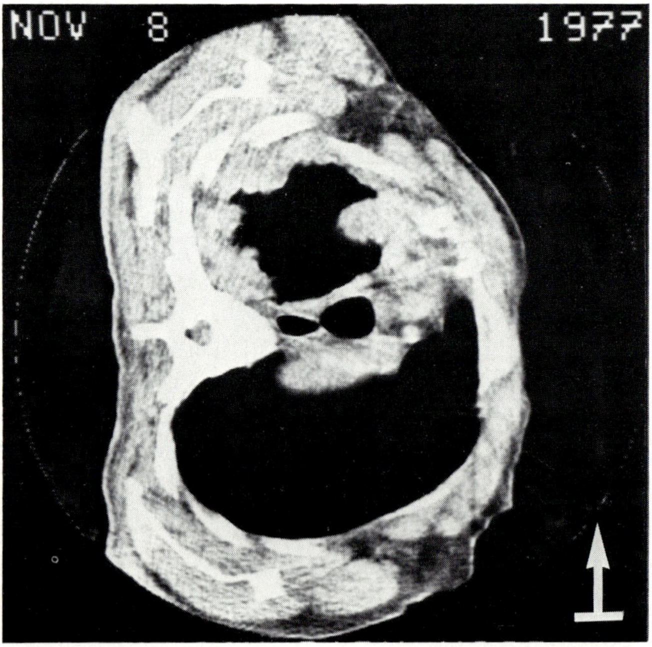

Fig. 13-13. Mesothelioma of the right hemithorax shown in the left decubitus position. Unlike a pleural effusion the "thickening" is unaltered by position.

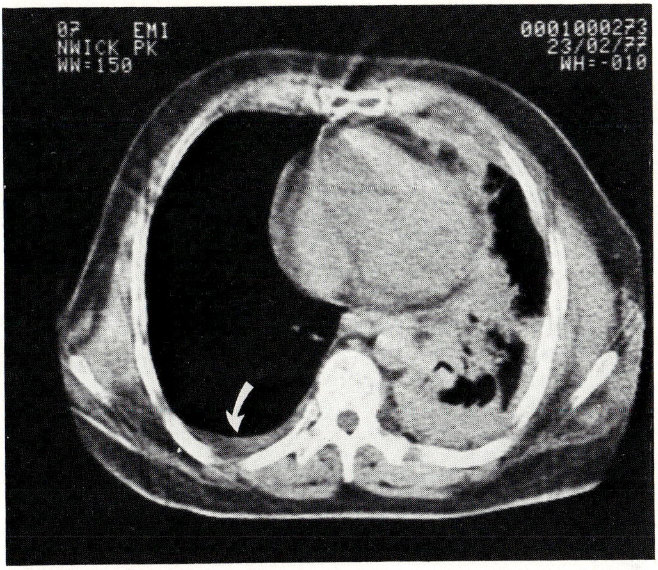

Fig. 13-14. Mesothelioma at the left base and a pleural effusion on the right (arrow).

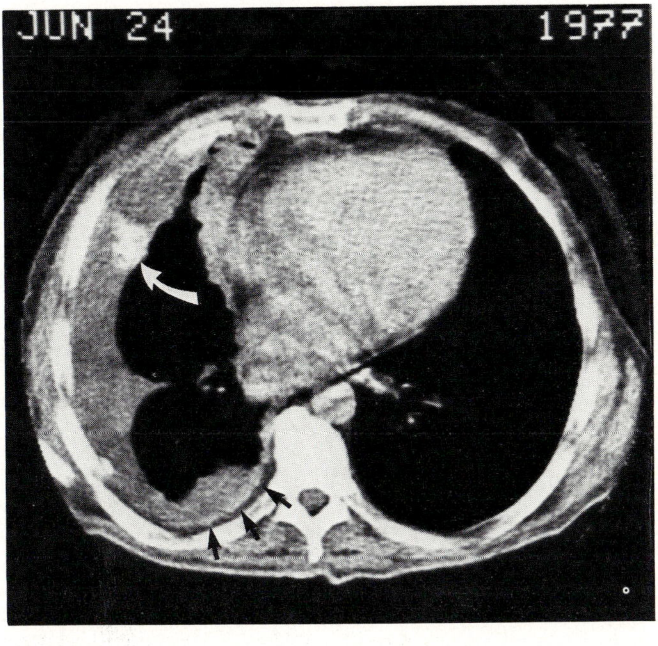

Fig. 13-15. Mesothelioma with a large calcified area (white arrow) and minimal residual basal calcification (black arrow).

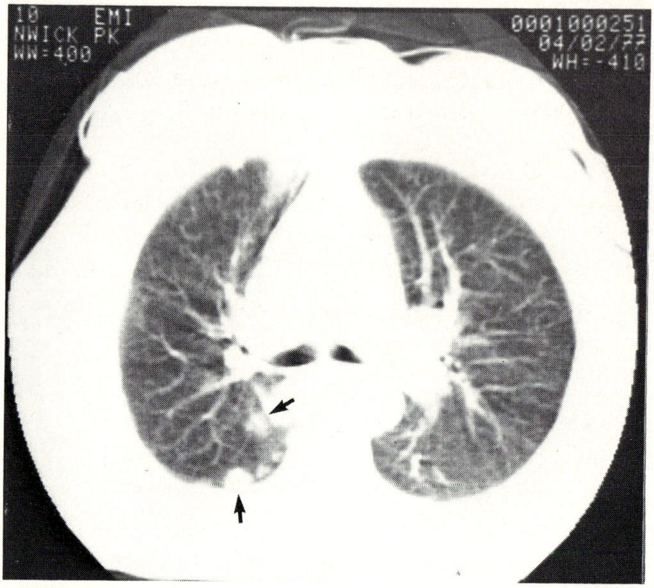

Fig. 13-16. Subpleural and intrapulmonary nodules in mesothelioma.

indicate metastases, are also apparent and have been noted in the contralateral lung as well.

A COMPARISON OF CONVENTIONAL CHEST RADIOGRAPHS AND CT

The findings in CT and conventional chest radiographs[16,17] show that, by and large, CT is a more sensitive indication of the disease process, but that there is major disagreement in a small number of cases.

Pleural plaques may be demonstrated on CT when they are still too small to be seen on chest radiographs. Furthermore, their presence is unequivocal since there are no confusing "companion shadows" and internally-protruding intercostal muscles are clearly visible. Calcified plaques and small calcifications in plaques can be clearly distinguished even when only 2–3 mm. in length.

Interstitial fibrosis is much more obvious on CT. When minimal interstitial changes are present on CT they are not visible on chest films, particularly when unilateral or adjacent to pleural plaques.

The chest radiograph has, however, a major advantage in showing thick fissures much more clearly than CT.

THE INCIDENTAL FINDING OF PLEURAL PLAQUES

In a number of cases pleural plaques were discovered in patients undergoing CT examinations for apparently unrelated conditions, particularly colon carcinoma. In several of these cases a clear-cut history of occupational exposure to asbestos was subsequently obtained. At present, the numbers involved are far too small to justify any generalized conclusions, but investigations are continuing. CT could certainly prove to be a method of establishing whether there is a significant correlation between asbestotic pleural plaque formation and abdominal cancer—in particular, colon carcinoma.

THE ROLE OF CT IN ASBESTOSIS AND MESOTHELIOMA DETECTION AND TREATMENT

However sensitive CT appears to be in detecting the changes associated with asbestosis, it is unlikely to replace chest radiography as a screening procedure, being less readily-available, more time-consuming and considerably more expensive. Furthermore, conventional chest radiography, with lateral and oblique views, detects the vast majority of changes. However, in cases of doubt or where medical–legal aspects are involved, CT is likely to produce a much more exact definition of the disease process and provide a more definite answer of normality.

CT is particularly valuable in monitoring the progress of mesothelioma and in assessing the effects of treatment in unexplained pleural effusions. The irregular pleural thickening of mesothelioma may be shown with CT, but diagnosis is much more likely to be made by needle biopsy.

SUMMARY AND CONCLUSIONS

The literature on asbestosis and mesothelioma recognizes the important role that chest radiographs have played in detection of exposure to asbestos; the abnormal radiological signs have been recognized and defined. There is, in general, substantial agreement between the radiology and the pathology. Interstitial fibrosis, however, when visible on chest radiographs, is associated with considerable impairment of lung function. Difficulties involved in the early detection of pleural plaques are recognized, and restrictive lung function can occur due to pleurisy *en cuirasse*.

CT shows most of the signs of asbestosis early and more clearly, but it is not applicable as a screening procedure, being too time-consuming and too expensive. However, in cases of doubt or for medical–legal purposes it could have an important role. It is a particularly important technique in demonstrating very early plaque formation and early interstitial fibrosis.

REFERENCES

1. Anton HC: Multiple pleural plaques: Part II. British J of Radiology 41:341–348, 1968
2. Cauna D, Totten RS, Gross P: Asbestos bodies in human lungs at autopsy. JAMA 192 (5):371–373, 1965
3. Edge JR, Choudhury SL: Malignant mesothelioma of the pleura in Barrow–inFurness. Thorax 33:26–30, 1978
4. Freundlich IM, Greening RR: Asbestosis and associated medical problems. Radiology 89:224–229, 1967
5. Frost J, Georg J, Moller PF: Asbestosis with pleural calcification among insulation workers. Danish M Bull 3:202–204, 1956
6. Gerbis H, Ucko M: Über Asbestosis. Dtsch Med Wochenschr 58:285, 1932
7. Gloyne SR: Pathology, Silicosis and Asbestosis. London, Oxford Medical Publications, 1938
8. Hourihane DO, Lessof L, Richardson PC: Hyaline and calcified pleural plaques as an index of exposure to asbestos: A study of radiological and pathological features of 100 cases with a consideration of epidemiology. British Med J 1:1069–1074, 1966
9. Hourihane DO: The pathology of mesotheliomata and an analysis of their association with asbestos exposure. Thorax 19:268–278, 1964
10. Hunter D: The Diseases of Occupations: Sixth Edition. London, Hodder and Stoughton, 1978
11. Hurwitz MD: Roentgenologic aspects of asbestosis. Am J of Roentgenology 85:256–262, 1961
12. Jacob G, Bohlig H: Die rontgenologischen Komplikationen der Lungenasbestose. Fortschr Geb Rontgenstrahlen 83:515–525, 1955
13. Kilivuoto R: Pleural calcification as a roentgenologic sign of non-occupational endemic anthophyllite—asbestosis. Acta radiol (Stockh) Suppl 194, 1960
14. Kreel L: The EMI whole body scanner: An interim clinical evaluation of the prototype. Br J Clin Equipment 4:220–227, 1976
15. Kreel L: Computed tomography of the lung and pleura: Seminars in roentgenology XIII (3):213–225, 1978
16. Kreel L: Computer tomography in the elevation of pulmonary asbestosis. Acta Radiol (Diagn) (Stockh) 17:405–412, 1976
17. Katz D, Kreel L: Computed tomography in pulmonary asbestosis. Clinical Radiology 30:207–213, 1979
18. Kruger E, Rostoski O, Saupe E: Uber lungenasbestose. Arch Gewer-be-path. Gewer Behyg 2:558, 1931
19. Lawson JP: Pleural calcification as a sign of asbestosis. Clinical Radiology 14:414–417, 1963
20. Leathart GL: Clinical, bronchographic, radiological & physiological observations in ten cases of asbestosis. Brit J Industrial Medicine 17:213–225, 1960
21. Merewether ERA, Price CW: Report on effects of asbestos dust on the lungs and dust suppression in the asbestos industry. London, HMSO, 1930
22. Sargent EN, Jacobson G, Wilkinson EE: Diaphragmatic pleural calcification following

short occupational exposure to asbestos. Am J Roentgenology Radium Ther Nucl Med 115:473–478, 1972

23. Schneider L, Wimpfheimer F: Multiple progressive calcification: pleural plaque formation. JAMA 189 (4):328–330, 1964
24. Seiler HE: A case of pneumoconiosis: Result of the inhalation of asbestos dust. British Med J 2:982, 1928
25. Selikoff IJ: Personal communication quoted by Sargent EN, et al., 1972
26. Simon G: Principles of Chest X-ray Diagnosis. London, Butterworths, 1971, p 151
27. Smith AR: Pleural calcification resulting from exposure to certain dusts. Am J Roentgenology 67:375–382, 1952
28. Solomon A: Radiology of asbestosis. Environ Research 3:320–329, 1970
29. Soutar CA, Simon G, Turner-Warwick M: The radiology of asbestos-induced disease of the lungs. Brit J of Diseases of the Chest 68:235–252, 1974
30. Wagner JC, Sleggs CA, Marchand P: Diffuse pleural mesothelioma and asbestos exposure in the North Western Cape Province. Brit J Industrial Med 17:260–270, 1960

Henry A. Anderson
Irving J. Selikoff

14 Asbestos-Associated Radiographic Changes Among Household Contacts of Amosite Asbestos Workers*

In growing numbers, toxic industrial agents are being detected in drinking water, urban air, and food sources. The halogenated hydrocarbons, [1,1,1-tri-chloro-2,2-bis (4-chlorophenyl) ethane] (DDT) and polychlorinated biphenyl (PCB) have spread into the general environment to such an extent that they can now be detected in the adipose tissue of many persons in the United States. Equally ubiquitous and widely used in industry is asbestos.

Asbestos pollution, a recently noted phenomenon, is associated with the rapid expansion of asbestos materials during and after World War II.[1] An extremely versatile mineral, the pervasiveness of its use is reflected in

*Research discussed in this chapter was supported by a Center grant from the National Institute of Environmental Health Sciences ES 00928 and a grant from the National Cancer Institute, CA 22791.

The authors are grateful for the valuable assistance given by Dr. Ruth Lilis, Dr. Susan Daum, Dr. AIF Fischbein and other colleagues in the Environmental Sciences Laboratory in conducting the clinical studies and interpreting the x-rays, and to our field survey staff, including Mrs. Dorothy Perron, Mr. Charles Nolan, Mrs. Rayla Margoles, Mrs. Stella Przybyla and Mrs. Shirley Levine. We wish to thank the staff of the Computer Center of The City University of New York for their support in providing computer time and assistance; Mrs. Selma Annenberg and Mrs. Valerie Josephson for preparation of tables and manuscript and Mr. Rupert Fuller for photographs of the chest x-rays.

the Department of Health, Education and Welfare's estimate that 1.5 to 2.5 million full- or part-time workers are currently exposed to asbestos and that 8 to 11 million workers have been exposed since the beginning of World War II.[2]

Asbestos fibers may be freed and enter the general environment while being processed or used in manufacturing, construction or demolition. Air in urban, as compared with isolated rural areas may have 10 to 1,000 times the concentration of such fibers.[3] Using electron microscope examination and tissue ashing techniques, chrysotile asbestos can be identified in the lungs of virtually all urban U.S. residents.[4]

Another specific pollution problem (which, however, can be more easily controlled or eliminated) is contamination of the home environment. Wives experience exposure to chemicals and dusts when laundering contaminated work clothes. Other household residents may also be exposed to the gradual accumulation of industrial materials shed daily from a laborer's dirty shoes and work clothes and subsequently circulated and suspended in the air. The potential health risk of such exposures is only beginning to be recognized.

Second to occupational exposure, household contact is the most frequently identified source of asbestos exposure among reported mesothelioma cases.[5] Vianna and Polan[6] reviewed 52 cases of mesothelioma among women in New York State; ten were known to have had husbands or fathers who had worked in an asbestos trade. Compared to a matched control population, an estimated relative risk factor of ten was calculated for women with this type of exposure. Despite the reports of *mesothelioma* among persons having household contact with asbestos workers, few attempts have been made to assess the prevalence of *other* asbestos-related diseases.

CHARACTERISTICS OF ASBESTOS-ASSOCIATED DISEASE

Asbestosis (parenchymal fibrosis, pleural fibrosis, pleural calcification) and malignancy (lung cancer, pleural and peritoneal mesothelioma, gastrointestinal cancer) are well recognized hazards of occupational exposure to asbestos. Epidemiologic investigations of these illnesses in heavily exposed occupational groups have defined the important relationships that characterize asbestos-associated disease. Intensity and length of exposure as well as amount of time elapsed from time of exposure were already apparent in Merewether and Price's 1930 report on asbestos.[7] They reported that individuals working in the less dusty areas of asbestos textile mills were less likely to develop parenchymal fibrosis than those working in more dusty areas (ten percent versus 34 percent). Sixty-one percent of individuals with more than 15 years' employment had fibrosis as compared with 20 percent among those employed less than 15 years. None of the workers employed for less than five years in either area showed evidence of fibrosis. Subsequent reports confirmed and refined these observations for both clinical asbestosis and, later, mortality from asbestos-associated malignancies.[8]

Even after excessive dust exposure, sufficient time must be allowed for this chronic disease to become manifest. From the same perspective, adverse effects of brief or low-level exposures are even less likely to become apparent rapidly. Insufficient elapsed time from first exposure, when evaluating exposures, will lead to underestimates of risk. Because duration of employment and elapsed time from onset parallel each other and provide a composite effect, independent effects are often difficult to appreciate. Seidman et al.[9] analyzed lung cancer deaths among individuals who had worked in an amosite asbestos factory for varying periods between 1941 and 1954, and had had no subsequent or previous asbestos exposure. They found that a group with only one month of exposure began to show excessive lung cancer deaths after 30 years had elapsed from first exposure. For those with more than one year employment, latency was shortened to 15 years. As the duration and/or intensity of exposure lessens, the period of latency of a particular effect increases.

RADIOGRAPHIC APPEARANCE OF ASBESTOS DISEASE

The ILO U/C International Classification of Radiographs of 1971[10] coupled with the set of standard x-ray films that define the abnormality categories in the Classification, now provide a common language and definition of radiographic abnormalities that should help reduce inter-reader variability and provide more reliable comparisons among epidemiological studies.

Radiodiagnostic characteristics (parenchymal opacities, pleural thickening, pleural calcification, pleural effusion) have played an important role in the recognition of asbestos diseases since the 1930s. Interstitial fibrosis initially appears as an increase of fine reticular markings especially in the lower lung fields. Such opacities, which appear predominately as "irregular opacities" but can also appear as "rounded opacities" in the ILO Classification are not entirely unique to asbestosis. However, given a documented asbestos exposure and the absence of other conditions such as rheumatoid lung, sarcoidosis, scleroderma, radiation fibrosis, Hamman-Rich Syndrome and chronic aspiration pneumonia, which share a similar radiographic appearance but differ in other clinical and past history parameters, such abnormalities can almost certainly be attributed to the asbestos exposure. If asbestos exposure is found concomitant with one of these other diseases, differential diagnosis may be difficult. Fig. 14-1 is an example of asbestosis. Often a minimal increase in opacities goes unnoticed unless standard normal films are used for comparison.

Pleural abnormalities as seen on the chest x-ray, are more unique to asbestos exposure than are the increased reticular markings. Other possible causes of lateral chest wall pleural thickening or discrete pleural plaques on the diaphragm or chest wall, such as post-traumatic pneumothorax or hemothorax, post-thoracotomy changes fibrin balls, or empyema residua, are usually apparent from past medical history and physical examination. A more difficult differential diagnosis is that of early pleural mesothelioma. Rapid enlargement of the pleural thickening is indicative of malignant pleural mesothelioma. Similarly, metastatic malignant disease to the pleura presents a more dynamic course. Fig. 14-2 demonstrates bilateral pleural thickening in the typical scalloped pattern. Fig. 14-3 demonstrates pleural thickening and a diaphragmatic plaque.

Pleural calcification, such as that seen in Fig. 14-4, is often indicative of past asbestos exposure. As with pleural thickening, other explanations for its presence—old tuberculosis infection or trauma, for example—are readily apparent in the past medical history. Less commonly reported

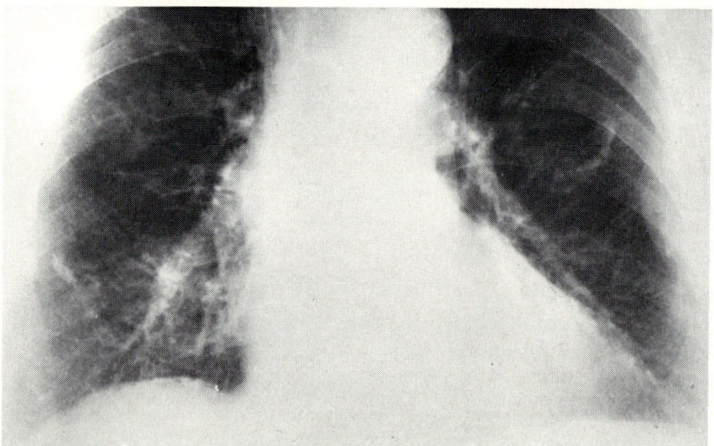

Fig. 14-1A. Sixty-seven year old wife of an amosite asbestos factory worker employed for two years (1942–1944). Never smoked cigarettes. ILO U/C Classification: irregular opacities s 1/1; bilateral chest wall pleural thickening, width b, extent 2; pleural calcification on right diaphragm and both chest walls, Grade 2.

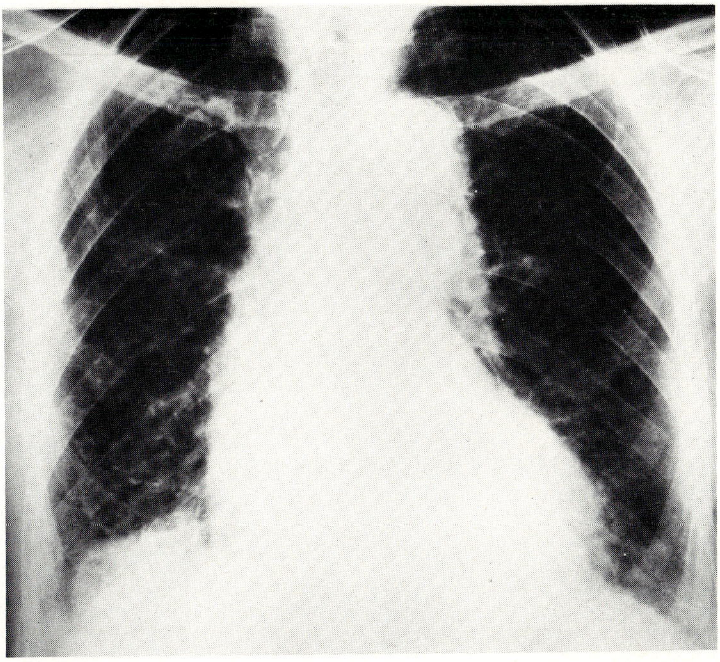

Fig. 14-1B. Sixty-seven year old wife of an amosite asbestos factory worker employed for 2½ years from 1943–1945. Never smoked cigarettes. ILO U/C Classification: irregular opacities s 2/2.

associations with calcification, such as mineral oil aspiration, must also be considered.

In combination, these abnormalities—parenchymal opacities (irregular or rounded) and pleural thickening or calcification—make the radiographic diagnosis of asbestosis virtually certain.

OCCUPATIONAL DISEASES AMONG NON-OCCUPATIONALLY EXPOSED INDIVIDUALS

The occasional appearance of overt disease among residents of neighborhoods in close proximity to factories and individuals having household contacts with workers directly involved in handling toxic materials has been recognized for more than 40 years. Polychlorinated biphenyls, beryllium, lead and asbestos have been responsible for diseases seen among individuals whose only known contact with the offending agent has been indirectly—via a member of or visitor to the household who had handled the material in an industrial setting.[11,12,13,14] The most

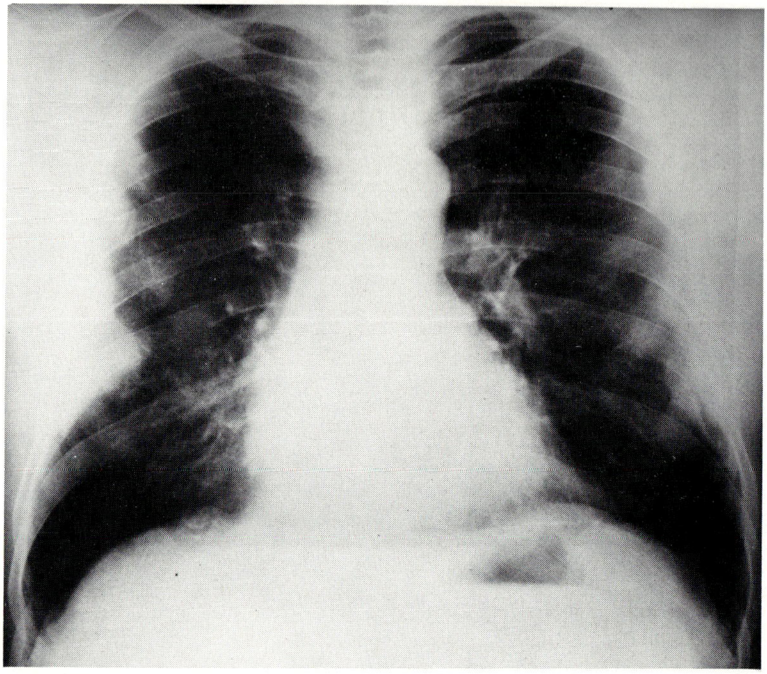

Fig. 14-2A. Forty-six year old son of an amosite asbestos worker employed for eight years from 1942 to 1950. Former cigarette smoker of 1½ packs per day. Employed as an engineer. ILO U/C Classification: irregular opacities s 1/0; bilateral chest wall pleural thickening, width C, extent 2; calcification on diaphragms Grade 1.

frequently described sources of home contamination are the chemicals and dust that adhere to shoes, hair and work clothes brought home for laundering. Some industries now provide change rooms and coveralls but many do not. Even when available, change rooms and showers frequently go unused because workers may not understand the potential long-term hazards and continue to inadvertently expose their unsuspecting families to the materials used and manufactured in their factories.

Case reports of overt disease among family contacts of workers have been frequently considered medical curiosities. The full extent of such risks is not known, for it is uncommon to inquire into the occupation and exposures of a patient's household contacts when investigating the symptoms of a disease. In all likelihood, most family exposure disease, especially with mild or sub-clinical manifestations which may only be contributory to a current health problem, goes unrecognized.

Because environmental exposures to asbestos are generally of low

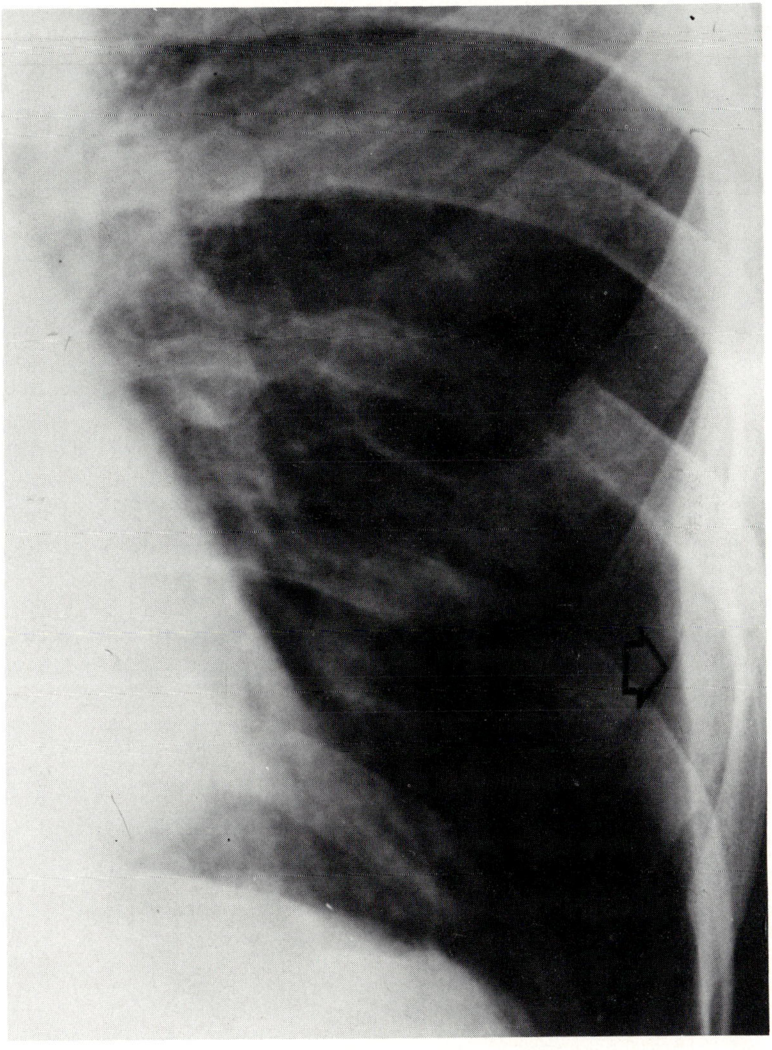

Fig. 14-2B. Thirty-one year old son of an amosite asbestos factory worker employed for six years (1948–1954). Two pack per day cigarette smoker. Employed in printing ink manufacturing plant. ILO U/C Classification: bilateral chest wall pleural thickening, width b, extent 2.

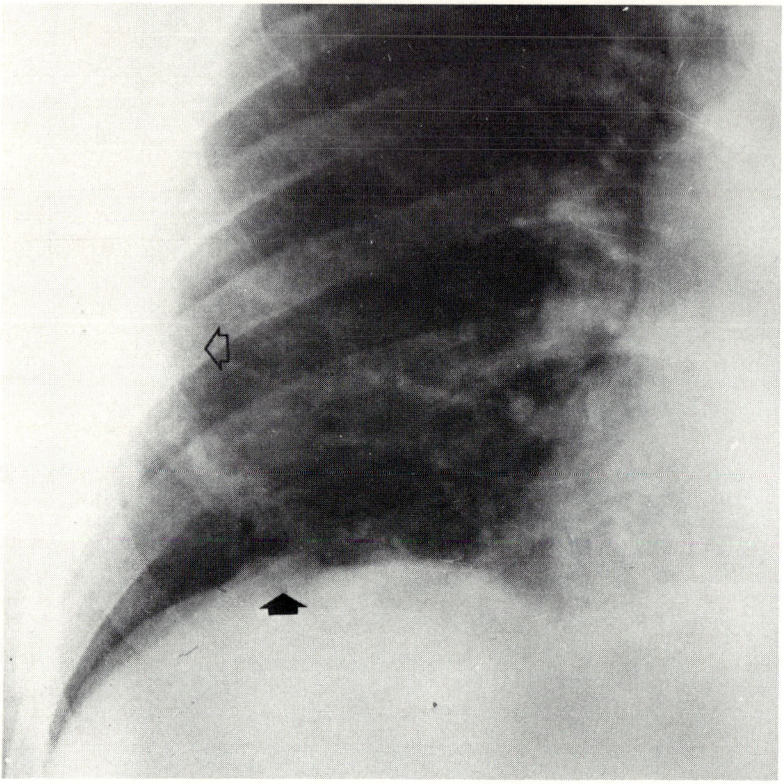

Fig. 14-3. Forty-six year old son of an amosite asbestos factory worker employed for six months in 1942–1943 (brother of individual in Figure 4). Never smoked cigarettes. Tire salesman for 32 years. ILO U/C Classification: irregular opacities p 1/1; bilateral pleural thickening extent 2; pleural plaques on both diaphragms.

intensity, effects would be expected to appear only after 20, 30 or more years. Unfortunately, because of this unusually long period of clinical latency, many of the consequences of today's exposures will not be detectable or quantifiable until well into the next century. On the other hand, health effects of environmental asbestos exposures that occurred in the 1940s would be expected to be seen now.

With the exception of pleural calcification, which was frequently reported as an incidental observation because of its striking appearance and novelty, few general surveys have provided data that can establish a general background prevalence of the x-ray abnormalities associated with asbestos exposure. Table 14-1 summarizes several large studies. In over 900,000 x-rays reviewed, pleural calcification was found in an average of

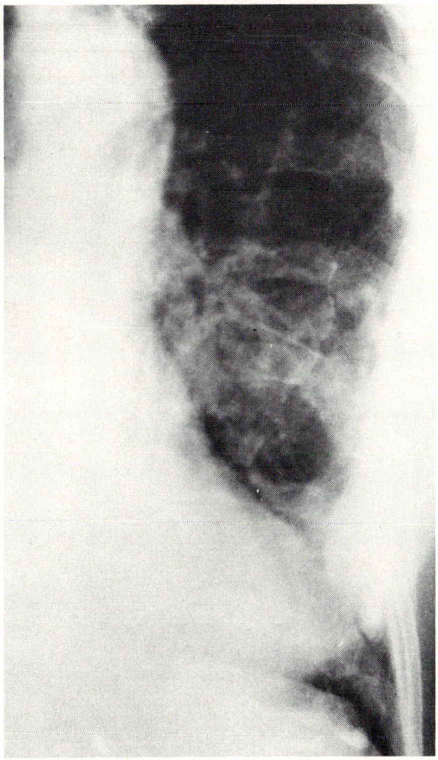

Fig. 14-4. Sixty-two year old wife of an amosite asbestos worker employed for two years, 1941–1943. One-half pack per day cigarette smoker. ILO U/C Classification: irregular opacities p 2/2; bilateral chest wall pleural thickening extent 2; bilateral chest wall and diaphragm calcifications Grade 3.

two of 1,000 x-rays. Pleural thickening and parenchymal fibrosis as described today, although accepted as uncommon, were not commonly reported; a broad base for statistical comparison is not, then, readily available.

Pleural calcification is noticeably more prevalent in surveys where non-occupational or environmental exposures to asbestos have been recognized. Table 14-2 summarizes several such environmentally exposed populations. The studies of Zolov and Bourilkov and Yazicioglu et al.[17,18] considered exposure from asbestos indigenous to the soil and rock outcroppings of the geographical areas examined. Kiviluoto[16] and Navratil[19] studied populations living in neighborhoods and districts with active asbestos mines and manufacturing facilities. Table 14-3 lists the spectrum seen in occupational groups. Comparing the three tables it is evident that when the prevalence of pleural calcification increases, asbestos exposure can be identified.

Radiographic abnormalities associated with asbestos exposure offer an opportunity to identify and evaluate past asbestos exposure in terms of one set of biologic effects, i.e., radiographic change. Unfortunately,

Table 14-1
Prevalence of Radiographic Abnormalities Among Survey Populations Without Easily Recognizable Asbestos Exposures

Author	Country	Total Examined	Pleural calcification	Parenchymal fibrosis
Floyd & Hepburn (1939)	U.S.A.	115,000	28 (0.02%)	Not reported
Neef (1963)	East Germany	111,069	36 (0.03%)	Not reported
Marsova (1964)	Czechoslovakia	44,549	241 (0.54%)	None
Hourihane (1966)	Great Britain	27,500	36 (0.13%)	7 (0.03%)
Raunio (1966)	Finland	631,000	1,516* (0.24%)	1

* Includes some with environmental exposure.

Table 14-2
Prevalence of Radiographic Abnormalities Among Survey Populations with Environmental and Neighborhood Asbestos Exposure

Author	Country	Total Examined	Pleural calcification	Parenchymal fibrosis
Kiviluoto (1960)	Finland	6,312	499 (7.9%)	Some
Zolov (1967)	Bulgaria	3,429	175 (5.1%)	7 (0.2%)
Yazicioglu (1976)	Turkey	5,989	288 (5%)	Not reported

Table 14-3
Prevalence of Radiographic Abnormalities Among Occupationally Exposed Workers in the United States

Author	Type of exposure	Number examined	Pleural calcification	Parenchymal fibrosis
Siegel (1943)	Talc workers	221	14 (6.3%)	31 (14%)
Selikoff (1965)	Insulation workers with >30 years exposure	315	137 (43%)	283 (90%)
	Insulation workers with <30 years exposure	802	13 (2%)	259 (32%)
Anderson (1978)	Insulation workers with >30 years exposure	113	37 (32%)	79 (70%)
	Insulation workers with <30 years exposure	539	24 (4%)	149 (20%)

radiological techniques are not sufficiently sensitive to detect asbestos-associated disease before a clinical latency period of 20, 30 or more years. Other means of determining earlier physiologic responses are needed.

RADIOGRAPHIC ABNORMALITIES AMONG HOUSEHOLD CONTACTS OF ASBESTOS FACTORY WORKERS

Navratil[19] studied factory workers, residents of a factory neighborhood, household contacts of the workers, and an unexposed control population in Czechoslovakia. Table 14-4 summarizes the results of that survey. Household contacts had a greater prevalence of pleural calcification than did the control. The population studied was small and only four

Table 14-4
Prevalence of Pleural Calcifications in Populations with Different Sources of Exposure to Asbestos in Czechoslovakia*

General non-exposed population	8,133	28 (0.34%)
Blood relatives of factory workers	114	4 (3.5%)
Neighborhood residents of asbestos factory	155	9 (5.8%)
Factory workers	755	42 (5.3%)

* Navratil et al. 1972.

abnormal individuals were reported. Similar exposures occurred in the United States. Since the 1930s the number has grown sufficiently to warrant investigation of this potential public health issue.

For more than 20 years workers employed for varying periods of time from 1941 to 1954 in a factory producing amosite asbestos products have been under clinical observation by one of us (IJS.) The group first employed (1941–1945) is known to have suffered excessive deaths due to lung, gastrointestinal, and mesothelioma malignancies, as well as asbestosis.[23] Table 14-5 summarizes the mortality experience of that group. In

Table 14-5
Expected and Observed Deaths Among 933 Amosite Asbestos Factory Workers Employed 1941–1945, Observed to December 31, 1977

	Deaths 1941–1977		
	*Expected**	*Observed*	*Ratio*
Total Deaths	368.62	594	1.61
Cancer all sites	73.35	195	2.66
Lung cancer	19.16	100	5.22
Pleural mesothelioma	a	8	—
Peritoneal mesothelioma	a	8	—
Gastrointestinal cancer	21.55	32	1.48
All other cancer	32.64	47	1.44
Asbestosis	a	30	—
Other non-infectious respiratory disease	8.47	19	2.24
All other causes	286.80	350	1.22

* Expected deaths based upon age-specific death rate data for New Jersey white males in corresponding years.

[a] Death rates not available, but these have been rare causes of death in the general population.

the course of periodic clinical evaluations of these workers, four pleural mesotheliomas were reported among their household contacts.[1]

In 1973, we began a clinical survey of the household contacts of these workers who could be identified as being resident in the workers' households during the period of their active asbestos employment. All identified individuals were invited to participate in a special clinical study. We have so far examined 776 of these household contacts. The examination included comprehensive occupational and residential histories, past and current medical histories, histories of current symptoms, smoking and respiratory questionnaires, physical examination, 14 in. × 17 in. postero–anterior and right and left oblique chest x-rays, and spirometry. Of the 776 examined, 685 had not had personal occupational exposure to asbestos and were household members at the time the factory workers were actively employed in the factory. The remaining 91 individuals were placed for analytical purposes in a separate category as outlined in Table 14-6.

For comparison purposes in the chest x-ray evaluation, a control population of urban New Jersey residents, living in the same community as the study population, was identified in the general medical clinic at the facility used to examine the workers and household members. Controls were matched for age and sex. Clinical records were reviewed, and none of the controls had recorded occupational or household contact with asbestos.

The chest x-rays of household contacts, factory workers and controls were interspersed and read without knowledge of exposure category. The ILO U/C Pneumoconioses Classification of 1971 was utilized by a panel of five experienced readers.

Table 14-6
Individuals Examined But Who Did Not Meet Study Criteria

Exclusion criteria	Number examined
Personal occupational exposure to asbestos*	51
Entered household after active worker asbestos employment ceased	40
Total	91

*	
Direct asbestos trade	19
Brake repair work	8
Dry wall taper	1
Shipyard trade	6
Job includes work with asbestos	16
Silica exposure	1
	51

Table 14-7 summarizes the overall results by exposure category. A film was classified as abnormal if one or more of the following abnormalities was recorded: irregular opacities of 1/0 or more; any lateral wall pleural thickening; any pleural calcification; pleural plaques on the diaphragm. It is interesting to note that of the children born shortly after the workers ceased active employment in the plant, but while the family still lived in the same house, six had abnormal x-rays. This would suggest that sufficient asbestos continued to be present in the home atmosphere to cause an increase of x-ray abnormality 30 years later.

As expected, individuals with personal occupational exposure to asbestos in addition to household exposure had the highest prevalence of abnormalities.

Table 14-8 summarizes the types of individual abnormalities seen among the 685 household contacts. Pleural abnormalities were predominant. No instances of pleural calcification were seen among the controls, while 8.5 percent of the study group had calcification present. In all abnormality categories, the household contacts had a statistically significantly higher rate of abnormality.

Given sufficient elapsed time from first exposure, it is apparent that for environmental and other low-level asbestos exposures, radiographic appearance of disease is predominantly pleural. In general, the presence of pleural change is of considerable significance and, when present, possible asbestos exposure should be investigated. The presence of the more "classical" appearance of asbestosis, with apparent parenchymal fibro-

Table 14-7
Prevalence of Radiographic Abnormalities Associated with Asbestos Exposure Among Household Members of Amosite Asbestos Workers

Exposure group	Total examined	One or more radiographic abnormalities present*	
New Jersey urban residents**	326	15 (5%)	$\chi^2 = 7.1$ $p < .01$ (rows 1–2)
Entered household after active worker employment ceased†	40	6 (15%)	
Household resident during active worker employment†	685	240 (35%)	$\chi^2 = 6.8$ $p < .01$ (rows 2–3)
Household resident and personal occupational asbestos exposure	51	23 (45%)	

* ILO U/C Pneumoconiosis Classification categories: irregular opacities 1/0 or greater; pleural thickening; pleural calcification; pleural plaques.

** No known direct occupational or household exposure to asbestos.

† No known direct occupational exposure to asbestos.

Table 14-8
A Matched Comparison Group: Chest X-ray Abnormalities Among 685 Household Contacts of Amosite Asbestos Workers and 326 Individual Residents in Urban New Jersey

Group	Total examined	Pleural thickening present	Pleural calcification present	Pleural plaques present	Irregular* opacities present
Household contacts of asbestos workers	685	146 (18.8%)	66 (8.5%)	61 (7.9%)	114 (16.6%)
Urban New Jersey residents	326	4 (1.2%)	0 (8.5%)	2 (0.6%)	11 (3.4%)

* ILO U/C Pneumoconioses Classification irregular opacities 1/0 or greater.

Table 14-9
Chest X-ray Abnormalities Among 685 Household Contacts of Amosite Asbestos Workers

Total examined	Number with only pleural abnormalities	Number with only irregular opacities	Number with both pleural and parenchymal abnormalities
685	126 (18%)	61 (9%)	53 (7.7%)

sis, is the exception rather than the rule after environmental exposures. In Table 14-9, the predominance of pleural abnormalities is further demonstrated. Pleural change was the only abnormality present in 18 percent of the cases. In nine percent, only irregular opacities were seen and in 7.7 percent both abnormalities were present. In over half of those with asbestos associated abnormalities, pleural change was the only evidence of exposure.

The actual extent and intensity of each household resident's asbestos exposure is unavailable. To help approximate a relative exposure dose index for each household contact, utilization was made of the employment history of the factory worker in whose household the contact resided. The resident factory worker for each household is referred to as the "index worker."

The importance of sufficient elapsed time from onset is demonstrated in Table 14-10. The length of index worker employment for both groups was roughly the same. Thirty-eight percent of the group with exposure beginning prior to 1945 had abnormalities, compared to 27 percent for those whose first exposure was after 1945.

Table 14-10
Prevalence of Chest X-ray Abnormalities in Household Contacts by Year of Onset of Exposure of Index Workers

Year of first exposure	Total examined	Number with abnormalities
Before 1945	403*	152 (38%)
1945 and after	244	67 (27%)

Prevalence of x-ray abnormalities significantly greater among those exposed before 1945 compared to those first exposed after 1945.

$$\chi^2 = 7.1 \quad p < .01$$

* Thirty-four individuals with more than ten years of exposure are excluded from this table. The distribution of duration of exposure of individuals in each of the groups was then identical.

Table 14-11
Prevalence of X-ray Abnormalities in Household Contacts by Duration of Employment of Index Amosite Asbestos Workers

Duration of employment	Number examined	Pleural abnormality present	Irregular opacities present	One or more abnormalities present
Less than 1 year	314	46 (15%)	46 (15%)	81 (26%)
1–5 years	288	90 (31%)	46 (16%)	110 (38%)
5–10 years	46	26 (57%)	14 (30%)	29 (63%)
10+ years	35	16 (46%)	8 (23%)	19 (54%)

Prevalence of abnormal chest x-rays is significantly greater among those with index workers with longer duration of employment.

$\chi^2 = 34.6 \quad df = 3 \quad p < .001$

Similarly, the importance of duration of exposure, in this case the length of the index workers' employment, is clearly seen in Table 14-11. Abnormalities were significantly more prevalent among those associated with index workers with a longer duration of employment. The most striking increment of abnormality prevalence is seen in pleural changes, which were three times as prevalent among those with ten years of exposure than among those with less than one year. These tables demonstrate the time dynamics for the appearance of radiographic abnormalities after this type of environmental exposure. Serial observations of this cohort will provide additional information concerning the interaction of length of exposure and lapsed time from onset of exposure. Tables 14-12, 13, and 14 give the distribution of parenchymal and pleural abnormalities recorded in ILO U/C Classification categories. In most cases, the abnormalities seen were in the lesser categories. Only two individuals had advanced parenchymal fibrosis of a category 2/2. Nineteen individuals had extensive pleural thickening and 10 had extensive pleural calcifica-

Table 14-12
ILO U/C Pneumonoconioses Classification of Irregular Opacities Among 685 Household Contacts of Amosite Asbestos Workers and 326 New Jersey Urban Residents

Total examined	0/0	0/1	1/0	1/1	1/2	2/2
685	406 (59%)	165 (24%)	47 (7%)	61 (9%)	4 (0.6%)	2 (0.3%)
326	288 (88%)	27 (8%	8 (3%)	3 (1%)	0 (0.0%)	0 (0.0%)

Table 14-13
ILO U/C Pneumonoconioses Classification of Pleural Thickening Seen Among 685 Household Contacts of Amosite Asbestos Workers*

Number examined	Extent 1			Extent 2		
	Width					
	a	b	c	a	b	c
685	61 (9%)	40 (6%)	8 (1%)	4 (0.6%)	11 (1.6%)	4 (0.6%)
Total		109 (16%)			19 (3%)	

* Extent 1 = Total length of pleural thickening does not exceed one-half of projection of one lateral chest wall.
Extent 2 = Total length of pleural thickening exceeds one-half of the projection of one lateral chest wall.
Width a = Up to 5 mm thick at widest part of any shadow
b = 5 mm to 10 mm thick at widest part of any shadow
c = over 10 mm thick at widest part of any shadow

tion. Figures 14-1–4 are examples of radiographs demonstrating the types of abnormalities seen.

Dyspnea is the most commonly reported symptom among occupationally exposed asbestos workers. Only 4.7 percent of the family cohort complained of dyspnea. However, those with abnormal x-rays had a significantly higher prevalence of this symptom than those with normal x-rays (7 percent versus 3 percent). Dyspnea was the only symptom statistically associated with abnormal chest x-rays.

Table 14-15 summarizes the clinical abnormalities found and their distribution in relation to x-ray findings. (Chest x-rays were interpreted after the physical examination had been completed.) Although in-

Table 14-14
ILO U/C Classification of Pleural Calcification* Seen Among 685 Household Contacts of Amosite Asbestos Workers

Total examined	Grade 1	Grade 2	Grade 3
685	27 (4%)	17 (3%)	10 (2%)

* Grade 1 = one or more areas of pleural calcification, sum of greatest diameters does not exceed about 2 cm.
Grade 2 = one or more areas of pleural calcification, sum of greatest diameters about 2–10 cm.
Grade 3 = one or more areas of pleural calcification, sum of greatest diameters exceeds 10 cm.

Table 14-15
Distribution of Symptoms and Physical Findings Among 685 Household Contacts of Amosite Asbestos Workers by Chest X-ray Findings

X-ray status	Total examined	Rales[1]	Dyspnea[2]	Cyanosis[3]	Clubbing[4]
Normal	445	14 (3.1%)	15 (3.4%)	0 (0.0%)	1 (0.2%)
Abnormal	240	21 (8.8%)	17 (7.1 %)	4 (1.7%)	4 (1.7%)
Total	685	35 (5.1%)	32 (4.7%)	4 (0.6%)	5 (0.7%)

A statistically higher prevalence of abnormal symptoms and physical findings was seen among individuals with abnormal chest x-rays than among those with normal chest x-rays.

[1] $\chi^2 = 10.1 \quad p < .01$
[2] $\chi^3 = 4.8 \quad p < .05$
[3] $\chi^4 = 7.5 \quad p < .01$
[4] $\chi^5 = 4.5 \quad p < .05$

frequently seen, rales, cyanosis and clubbing were statistically more prevalent among those with abnormal x-rays.

DISCUSSION

The widespread use of asbestos and subsequent release and accumulation of fibers in non-work environments did not occur on a large scale until the mid-1940s. Highly exposed occupational groups were the first to be known to have increased risk of asbestos associated illnesses (asbestosis, pleural and peritoneal mesothelioma, lung cancer). Occupational exposures in the 1940s, 1950s and 1960s have generally been described as excessive. This is certainly true for the occupational groups studied from which clinical latency periods of 15 to 30 years were established.

Appearance of disease has been shown to depend upon duration and intensity of exposure. The greater the exposure, the sooner the disease could be expected to appear and, conversely, the shorter and less intense the exposure, the longer the time before appearance of disease could be demonstrated. Asbestos exposure in the 1940s, which might be expected to have had a clinical latency period up to 40 or more years, only now and in the next ten years may be detected. Household contacts of workers would then constitute a large population whose latency periods would be expected to be longer than those of the workers themselves, due to exposures greater than those of the general population but less than those of the index workers.

Using one measure of asbestos effect, the chest x-ray, we have seen in one well-defined group of 685 household contacts of amosite factory workers that x-ray abnormalities characteristically seen after occupational asbestos exposure, are common. As in occupational groups, an increased duration of exposure was associated with a higher prevalence of abnormalities. As other investigators of environmental exposure asbestos disease have also reported, pleural abnormalities predominated.

We do not yet know the full extent of the disease risk that will be experienced by the other household contacts. Prospective observation of this young cohort (75 percent under age 50) and other similar groups will determine whether an unusual malignancy risk exists in addition to the demonstrated x-ray abnormalities. Continued observation will also help assess whether the presence or absence of pleural disease is of prognostic value in assessing future health risk.

Clinicians and radiologists need to become aware of the possible significance of pleural disease unaccompanied by evidence of parenchymal fibrosis. The presence of such abnormalities should be recorded and reported to the patient. Possible history of exposure to asbestos should be sought. Among household contacts we examined, only a few were aware that they had previously had an abnormal x-ray, although on review abnormalities were often present in past films, when these were available. None had been queried regarding prior exposure to asbestos.

REFERENCES

1. Selikoff IJ: Asbestos disease in the United States, 1918–1975. Rev Fr Mal Respir 4:7–24, 1976
2. Califano Jr JA: Statement. Washington DC, Dept HEW, April 26, 1978
3. Selikoff IJ, Nicholson WJ, Langer AM. Asbestos air pollution. Arch Environ Health 25:1–13, 1972
4. Langer AM, Selikoff IJ, Sastre A: Chrysotile asbestos in the lungs of persons in New York City. Arch Environ Health 22:348–361, 1971
5. Anderson HA, Lilis R, Daum SM, Fischbein AS, Selikoff IJ: Household contact asbestos neoplastic risk. Ann NY Acad Sci 271:311–323, 1976
6. Vianna NJ, Polan AK: Non-occupational exposure to asbestos and malignant mesotheliomas in females. Lancet 1:1061–1063, 1978
7. Merewether ERA: Annual Report, Chief Inspector of Factories and Workshops for England and Wales. London, HM Stationery Office 1933–1934, p 63
8. Selikoff IJ, Lee DHK: Asbestos and Disease. New York, Academic Press, 1978
9. Seidman H, Lilis R, Selikoff IJ: Short-term asbestos exposure and delayed cancer risk. Unpublished presentation, Third Symp Detect Prev Cancer, 1976
10. ILO U/C International Classification of Radiographs of Pneumoconioses. Geneva, International Labour Office, Occupational Safety and Health Series, 1971
11. Selikoff IJ, Churg J, Hammond EC: Asbestos exposure and neoplasia. JAMA 188:22–26, 1964

12. Neef W: Beitseitige Pleuraverkalkungen. Alter Fortschr Geb Roentgenstr Nuklearmed 99:632–638, 1963
13. Marsova D: Beitrag zur Atiologie der Pleuraverkalkungen. Z Tuberk 121:329–334, 1964
14. Hourihane DO'B, Lessof L, Richardson PC: Hyaline and calcified pleural plaques as an index of exposure to asbestos. Br Med J 1:1069, 1964, 1974, 1966
15. Raunio V: Occurrence of unusual pleural calcification in Finland. Ann Med Intern Fenn 55 (Suppl 47), 1966
16. Kiviluoto R: Pleural calcification as a roentgenologic sign of non-occupational endemic anthophyllite-asbestosis. Acta Radiol Suppl 194:1–67, 1960
17. Zolov C, Bourilkov T, Babadjov L: Pleural asbestosis in agricultural workers. Environ Res 1:287–292, 1967
18. Yazicioglu S: Pleural calcification associated with exposure to chrysotile asbestos in southeast Turkey. Chest 70:43–47, 1976
19. Navratil M, Trippe, F: Prevalence of pleural calcification in persons exposed to asbestos dust, and in the general population in the same district. Environ Res 5:210–216, 1972
20. Siegal W, Smith AR, Greenburg L: The dust hazard in tremolite talc mining, including roentgenologic findings in talc workers. Am J Roentgenol Radium Ther [NS] 49:11–29, 1943
21. Selikoff IJ: The occurrence of pleural calcification among asbestos insulation workers. Ann NY Acad Sci 132:351–367, 1965
22. Anderson HA, Selikoff IJ: Pleural reactions to environmental agents. Federation Proceedings 37(11):2496–2500, 1978
23. Selikoff IJ, Hammond EC, Churg J: Carcinogenicity of amosite asbestos. Arch Environ Health 25:183–186, 1972

E. Nicholas Sargent
W. K. C. Morgan

15
Coal Workers' Pneumoconiosis

The first description of the morbid anatomy of coal workers' pneumoconiosis (CWP) was published in 1831 by Gregory.[1] However, no real understanding of the various pathophysiological effects that result from the inhalation of coal dust emerged until the last two to three decades. In the early part of this century, it was observed that coal miners developed radiographic abnormalities that were indistinguishable from those seen in men exposed to silica. Since there is nearly always a small quantity of free silica present in coal mine dust, it was assumed that the silica was responsible for the development of the radiographic opacities in the chest film, and to this day many Europeans still refer to the lung disease that occurs in coal miners as silicosis.

The observation that similar radiographic appearances occurred in coal trimmers first suggested that coal dust in the absence of silica could lead to radiographic abnormalities.[2] A coal trimmer was a special type of stevedore who was responsible for seeing that the coal, which was being loaded into the holds of ships, was evenly distributed. This prevented the ship from developing a list when it put to sea. The coal that was loaded in this fashion had been washed, and was therefore almost free from silica. Thus, it appeared that the presence of silica was unnecessary for the x-ray opacities that were observed in coal miners and trimmers to develop. Further evidence in favor of this point of view came when it was shown that at postmortem, the lungs of coal trimmers who in life had been observed to have opacities on the radiograph, bore no more free silica than did the general population. Subsequently, the inhalation of pure carbon was shown to produce a condition that could not be distinguished either radiologically or pathologically from coal workers' pneumoconiosis.[3]

During the 1930s it was observed that British, and, in particular Welsh coal miners had a death rate from respiratory disease that far exceeded that of the general population. As a result the Medical Research Council of Great Britain organized the Pneumoconiosis Research Unit to investigate and characterize the cause of this increased mortality in coal miners. Following the pioneering work carried out at the Pneumoconiosis Research Unit, which was later supplemented by other studies from Germany, South Africa, Belgium, the USA and elsewhere, a much better understanding of the etiology of respiratory disease in coal miners came to exist.

PATHOLOGY

When coal dust is deposited in the alveoli, it is taken up by the alveolar macrophages, some of which may migrate to the terminal bronchiole. Subsequently, the macrophages are swept up by the mucocilliary escalator to the glottis and either swallowed or expectorated. Other macrophages may migrate with their dust burdens into the interstitium of the lung, and from thence to the lymphatics and regional lymph nodes. Many die, however, and deposit their dust burden. When dust inhalation is prolonged and severe, the clearing mechanisms are overwhelmed and the dead and dying macrophages start to aggregate around the proximal divisions of the respiratory bronchioles. There they discharge their coal dust content. Subsequently, a fine reticulin fibrosis develops around the bronchiolar mantle of coal dust. Later on, the smooth muscle in the bronchiolar wall atrophies and the wall dilates, owing to the mechanical stresses that are exerted upon it. This dilatation, as well as the dilatations of adjacent alveoli, is known as focal emphysema. Often incorporated in the coal mantle is the adjacent bronchiolar artery; occasionally, there is a minor loss of the capillary bed from this encroachment (Fig. 15-1).

Simple coal workers' pneumoconiosis appears in a gross specimen as pin head-sized black opacities, some of which may have a stellate appearance. These aggregates are often referred to as the coal macule and consist for the most part of accumulations of coal dust and a very fine surrounding reticulin fibrosis. As the category of simple coal workers' pneumoconiosis advances from 1 to 2, so the size of the macules increases; often a translucency develops around the center of the aggregate due to a localized focal emphysema (Fig. 15-2).

Complicated pneumoconiosis, or progressive massive fibrosis, appears as large black amorphous masses which are usually situated in one

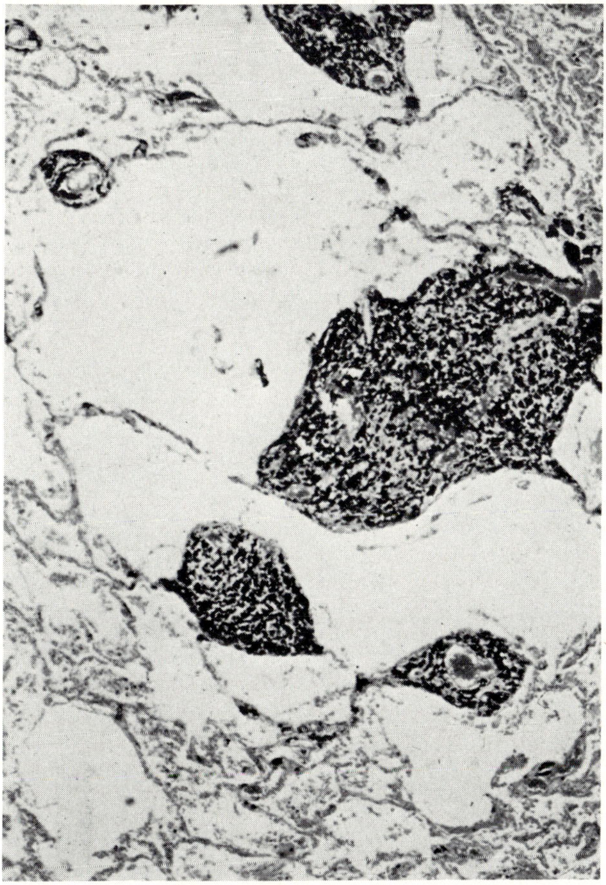

Fig. 15-1. Microscopic section of lung of coal miner. Coal macules surrounded by localized focal emphysema. Coal also deposited around small blood vessels.

or both upper lobes. The remainder of the lung usually shows changes typical of simple coal workers' pneumoconiosis as well as quite severe dilatation and destruction of alveoli resulting from panlobular emphysema (Fig. 15-3).

Progressive massive fibrosis begins as a 1 cm. mass that slowly enlarges. Unlike silicosis, in which the large conglomerate lesion is formed by the aggregation of multiple smaller nodules, the lesion of coal workers' pneumoconiosis consists of an amorphous black mass (often with a liquid core) which is surrounded by collagenous fibrous tissue. The center of the lesion of progressive massive fibrosis, however, is not

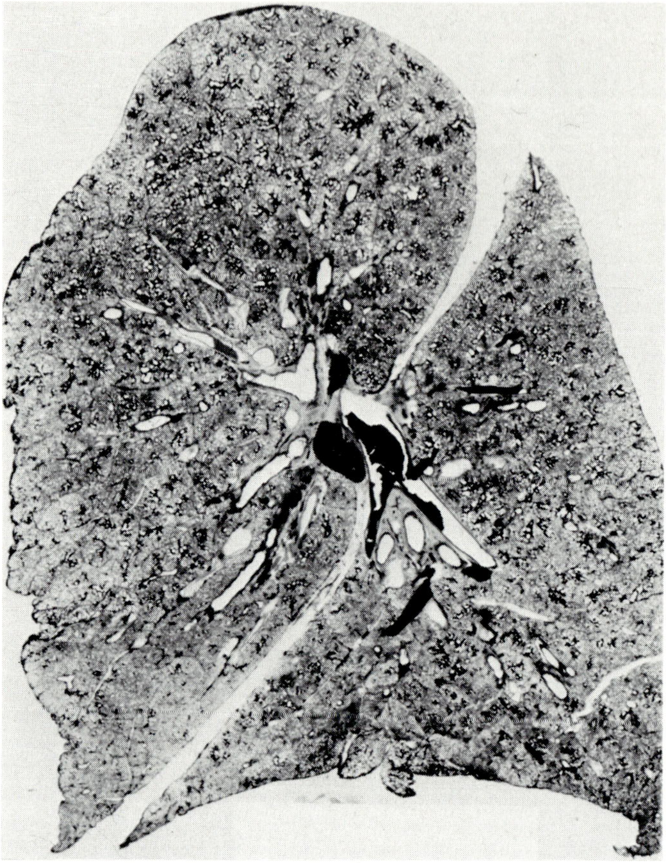

Fig. 15-2. Gough section of lung of coal miner. Pinhead-sized black opacities (coal macules) surrounded by localized areas of focal emphysema. Although the entire lung is involved, the areas of involvement show a greater profusion of opacities in the upper and middle thirds of the lung. Superimposition of microscopic macules and larger macroscopic macules results in the small rounded opacities seen on the chest radiograph.

composed of fibrous tissue. The masses may undergo cavitation from either ischemic necrosis or from tuberculous infection, although the latter has become increasingly uncommon. As the masses enlarge they destroy the vascular bed, and it is not unusual to see segmental and lobar arteries incorporated into the mass. The adjacent bronchi are similarly affected. Pulmonary hypertension often develops in progressive massive fibrosis, especially when stages B and C (described under Radiographic Classification) are reached. The severity of pulmonary hypertension is related to the size of the conglomerate large opacities.

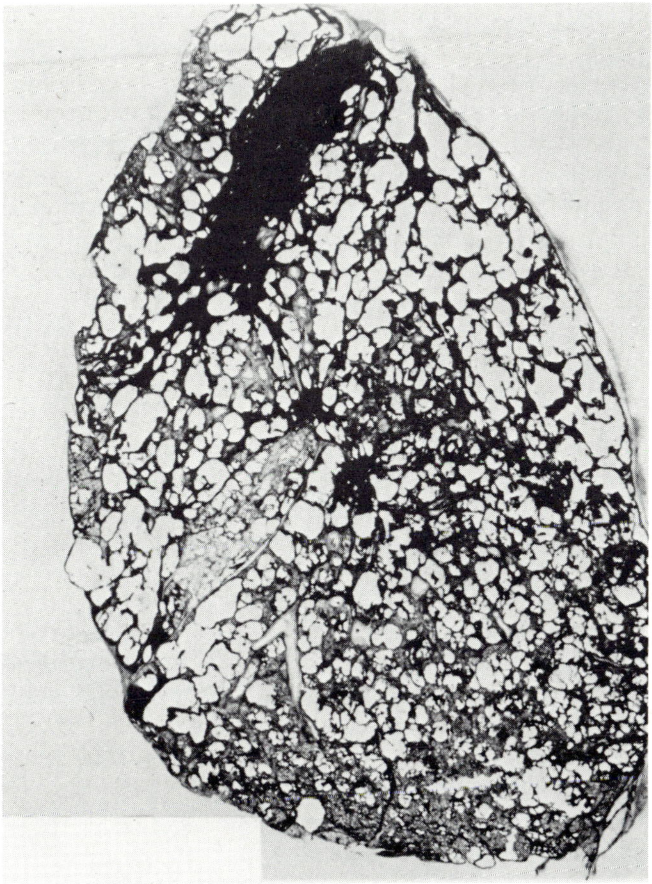

Fig. 15-3. Gough section of lung of coal miner with complicated pneumoconiosis. Large opacity in upper third of section. Several smaller large opacities in the middle third of the section. Extensive surrounding panlobular emphysema and marked destruction of the pulmonary tissues secondary to progressive massive fibrosis.

RADIOGRAPHIC CHANGES ASSOCIATED WITH COAL WORKERS' PNEUMOCONIOSIS

Necessary for establishing a diagnosis of coal workers' pneumoconiosis are a suitable history of exposure to coal dust (usually at least ten years or more underground) and certain relatively characteristic abnormalities on the chest radiograph. Coal workers' pneumoconiosis is separated into simple and complicated forms according to the appearance of the chest film.

Simple coal workers' pneumoconiosis is diagnosed and classified according to the number, size and shape of small opacities present in the chest radiograph. Such opacities may occur anywhere in the lungs, although it is commonly stated that they are seen most frequently in the upper lung zones—a dictum that is for the most part true. (This is in contrast to the changes that occur in asbestosis, which are seen predominantly in the lower lung zones.) The small opacities are more commonly rounded than irregular, although either, or a combination, may be present. The radiographic classification currently in use, both for international comparability of statistics and for compensation purposes in the United States, is the latest ILO/UC 1971 classification, which can be used for classifying all of the pneumoconioses including asbestosis.[4,5]

DETAILS OF COMPLETE RADIOGRAPHIC CLASSIFICATION

Small Rounded Opacities

These opacities are roughly rounded, but if magnified, their margins may appear poorly defined and irregular.* They are classified according to their approximate diameters: *p* up to 1.5 mm., *q* between 1.5 and 3 mm., and *r* between 3 and 10 mm. Although mixtures of *p, q* and *r* can occur, classification is based on the predominant diameter of the opacity. These opacities are usually not seen in the coal worker until ten years after the initial exposure. These three groups comprise what is classified as simple pneumoconiosis. (Any opacity greater than 1 cm. in diameter is no longer classified as a small opacity.) Unlike complicated coal workers' pneumoconiosis, the rounded opacities of simple coal workers' pneumoconiosis, which are a reaction to dust alone, do not progress in the absence of further dust exposure.

If a miner initially develops opacities of the *p, q* or *r* type, with continued exposure he tends to get more of the same size opacity rather than progressing from a *p* to a *q* to an *r*. With increasing numbers of opacities, the upper and middle lung zones lose their predominance and all lung zones become involved. Without exception, *q* opacities occur most frequently. Radiographically, it is impossible to distinguish the opacities that occur with pure coal dust from pure silica dust, or with mixtures of the two dusts.

---

* ILO/UC International Classification of Pneumoconiosis 1979. Switzerland, Occupational Safety and Health Series International Labour Office, 1980 (in press). A new modified classification describing predominance of shape from rounded to irregular, with new standard films, will be available in 1980.

For descriptive purposes each lung is divided into three zones: the upper, middle and lower lung zones. In early cases most small opacities are found radiographically in the upper and middle lung zones. Gough sections will show that there are small opacities in the lower lung zones as well, although these are usually not visible on a radiograph at early stages. This is probably because relatively few opacities are distributed throughout the greater volume of surrounding normal lung tissue at the lung bases. However, with increasing exposure to coal dust, the lower lung zones become more extensively involved: the amount of normal lung tissue decreases, and the small opacities become more readily visible.

The twelve point scale devised by Liddell & May is based on the acceptance of a continuum of change from no dust to maximal dust.[6] Liddell's elaboration allows for the retention of the major categories, namely, 0, 1, 2, and 3, but provides a means of rendering more sensitive the old ILO classification. Its main application is in epidemiological surveys in which environmental measurements are being compared and related to medical and other biological indices—in particular, to chest radiographs. When using the 12 point scale, the interpreter should first look at the unknown film and match it as nearly as possible with one of the standard mid-category films. Standard radiographs exist only for the mid categories 0/0, 1/1, 2/2 and 3/3. Figs. 15-4, 5, and 6 are examples of categories 1/1, 2/2, and 3/3. If the interpreter thinks that the film very closely resembles a mid-category standard film, then he should classify the film as 0/0, 1/1, 2/2 or 3/3, as the case may be. If he also happens to consider another category, deciding that the film does not match any of the standard films, he records this "other" category. Thus, category 0/- is a barn door normal; this implies that under no circumstances could the film be considered anything but normal. On the other hand, a reading of 1/0 means that the interpreter, after considering category 0, decided that the film was a category I, but showed fewer opacities than the standard 1/1 film. Similarly, a 2/3 reading means that the interpreter considered category 3, but eventually decided that it was still a category 2 although the opacities were more profuse than in category 2/2.

The concept of profusion is based on averaging all of the zones predominantly involved. It is fraught with errors, however, primarily because it permits a radiograph of a disease involving all six zones to have an average lower than one that, for example, involves only two zones, even though the profusion in these two zones is less than or equal to the maximal profusion in any given zone of the roentgenogram. This is an important cause of interobserver error. As a matter of fact, it has become apparent that many experienced interpreters tend to record the zone of maximal profusion and ignore the principle of averaging. This problem is being addressed currently at meetings where ILO classification revisions are a topic of discussion (see footnote p. 280).

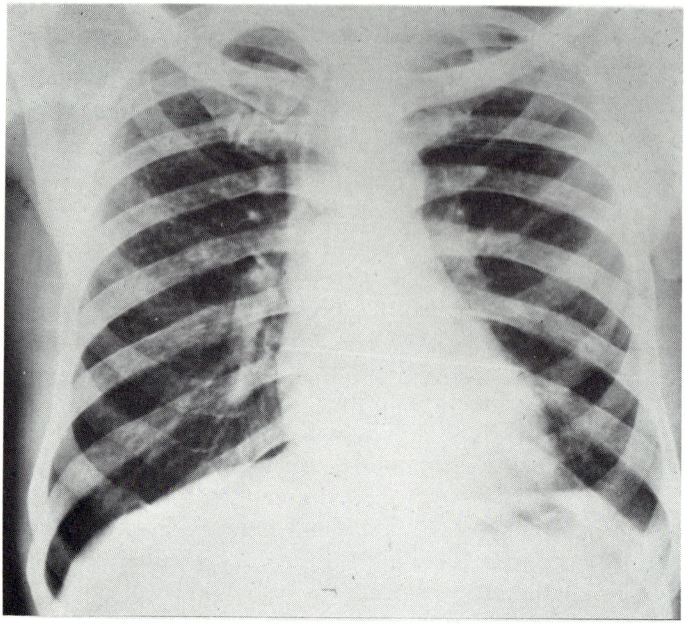

Fig. 15-4. Chest radiograph. Small rounded opacities (*r*, 3-10 mm. in diameter) in the upper and middle lung zones on the right, with a few opacities in the upper and middle lung zones on the left, resulting in a profusion of *r* 1/1. No involvement of the lower thirds of the lungs.

Furthermore, in a large percentage of subjects with pneumoconiosis (whether derived from silicosis, coal workers' pneumoconiosis, asbestosis, or a mixture of dusts) both rounded and irregular opacities may be seen. In such cases it is difficult to evaluate accurately the profusion of each, as is recommended. The possibility that all opacities be recorded, ignoring whether they are rounded or irregular, might be a solution (see footnote p. 280).

Small Irregular Opacities

These opacities are most common in cases of asbestosis, where they are customarily seen at the bases of the lungs. However, they are occasionally present in coal workers' pneumoconiosis, and if so, will appear in the upper lung zones as well. Since no measurements are available, one must use the ILO standard films for comparison. The small, irregular opacities are divided into three types, according to their thickness and texture: *s*—very fine irregular, linear or hairlike opacities; *t*—medium irregular opacities; and *u*—coarse, irregular or blotchy shadows. Most

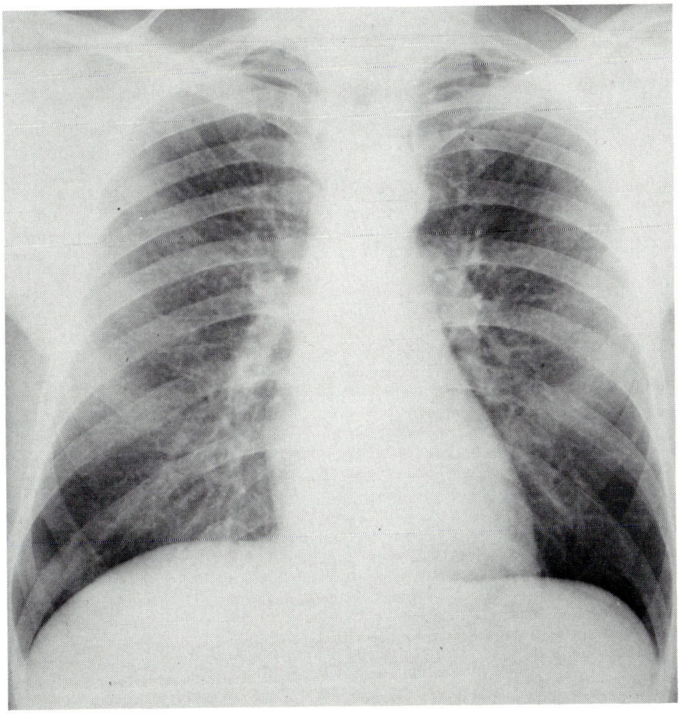

Fig. 15-5. Chest radiograph. Small rounded opacities (*q*) 2/2 profusion. These opacities are smaller than the *r* opacities and do not exceed 3 mm. in diameter on the average. It is common to find varying diameters in individual rounded opacities, but one judges the average size of the predominant opacities. Although the upper and middle lung zones are mainly involved in this patient, there are a few opacities in the lower lung zones as well.

films that were formerly described as having linear, reticular or blotchy irregular opacities are now classified as showing irregular opacities. Studies in Great Britain[7] have indicated that a positive correlation exists among irregular opacities, the extent of emphysema, and the impairment FEV_1. No such positive correlation was observed for rounded opacities.

The category of profusion for irregular opacities is similar to that described for small rounded opacities. Profusion is determined by averaging the opacities in the affected zones, but if there are marked disparities among the zones involved, averaging is done over the predominantly affected zones. When both rounded and irregular opacities are present the extent of profusion for each type is recorded separately. Following this, an attempt is made to record the "combined profusion" of both types. This is done by examining the film, but refraining from distinguishing

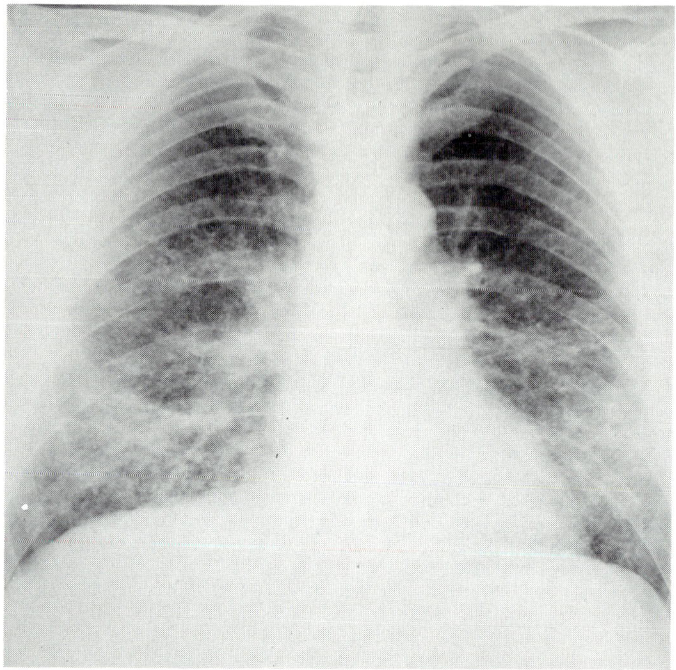

Fig. 15-6. Chest radiograph. Small rounded opacities (*p*) with a profusion of 3/3. The small opacities are like grains of sand and the average size is 1-1.5 mm. Although a few *q* and *r* opacities may be present, one judges the predominant size of the opacity. All lung zones are involved. Note that, as the profusion of *p* opacities increases, there is confluence of the rounded opacities. These may appear as linear shadows, particularly at the bases. In these instances, it may be impossible to distinguish between rounded and irregular opacities and, therefore, both types of opacities should be recorded.

between rounded or irregular opacities. Fig. 15-7 shows a coal worker with both rounded and irregular opacities.

Large Opacities

Any opacity greater than a centimeter in diameter is classified as complicated pneumoconiosis or progressive massive fibrosis. This condition is subdivided into stages (categories A, B and C) according to the size of the large opacities. Category A: An opacity whose greatest diameter is between one and five cm., or several such opacities, the sum of whose greatest diameter does not exceed 5 cm. Category B: An opacity whose combined diameter is greater than 5 cm., but whose combined area is less

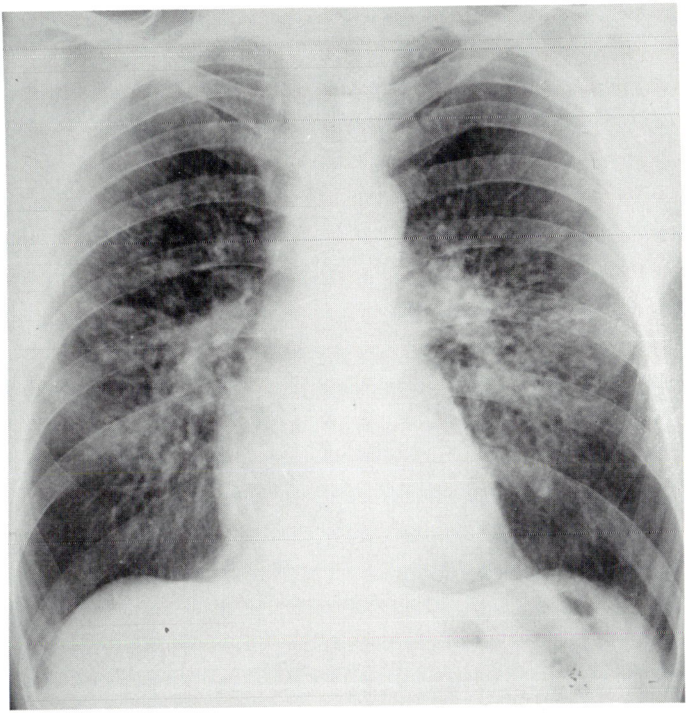

Fig. 15-7. Chest radiograph. Both rounded and irregular opacities are seen. Present are *r* opacities (profusion 2/2) and *u* irregular opacities (profusion 1/2). The upper and middle lung zones are predominantly involved, although there are a few opacities in the lower lung zones as well. In this particular case, both rounded and irregular opacities should be recorded, as well as a combined profusion.

than one-third of the upper lung. Category C: An opacity whose area exceeds one-third of the lung. Such opacities are also subdivided into WD (well-defined) and ID (ill-defined) types. Note that an opacity must be a centimeter or larger in size in order to be classified as a large opacity. Complicated pneumoconiosis is usually seen with a background of category 2 or category 3—i.e., one of the higher categories—of simple coal workers' pneumoconiosis (Fig. 15-8). Unlike simple pneumoconiosis, progressive massive fibrosis may develop after coal dust exposure has ceased and may progress in the absence of further exposure.

When Stage 3 progressive massive fibrosis develops, the affected lobe may shrink to one quarter of its size as a result of ischemic necrosis of the large opacities or fibrotic contraction. This leads to compensatory overdistension in the remaining lung lobes. The end result is that the small opacities present in the part of the lung that is not involved by the

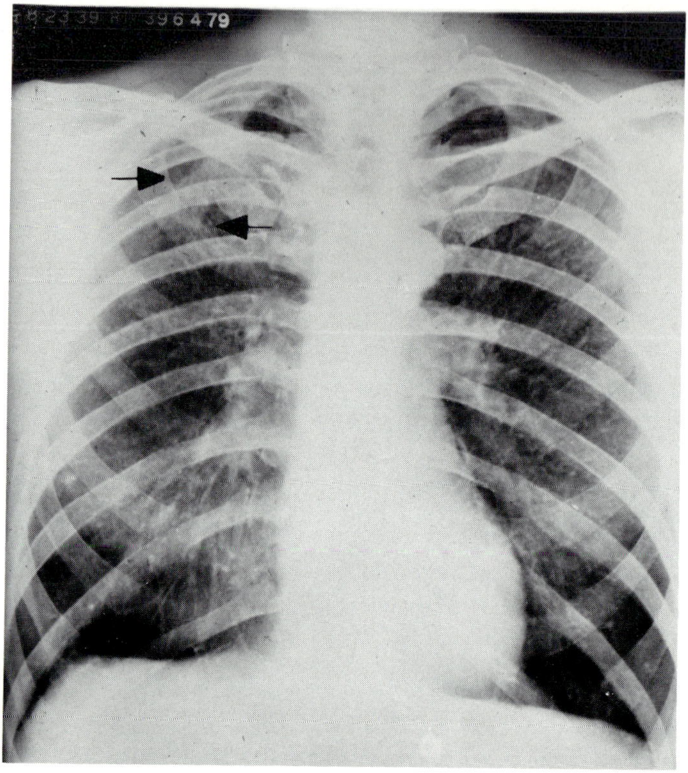

Fig. 15-8. Chest radiograph. Single large opacity in upper third of right lung (arrow), category A. This type of opacity is usually associated with complicated pneumoconiosis resulting in pulmonary fibrosis. It is usually seen with a background of small rounded opacities. Note background of small rounded opacities, *q* 2/2, in all lung zones but predominantly in the upper and middle lung zones.

conglomeration will become more widely separated and appear less profuse than previously. Furthermore, complicated pneumoconiosis is usually associated with a large amount of bullous emphysema, which will often cause disappearance of the small opacities on the radiograph. As the fibrosis increases it usually becomes associated with severe pulmonary tissue destruction, hilar distortion, and advanced emphysematous changes (Fig. 15-9).

The large opacities are more common in the upper and middle lung zones but can occur in the lower zones as well. Radiographically the large opacities resulting from exposure to pure coal, to pure silica or to coal and silica mixtures are indistinguishable. The only difference, as noted in Chapter 16, is that in cases of pure silicosis or high silica content the large

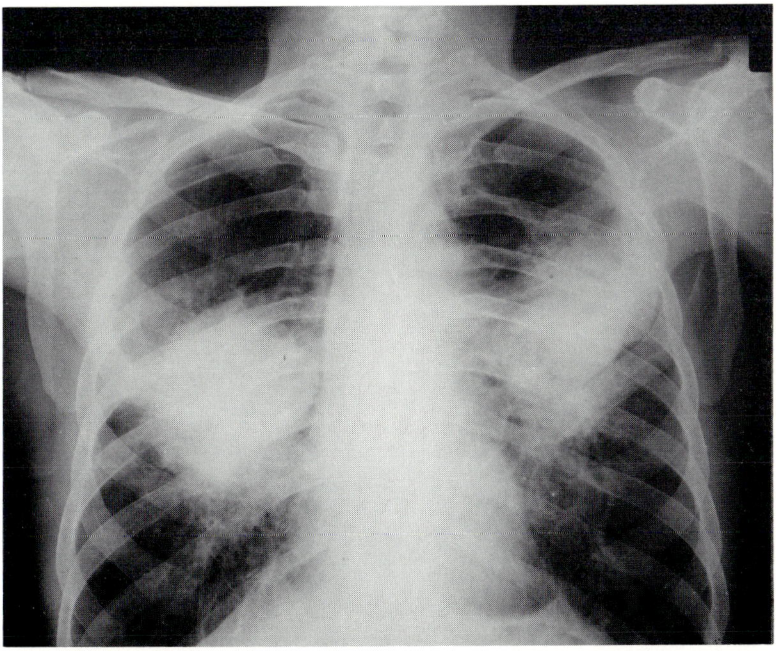

Fig. 15-9. Chest radiograph. Advanced, complicated coal workers' pneumoconiosis with progressive massive fibrosis. Two extremely large opacities involving the mid zones bilaterally with advanced pulmonary emphysema associated hilar distortion. In advanced, complicated pneumoconiosis the background of small rounded opacities tends to disappear as they are incorporated into the large fibrotic masses. In addition, the small rounded opacities tend to be obscured by the surrounding emphysematous lung.

opacities tend to be larger in size and of the C variety. Using conventional tomography, the large opacities are relatively flat and are not as thick as opacities that are seen in tuberculosis or carcinoma of the lung. Cavitation occurring in a large opacity is a reflection of poor blood supply (Fig. 15-10). Here it is difficult to distinguish from cavitating neoplasms or cavitating tuberculosis without the help of correlative clinical and laboratory findings. (See further discussion in Chapter 16.) Bronchography is of no value since bronchial obstruction occurs in large opacities due to distortion without any associated neoplasia. Computerized axial tomography demonstrates the extent of the large opacities in three dimensions and also reveals calcifications to better advantage. It may be of value in demonstrating additional areas of involvement, to differentiate between possible neoplasms (Figs. 15-10, 11, and 12).

The relationships between lung dust, work history, pathological stage

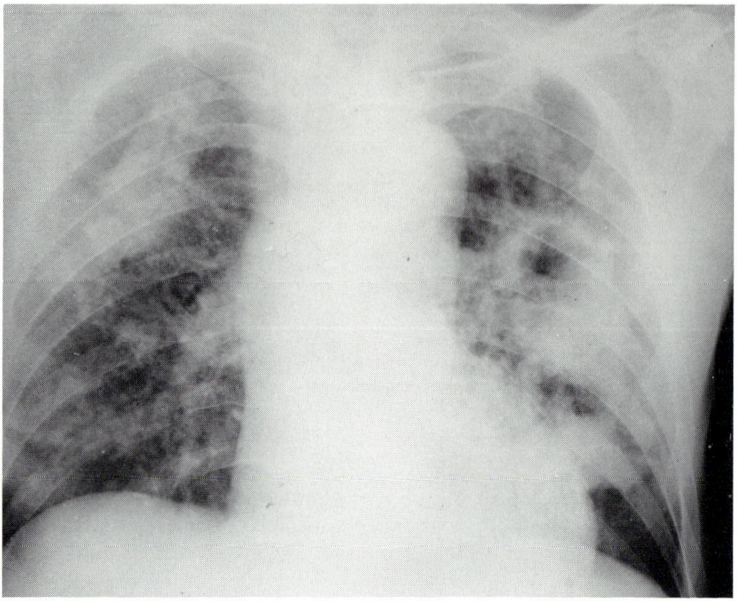

Fig. 15-10. Chest radiograph. Note background of small rounded opacities, *q* 2/2. Large opacity involving the upper two lung zones on the right. Cavitating large opacity in the left middle lung zone. No evidence of neoplasia and no evidence of pulmonary tuberculosis at post mortem. The cavitation of the large opacity in the left mid lung zone resulted from ischemic necrosis secondary to compromise of the blood supply. Radiographically, the cavitating large opacity is indistinguishable from neoplasia or cavitating inflammatory disease.

of disease and radiographic category have been studied by a number of investigators.[8-12] It is now apparent that dust found in the lungs of coal miners consists mainly of coal, quartz, mica and kaolin.

Analyses of the lungs of deceased miners have shown that the higher the rank of coal mined, the higher the coal content and the lower the free silica content of the lungs. Rank is a geological term used to describe the mineral characteristics of coal. The higher-ranked coals such as anthracite tend to be more dense, have a higher carbon content, give off more BTUs per gram when burned, and contain less volatile matter. At the other extreme, lignite, the lowest ranked coal, liberates less heat when burned, but contains a greater volume of volatile material. Weight for weight, coal contributes less to radiographic category than do quartz and the other constituents of coal mine dust (e.g., mica and clay). Iron is also present in excess in pneumoconiotic lungs, the amount being such that it cannot be accounted for by the inhalation and deposition of exogenous

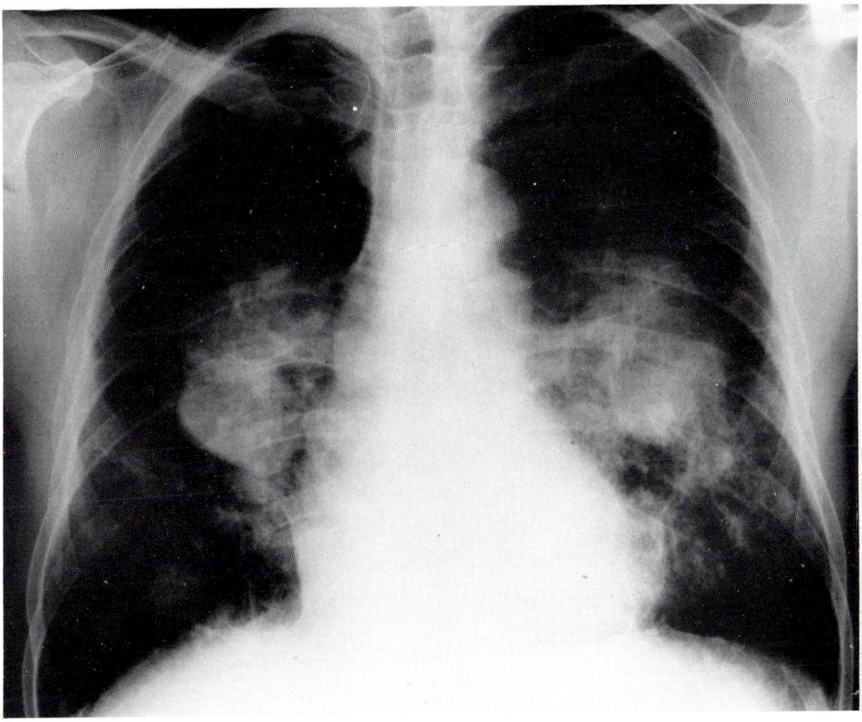

Fig. 15-11. Chest radiograph. Large opacities bilaterally with progressive massive fibrosis in a coal worker. Small opacities have disappeared and incorporate into the large fibrotic masses. Poorly defined calcification on left.

iron. Its source, then, must be assumed to be endogenous. The iron content of the lungs increases with the number of years spent underground and with the coal content of the lungs. The lungs of subjects dying with progressive massive fibrosis usually have about the same weight of coal dust as do the lungs of subjects with categories 2 and 3 simple coal workers' pneumoconiosis.

It has often been suggested that coal dust, or at least the carbon in coal dust, cannot account for the opacities present in the lung. Some persons feel that the formation of radiographic opacities is mainly a consequence of the collagen and fibrous protein content of the lungs, and, indeed, there may be an element of truth in this claim. Nevertheless, one outstanding factor that emerges from most studies is the excellent relationship between coal dust content of the lung and radiographic category.[10] The chest film, therefore, despite drawbacks in interpretation, remains the only feasible method of determining and quantifying dust exposure in life.

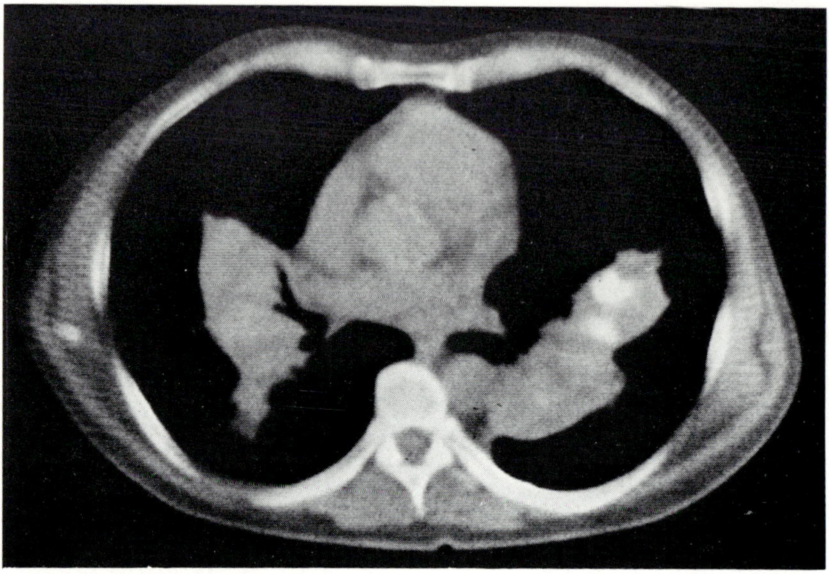

Fig. 15-12. CAT section. Large fibrotic masses well outlined. Calcification in left better seen with tomography.

Caplan's Syndrome

In 1953 Caplan first described rheumatoid nodules in the lungs of coal miners.[13] The condition is now referred to as Caplan's syndrome or rheumatoid pneumoconiosis. The opacities seen on the radiograph tend to be rounded and peripherally situated. They occur most often on a background of category 0 or 1 simple coal workers' pneumoconiosis (Fig. 15-13) and may develop within a period of only a few weeks. The rheumatoid nodules vary from 0.5 to 5 cm. in diameter and most often develop concomitantly with joint manifestations of rheumatoid arthritis. Infrequently, they may even precede the arthritis by several years. Fresh crops of nodules may appear at intervals (while others may have disappeared) and often portend an exacerbation of the arthritis. Calcification within the nodules is fairly frequent, and pleural effusions may occur. The rounded rheumatoid nodules may occur in some instances along with the typical larger opacities of progressive massive fibrosis. There is a definite association between the nodules occurring in the lung and the nodules that may be found in the elbows and Achilles tendons. Only subjects with a classic appearance of Caplan's syndrome were found to have rheumatoid factor in their serum.[14]

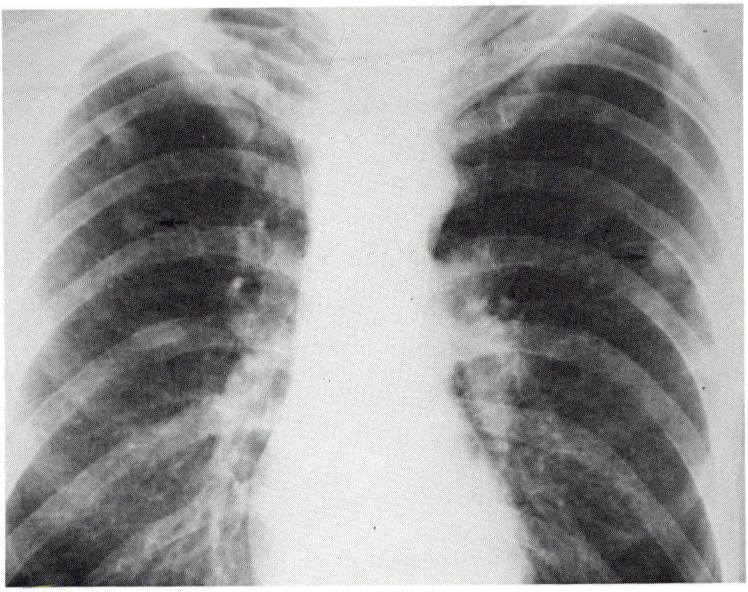

Fig. 15-13. Chest radiograph. Several large nodules in both upper lung zones, ranging in size from 1-2 cm. in diameter (arrows). Calcification in nodule in left middle lung zone (arrow). Background of small rounded opacities (R 1/1). The larger nodules were due to rheumatoid nodules. Frequently, new rheumatoid nodules appear while others disappear, and cavitation may occur. The appearance of fresh crops of nodules often portends an exacerbation of the patient's rheumatoid arthritis. Subjects with classic appearance of the nodules usually have rheumatoid factor in their serum.

SYMPTOMS AND SIGNS

Simple coal workers' pneumoconiosis has neither symptoms nor signs. It is often accompanied by industrial bronchitis, which may lead to the presence of cough, sputum, and a few scattered wheezes. Industrial bronchitis, in contrast to coal workers' pneumoconiosis, is a response to the deposition of dust particles in the conducting airways. It is characterized by hypersecretion and mucous gland hypertrophy, and is pathologically similar to the chronic bronchitis seen in cigarette smokers. However, the marked atypia and metaplasia that occur in cigarette smoke-induced bronchitis are not seen in industrial bronchitis, nor is industrial bronchitis associated with emphysema.[15]

Complicated coal workers' pneumoconiosis is a more serious condition, and in categories B and C leads to marked shortness of breath.

Cough and sputum are also often present, but again are probably related to coincidental concomitant industrial bronchitis. In the more advanced stages, there may be signs of consolidation of the lungs; in this regard the upper lobes are most commonly affected. Contraction of the upper lobes with tracheal deviation is frequent, and may be associated with bronchial breathing. Signs of pulmonary hypertension develop at a later stage, and there may be an obvious right ventricular gallop as well as overt cor pulmonale. Nonetheless, in most subjects with progressive massive fibrosis, there is a complete absence of signs, other than a few scattered wheezes. Exceptionally, when one of the larger conglomerate opacities undergoes ischemic necrosis and cavitates, the patient may cough up several ounces of a jet black sputum, a symptom that may be referred to as melanoptysis.

PHYSIOLOGICAL ABNORMALITIES

Simple coal workers' pneumoconiosis has no effect on ventilatory capacity, and higher categories of the condition are not associated with declines in the FEV_1 or FVC.[16] Nonetheless, when a population of coal miners is compared to a control group of nonminers, the miners, for the most part, have been shown to have a lower ventilatory capacity and more cough and sputum. These changes cannot be attributed to either simple coal workers' pneumoconiosis or progressive massive fibrosis, since both the respiratory symptoms and the reduction in ventilatory capacity occur as frequently in miners with clear chest films. There is now enough evidence to indicate that the decrease is due to industrial bronchitis.[15] Higher categories of simple coal workers' pneumoconiosis, i.e., categories 2 and 3, are sometimes associated with minor abnormalities in the distribution of inspired gas. Thus, the alveolar arterial gradient for oxygen, (A-a) O_2, may be widened; in addition, the arterial partial pressure for oxygen may be minimally reduced. Similarly, subjects with categories 2 and 3 simple coal workers' pneumoconiosis may demonstrate frequency dependence of dynamic compliance, but the presence of the latter phenonenon is independent of whether the subjects have bronchitis.[17] The higher categories of simple coal workers' pneumoconiosis are occasionally associated with minor reductions in the diffusing capacity, especially when the punctate type of opacity predominates in the chest x-ray.[17]

Simple coal workers' pneumoconiosis may lead to minor reductions in elastic recoil and to comparable slight decreases in static compliance.[18] Such changes are probably a consequence of focal emphysema, which accompanies simple coal workers' pneumoconiosis and is characteristic of the higher categories. These impairments are slight, in that focal emphysema is not associated with a significant loss of the alveolo-capillary surface.[15] Owing to the minor loss of elastic recoil, the residual volume of the functional residual capacity tends to be slightly larger than normal in subjects who have simple coal workers' pneumoconiosis, but here again the changes are small.[17]

In many instances the effects of progressive massive fibrosis on pulmonary function are difficult to separate from those of coincident unrelated heart and other pulmonary diseases. There is, however, ample evidence to suggest that, in progressive massive fibrosis the ventilatory capacity is definitely reduced; the extent of this reduction is related to the size of the larger opacity. With category A, a normal FEV and FVC are the rule, and it is only when categories B and C are reached that impairment becomes obvious. Thus, complicated pneumoconiosis, at least in stages B and C, leads to a reduction in ventilatory capacity, a low diffusing capacity, abnormalities of gas exchange, a low arterial oxygen tension and pulmonary hypertension. In addition, in some miners with progressive massive fibrosis, the lungs tend to be stiffer than normal. Static compliance, then, is often reduced, as is specific compliance, while the pulmonary recoil pressure at total lung capacity is often increased.

PROGNOSIS

The modern coal miner has a normal life span. While simple coal workers' pneumoconiosis has no effect on life expectancy, complicated pneumoconiosis, in particular stages B and C, leads to morbidity and premature death.[19] But it must be remembered that only between 30 and 40 percent of subjects with progressive massive fibrosis show progression. In this regard the effects of progressive massive fibrosis on life expectancy are counterbalanced by the lower incidences of lung cancer and heart disease that occur in coal miners. Industrial bronchitis is also prevalent in coal miners and, in itself, can lead to a minor degree of ventilatory impairment, but it is not associated with an increased mortality.

PREVENTION AND CONTROL OF COAL WORKERS' PNEUMOCONIOSIS

Several studies have shown that the progression of coal workers' pneumoconiosis is related to the dust levels that prevail in the coal mines, and that, with adequate dust control, both the prevalence and incidence of coal workers' pneumoconiosis will decline. Dust control is best effected by adequate ventilation and by the use of equipment designed to generate less dust. Dust control is important in that, if effective, it will prevent the development of the higher categories of simple coal workers' pneumoconiosis, which in turn will lead to a reduced incidence of progressive massive fibrosis. Jacobsen has derived mathematical models to predict the likelihood of the development and progression of simple coal workers' pneumoconiosis.[20] Based on his calculations, if the dust level is kept below 3.5 g/cu. meter, less than three percent of those exposed for 35 years will go on to develop category 2 or category 3 simple coal workers' pneumoconiosis.

REFERENCES

1. Gregory JC: Case of peculiar black infiltration of the lungs resembling melanosis. Edin Med Surg J 36:389, 1831
2. Collis EL, Gilchrist JC: Effects of dust upon coal trimmers. J Ind Hyg 10:101–110, 1928
3. Watson AJ, Black J, Doig AT, et al: Pneumoconiosis in carbon electrode makers. Brit J Ind Med 16:274–285, 1959
4. IV International Pneumoconiosis Conference. Bucharest, International Labor Office, Working Group on Definition of Pneumoconiosis, September 29 to October 2, 1971
5. International Labour Office/Union International Contre Cancer: International classification of radiographs of the pneumoconioses. Med Radiogr Photogr 48:65–110, 1972
6. Liddell FDK, May JD: Assessing the radiological progression of simple pneumoconiosis. London, National Coal Board Medical Service, 1966
7. Lyons JP, Ryder AC, Campbell H, et al: Significance of irregular opacities in the radiology of coal workers' pneumoconiosis. Br J Ind Med 31:36–44, 1974
8. Caswell C, Bergman I, Rossiter CE: The relationship of radiographic appearances in simple pneumoconiosis of coal workers to the content and composition of the lung, in Walton WH (ed): Inhaled Particles, Vol 2, No 3. London, Unwin Bros, 1971, p 713
9. Bergman I, Caswell C: Lung dust and lung iron contents in coal workers in different coal fields in Great Britain. Br J Ind Med 29:160–168, 1972
10. Rossiter CE: Relations of lung dust content to radiological changes in coal workers. Ann New York Acad Sci 200:465–478, 1972
11. Nagelschmidt G: The study of lung dust in pneumoconiosis. Am Ind Hyg Assoc J 26:1–7, 1965
12. Rivers D, Wise ME, King EJ, et al: Dust content, radiology and pathology in simple pneumoconiosis of coal workers. Br J Ind Med 17:87–108, 1960
13. Caplan A: Certain unusual radiological appearances in the chest of coal miners suffering from rheumatoid arthritis. Thorax 8:29–37, 1953
14. Lippman M, Eckert HL, Hahon W, et al: The presence of circulatory antinuclear and rheumatoid factors in United States coal miners. Ann Intern Med 79:807–811, 1973
15. Hankinson JL, Reger RB, Morgan WKC: Maximal expiratory flows in coal miners. Am Rev Respir Dis 116:175–180, 1977

16. Morgan WKC, Handelsman L, Kibelstis J, et al: Ventilatory capacity and lung volumes of U.S. coal miners. Arch Environ Health 28:182–189, 1974
17. Morgan WKC, Seaton A: Occupational Lung Diseases. Philadelphia, WB Saunders Company, 1975, pp 149–215
18. Seaton A, Lapp NL, Morgan WKC: Lung mechanics and frequency dependence of compliance in coal miners. J Clin Invest 51:1203–1211, 1972
19. Ortmeyer CE, Costello J, Morgan WKC, et al: The mortality of Appalachian coal miners, 1963 to 1971. Arch Environ Health 29:67–72, 1974
20. Jacobsen M: Progression of coal workers' pneumoconiosis in Britain in relation to environmental conditions underground: Proceedings of Conference in Technical Measures. J Dust Prevention & Suppression in Mines (Luxembourg) Oct 1972

E. Nicholas Sargent
W. K. C. Morgan

16
Silicosis

Silica is one of the most widespread elements found on earth. Aside from the sands of the desert and seashore, silica is found in numerous rock formations including sandstone, granite, and many other metal-containing ores. It exists in three forms: crystalline, amorphous, and, in combination with other elements, as a silicate. Crystalline silica is composed of silicon dioxide (SiO_2) in the form of a tetrahedron. The most frequently encountered crystalline form of silica is quartz, but other crystalline forms exist, including tridymite, cristobalite, and stishovite. The fibrogenic potential of the various forms of crystalline silica varies greatly, ranging from the most fibrogenic, cristobalite and tridymite, to the moderately fibrogenic quartz, and, at the other extreme, the nonfibrogenic stishovite. Amorphous silica is probably non-fibrogenic despite claims to the contrary.[1] Finally, combined silica in the form of silicates varies greatly in its fibrogenic properties, but for the most part tends to be less fibrogenic than free crystalline silica.

AFFECTED OCCUPATIONS

The disease produced by the inhalation of silica is popularly known as silicosis. It is found in association with a number of industries, in particular, heavy metal mining, which includes the mining of gold, silver, tin, iron and copper. Coal mining, under certain circumstances, may also involve considerable exposure to free silica. Subject to most frequent exposure are workers who sink the shafts of portals for the mine, "hard headers," who develop the new mine faces, and transportation employees whose work includes dusting sand on the rails in order to provide traction. Silicosis also occurs in graphite miners, slate quarriers, and uranium miners. The use of finely divided sand in various industrial processes, such as the manufacture of refractory bricks, ceramics and pottery, also poses a risk to those exposed. Silicosis has been found in iron and steel foundry workers who pour molten metal into molds. The molds are made of a mixture of sand and clay, and the high temperature tends to fuse some of the silica onto the metal surface. This fused silica in turn must be removed by fettling. The disease is therefore found in men working as casters and fettlers. Sandblasters are particularly likely to develop silicosis; many countries have in fact banned this practice. Finally, miners of bentonite and diatomite are often exposed to appreciable concentrations of free silica in their work environments.

Thus, it is apparent that large numbers of workers in a variety of industries are still exposed to the hazards of respirable silica dust. Silicosis probably remains the most prevalent pneumoconiosis in the United States and Canada. Nevertheless, because of the many different ways in which silica exposure can occur, prevalence rates in the various occupations are difficult to obtain. In the United States there seems little doubt that the metal mining industry is the most important single source of silicosis; the same is probably also true of Canada.

PATHOGENESIS AND PATHOLOGICAL CHANGES

Following deposition in the lung, silica particles are ingested by the alveolar macrophages and pass into the macrophages' phagosomes. Lysozymes are drawn from the macrophage cytoplasm by the silica particles. The lysozymes pass into the phagosomes, whose disruption they later will bring about. The phagosomal contents, which by now include numerous enzymes, leak into the cytoplasm. This leads to the death of the macrophage and the subsequent release of enzymes and other fibrogenic substances, along with ingested silica particles. It is the breakdown of the macrophage and the release of the products and enzymes it contains that lead to the fibrogenic response, rather than silica itself. Silica particles are now available for reingestion by other macrophages and the entire process is repeated. Herein lies the explanation for the progressive nature of silicosis, and why the disease often progresses after dust exposure has ceased.

Exceptionally, when the clearing mechanisms are overwhelmed and there are insufficient macrophages to ingest all the deposited silica particles, the role of the macrophage is taken over by type 2 pneumocytes. When this occurs, the pneumocytes disintegrate and liberate lamellar bodies and lipids into the alveoli, thereby leading to a localized form of alveolar proteinosis. If the number of silica particles is so great that most are taken up by type 2 pneumocytes, then a generalized form of alveolar proteinosis may occur. This generalized alveolar proteinosis is seen almost entirely in cases involving sandblasters or individuals exposed to massive quantities of free silica. An excellent description of the pathogenesis of silicosis has been given by Wagner.[2] Provided that the clearing mechanisms are not overwhelmed, the macrophages slowly remove the silica particles from the alveoli and transport them via the lymphatics to the regional nodes. Moving along in the lymphatics with the macrophages are the enzymes and lipids that have been formed as a result of the breakdown of macrophages. When the enzymes and lipids arrive in the lymph tissue aggregates, they engender a proliferative fibrogenic response. In many instances the adjacent arteriole supplying the respiratory bronchiole or acinus is incorporated in the process, and the collagenous fibrosis that is deposited occludes and obliterates the vessel. As necrotic nodules develop and enlarge in the lymph nodes, the centers often undergo ischemic necrosis, so that the cellular elements aggregate at the periphery of the node along with the silica particles. The center of the node seldom contains any silica particles. Following prolonged exposure to silica, distal lymph gland involvement occurs, and the hilar, as well as the cervical and abdominal aortic nodes may become involved.

Macroscopically, simple silicosis is characterized by the presence of multiple grayish nodules distributed throughout the lungs, with the highest concentration, however, in the upper lobes (Fig. 16-1). In some instances the nodules undergo calcification. The lymph nodes of the lung itself are often enlarged and sometimes calcified, as are the hilar and regional nodes. The nodules themselves appear to be whorled and the center is often necrotic. Conglomeration occurs when several nodules merge into one another and become confluent. The confluent area then usually extends slowly. As it does so, it incorporates adjacent pulmonary vessels and airways into the mass, thereby destroying them. The conglomerate area occasionally undergoes ischemic necrosis with cavitation, but tuberculosis is also seen; this likewise may be associated with cavitation. Microscopically, the silicotic nodule arises in or around the respiratory bronchiole and adjacent to the supplying bronchiolar artery. The nodule consists of hyalin fibers, which are often centrally situated and associated with some ischemic necrosis. As mentioned earlier, the nodules present a concentric arrangement, with fibroblasts and reticulin fibers at the periphery (Fig. 16-2). The silica particles can be detected with polarized light, under which circumstances they appear as birefringent crystals; this technique does not, however, distinguish silica from silicates.

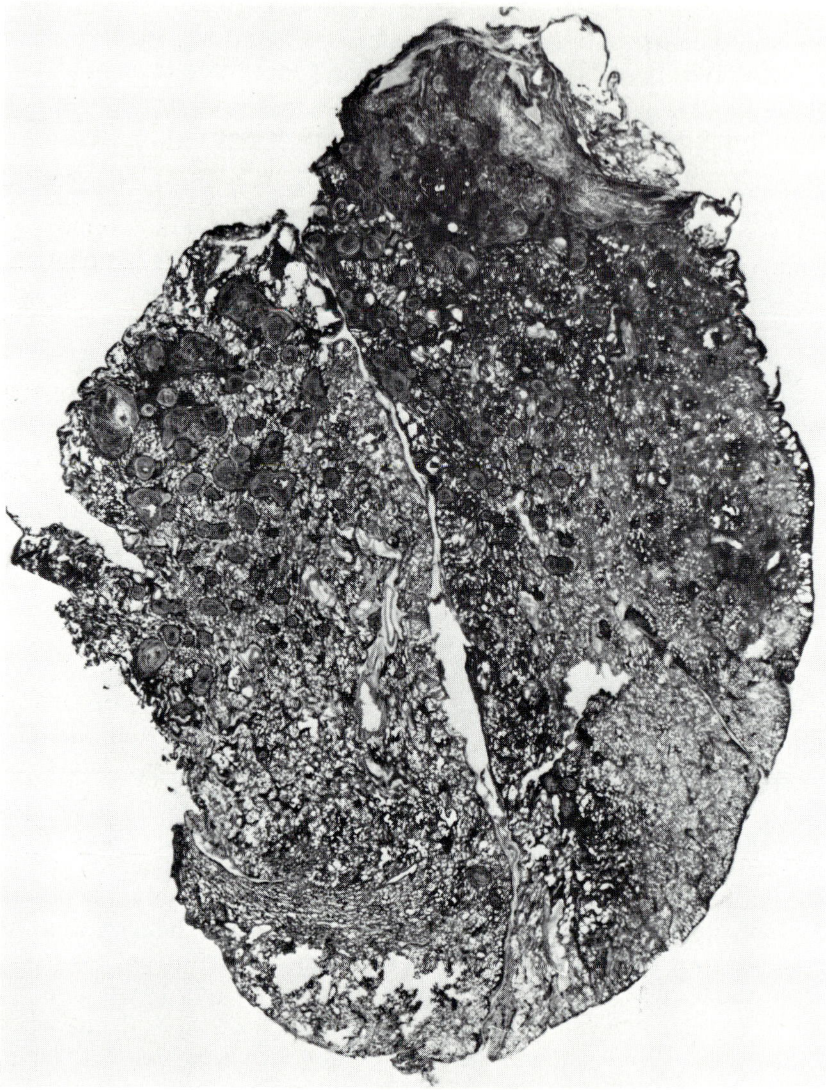

Fig. 16-1. Gough section of lung of hard rock miner. Large macroscopic silicotic nodules distributed mainly throughout the upper and middle thirds of the lung. (The lower portions of the lung are involved to a lesser extent.)

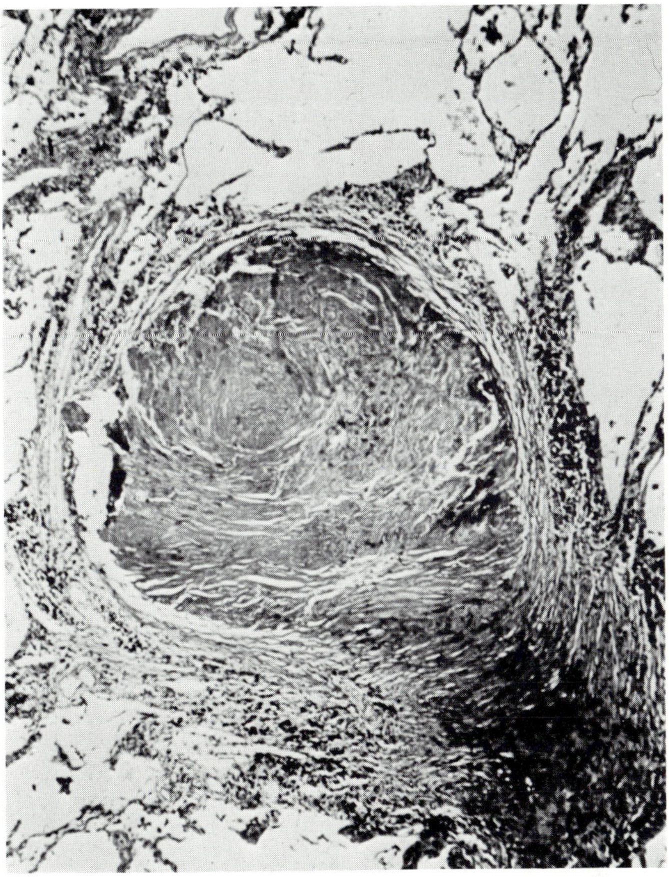

Fig. 16-2. Microscopic section of lung. Silica macule showing whorled collagenous fibers. Unlike coal, silica is much more fibrogenic with a great deal more surrounding fibrosis and scar type emphysema. However, radiographically the silica macule and the coal macule are indistinguishable. Superimposed microscopic macules and larger macroscopic macules appear as small rounded opacities on the radiograph.

RADIOGRAPHIC CHANGES

Radiographically, silicosis can be classified as simple or complicated. Either of these forms can be associated with rheumatoid nodules in the lung (similar to Caplan's syndrome), and silicotuberculosis. The radiographic classification of these abnormalities is described in detail in Chapter 15. The silica-related abnormalities are radiologically indistinguishable from those of coal workers' pneumoconiosis, regardless of the silica content of the coal dust. At present, the opacities seen in simple silicosis are classified according to the ILO/UC International Classification of Radiographs of Pneumoconioses (1971).[3,4] (See Chapter 15.) The classification is being revised and refined to the extent that profusion and the description of small opacities will be further simplified.*

In classical silicosis the radiographic changes usually occur ten or more years after the initial exposure to silica dust. A major requisite in making the roentgen diagnosis of pneumoconiosis, particularly when small opacities, such as those of silicosis, are to be examined, is a high quality radiograph. Incomplete radiographic studies, inadequate exposures, or poor quality films preclude the accurate detection of small rounded opacities. On the other hand, there is a tendency for inexperienced observers to overinterpret suspected nodularity, or to completely overlook nodules that are present, particularly if they are unfamiliar with the normal chest x-ray. The silicotic nodules are not uniform in size and shape and are not as diagnostic as one might hope. They are rounded but may often appear somewhat irregularly rounded or even irregularly linear. A comparative study of pneumoconiotic lesions in bituminous coal miners and metal miners showed that although more positive roentgenograms were seen for coal miners than for metal miners, the size and extent of the small opacities were similar in the two occupational groups.[5] The report is somewhat at variance with previous observers, who considered the small opacities of silicosis to be on the average larger (i.e., category *r*) and denser than those of coal workers' pneumoconiosis. Fig. 16-3 is an illustration of classical silicosis with *r* opacities (profusion 3/3). The nodules may occasionally calcify.

Calcification of the peripheries of hilar lymph nodes, which may occur in silicosis, is known as *eggshell calcification* (Fig. 16-4). When it occurs in coal workers it is due not to the coal dust, but to the silica content. Eggshell calcification is usually found against a background of small rounded opacities, but in rare cases has been found to occur with no other radiographic findings. Eggshell calcifications in association with tuberculosis, coccidioidomycosis, histoplasmosis and other fungi, sarcoidosis, and irradiated lymphomas have also been described, but when they are found in subjects that have been exposed to dust, silicosis should be the first consideration.

Radioactive nuclides may also be of limited value in diagnosing patients with suspected silicosis—limited, because Gallium 67 accumulates not only in inflammatory focal disease processes, but also in certain neoplasms. The lesions of pneumoconiosis consist in part of proliferating

---

* See footnote p 280.

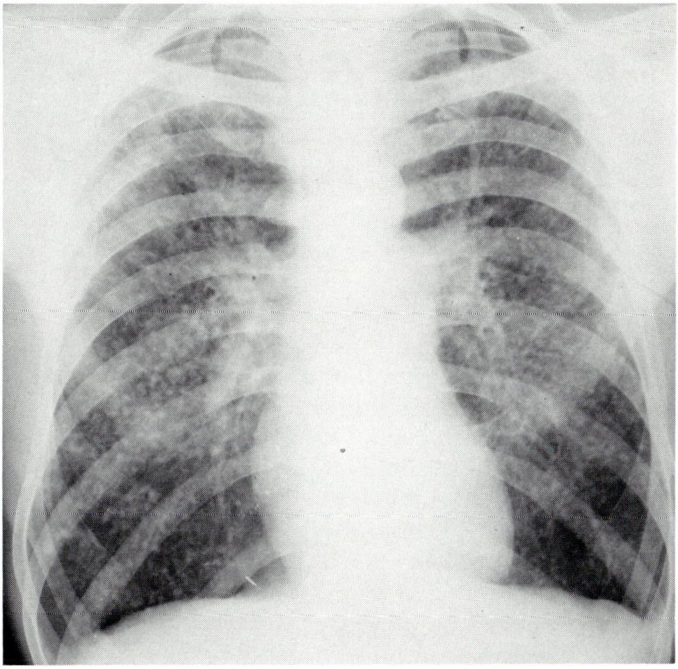

Fig. 16-3. Chest radiograph. Classical silicosis. Small rounded opacities varying in size from 3.0 to 10 mm. All lung zones are involved (profusion *r* 3/3). Associated depression of the leaves of the diaphragm secondary to pulmonary emphysema. Enlargement of the central pulmonary vessels as well as the main pulmonary artery due to cor pulmonale (history of heavy smoking).

and metabolically active cells, and pulmonary studies have shown that Gallium 67 concentration is abnormally increased in all patients with overt silicosis and asbestosis.[6] Although the findings are nonspecific, two distinct patterns are noted: a diffuse peripheral concentration and a central hilar concentration. The spatial extent of Gallium 67 uptake is substantially greater than that of the observed radiologic abnormalities in about one third of the patients. Reduction of pulmonary radiogallium concentration in sequential studies of pneumoconiosis patients may indicate at what point the disease process is halted.

Complicated silicosis is present when conglomerate masses 1 cm. in diameter or greater are present. The classification of conglomerate masses, or large opacities, is described in detail in Chapter 15. The opacities are indistinguishable from those caused by coal dust, but the average size of large opacities has been found to be greater among metal miners than among coal miners.[5] These lesions occur predominantly in the upper and

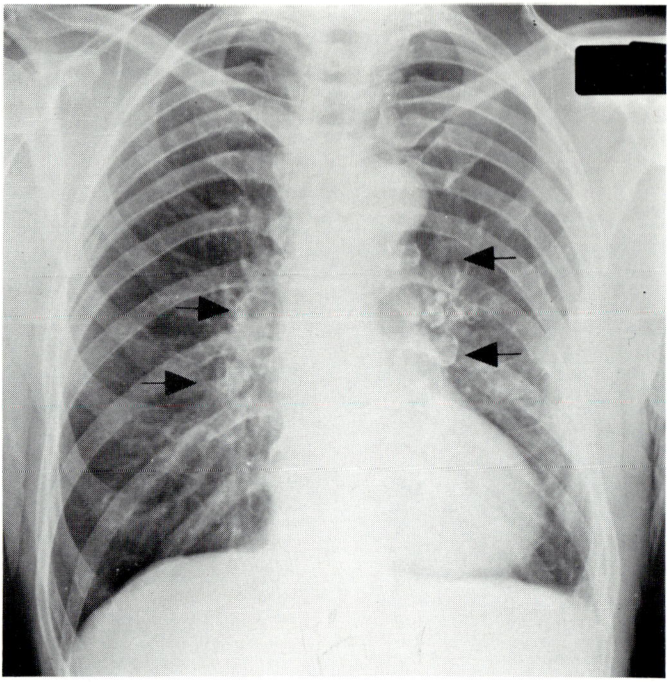

Fig. 16-4. Chest radiograph. Circular peripheral calcifications in lymph nodes. Characteristic of eggshell calcifications of silicosis in both hilar regions (arrows). This type of calcification should be considered due to silicosis, unless proven otherwise.

middle lung zones. They commence as ill-defined conglomerations of several small nodules that may be in one of several areas and slowly become both denser and better defined. In the advanced stage, they appear as large, often sausage-shaped masses and are often surrounded by large areas of bullous emphysema. The walls of the bullae contain strands that extend into the mass.

In patients with conglomerate masses, it is often difficult to determine whether or not a neoplasm is present. Examined tomographically, non-cavitating conglomerate masses appear relatively thin in one plane and rather flat as compared with neoplastic lesions. The development of a pulmonary osteoarthropathy may lead one to diagnose a neoplasm instead of a conglomerate mass. The osteoarthropathy will often disappear with removal of the primary neoplasm. Pulmonary angiography cannot distinguish between neoplasms and conglomerate masses. It may, however, enable one to demonstrate the adequacy or inadequacy of the pulmonary vascular tree and allow a better determination of physiological impairment. Bronchography is of little value in that the large conglomerate masses will often show bronchial obstruction that is not due to a neoplasm. However, if surgical procedures are anticipated, angiography and bronchography might be of value in demonstrating areas of compressed lung that are adjacent to fairly good lung tissue.

The conglomerate masses of silicosis (or of coal workers' pneumoconiosis) may become necrotic in the center and excavate, and the patient may cough up large amounts of unusual material. Large opacities that cavitate merely reflect a compromised blood supply and are not necessarily associated with pulmonary tuberculosis or neoplasia.

The development of conglomerate silicosis leads to scarring and retraction of the hila. The density per unit area of the small regular opacities that are present becomes lower as the conglomerate masses migrate towards the hila. This is a result of the overdistension of the remaining lung, so that the number of opacities decreases as the surrounding lung overexpands. Such changes are usually seen only in late stages B and C complicated simple silicosis (Fig. 16-5). The chest film often shows bullous changes, and there is little doubt that traction from the fibrotic masses is largely responsible for these changes.

When tuberculosis develops in a subject with complicated silicosis there is no characteristic radiographic appearance. Conglomerate fibrotic lesions may extend and may cavitate from either ischemic necrosis or tuberculosis, but radiographically the cause of the cavitation cannot be distinguished. It is easier to recognize tuberculosis when it complicates simple silicosis because fluffy, soft apical infiltrates often appear relatively quickly and can be distinguished from the more densely contracted masses of conglomerate silicosis. Even so, examination of the sputum remains the only certain way of diagnosing tuberculosis in a silicotic.

Caplan's syndrome may occur in silicosis as well as in coal workers' pneumoconiosis (see Chapter 15). Many prefer the term "rheumatoid pneumoconiosis" to Caplan's syndrome, since similar nodules occur in asbestosis, silicosis and other such diseases. The Caplan nodule microscopically resembles the nodules that are found on the elbow in classical rheumatoid arthritis. Rheumatoid pneumoconiosis may appear on a background of early silicosis; it may also occur when there is exposure but no radiographic evidence of the disease. The nodules frequently appear in crops that form over a relatively short period. When Caplan nodules appear in silicosis, they have the same radiographic appearance as they do in other diseases, with the exception that their propensity for undergoing calcification is greater.

Diatomaceous earth pneumoconiosis occurs primarily in association with a process in which large amounts of crystobalite, which is particularly fibrogenic, are formed. Pulmonary changes often develop in mill

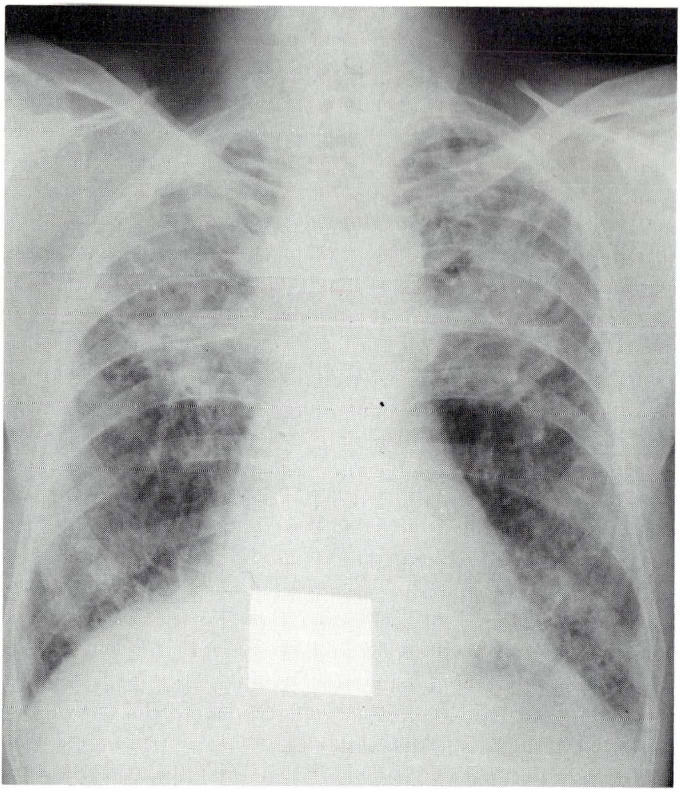

Fig. 16-5. Chest radiograph. Large opacities involving both the upper and middle lung zones (Category C). Progressive massive fibrosis. Compensatory emphysematous changes in the lower halves of both lungs. Marked hilar distortion. Background of *q* opacities in the lower lung zones, many of which are only faintly seen due to obscuration by the associated emphysematous changes. Small rounded opacities in the upper lung zones are not visualized due to incorporation into the large fibrotic masses.

and maintenance workers involved in the processing.[7,8] Diatomite pneumoconiosis is characterized by fine, linear or irregular opacities and fine, rounded opacities—either alone or in combination (Fig. 16-6)—located predominantly in the upper lung zones. The changes are radiographically indistinguishable from silicoses that have developed from other causes, but they appear earlier (in many cases after less than ten years of exposure). The nodules seem to be of lesser contrast radiographically and they rarely become as dense as other silicotic nodules. Mediastinal, hilar and diaphragmatic distortion as well as advanced emphysematous changes associated with cor pulmonale are not infrequent complications in the terminal phases of diatomite pneumoconiosis (Fig.

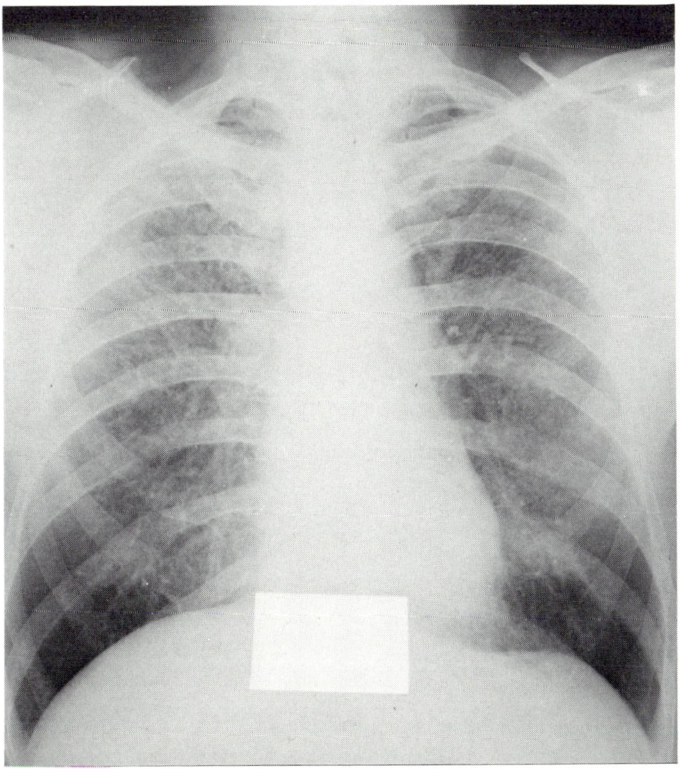

Fig. 16-6. Chest radiograph. Diatomaceous earth worker (milling operation). Small rounded opacities (*p* 2/2) and irregular opacities (*s* 2/2) involving mainly the upper and middle lung zones. Small rounded opacities of the *p* variety are often overlooked (and are difficult to reproduce in photographs). They vary between 1.5 mm. in diameter and often appear as a faint background haze until they become more numerous. The changes following diatomaceous earth workers' exposures usually occur earlier (five to ten years after exposure) than do changes in miners who are exposed to silica. (The changes usually occur after ten or more years.)

16-7). They may occur even when relatively small areas with larger opacities are involved. Hilar or mediastinal adenopathy usually never occurs with diatomaceous earth pneumoconiosis, and eggshell calcifications are seldom if ever found.

ACUTE SILICOSIS

Acute silicosis should, by now, have been eradicated; unfortunately, sporadic cases still occur.[9]

The acute form of silicosis occurs in subjects exposed to high levels

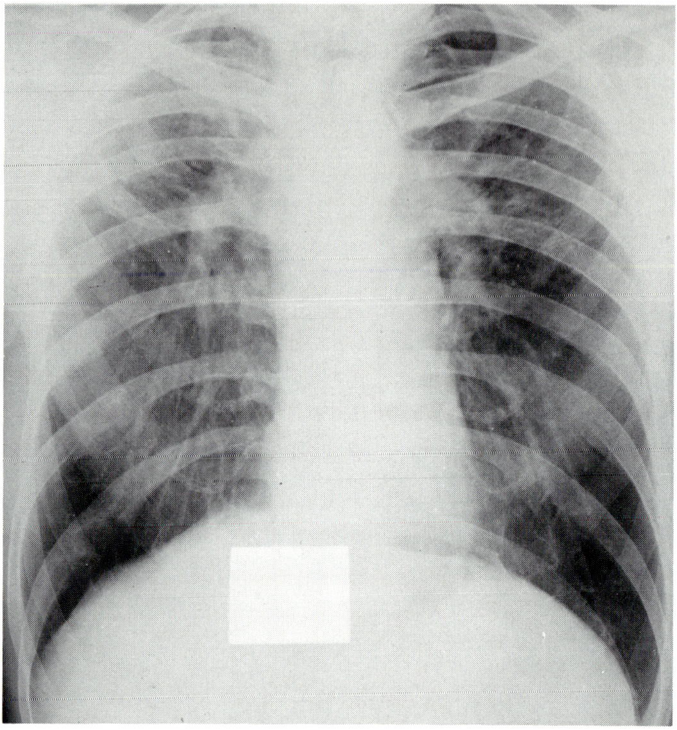

Fig. 16-7. Chest radiograph. Diatomaceous earth worker with complicated pneumoconiosis and progressive massive fibrosis. Marked hilar distortion, advanced emphysematous changes, and disappearance of small opacities, mostly secondary to the surrounding advanced emphysematous changes. Ill-defined large opacity in the right upper lung zone. The advanced surrounding changes occur even when relatively small areas of involvement with large opacities are present. (Eggshell calcifications are seldom, if ever, found.) Hilar or mediastinal adenopathy never occurs with diatomaceous earth pneumoconiosis. Cor pulmonale is a frequent complication in the terminal stage of the disease.

of respirable silica over a relatively short period of time (six to eight months) and is almost entirely limited to sandblasters and tunnelers. The subject often presents with high fever, a productive cough, and severe weight loss; as a result, his condition is sometimes mistaken for tuberculosis or a fungal disease. The initial impression is often reinforced by radiographic appearances. Physical signs are stiff lungs with tachypnea, indications of consolidation, and scattered crackles and wheezes. The chest film frequently shows areas of consolidation, and the nodules typical of classical silicosis are either absent or scanty. Tuberculosis and infection by other atypical mycobacteria are frequently seen as complications. Medical treatment is futile, although lung transplantation has been tried with a survival rate of ten months in one subject.[9A] Pathologically, the lungs are firm and consolidated. The alveolar walls are infiltrated with plasma cells, lymphocytes, and some fibroblasts. The alveoli are crammed with a PAS staining material which resembles that seen in pulmonary alveolar proteinosis (Fig. 16-8). Silicotic nodules are few.

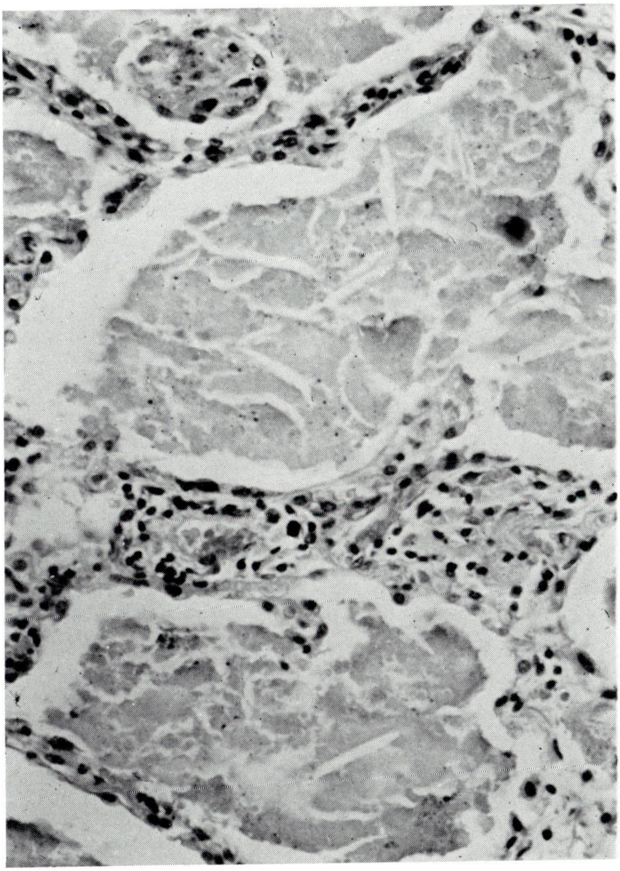

Fig. 16-8. Microscopic section of lung. Patient with acute silicosis. Alveoli filled with proteinaceous material. This often results in characteristic x-ray changes of "air bronchogram." The surrounding alveolar walls are infiltrated with plasma cells, lymphocytes, and some fibroblasts. Silicotic nodules are infrequently seen. (With permission of Paul M. Suratt, M.D., Charlottesville, West Virginia.)

Acute silicosis differs clinically and radiographically from classical silicosis (Fig. 16-9). The chest film often shows lobar or segmental consolidation, usually of the upper zones. On occasion it may resemble pulmonary edema with typical perihilar "bat's wing" shadows. An air bronchogram is usual, but often there is a superimposed nodular process. Peripheral air trapping, bullae formation, loss of lung volume and distortion of hilar and mediastinal structures are common features indicative of pulmonary fibrosis without specific differential diagnostic values. Pneumothorax may occur and, although there is an increased instance of

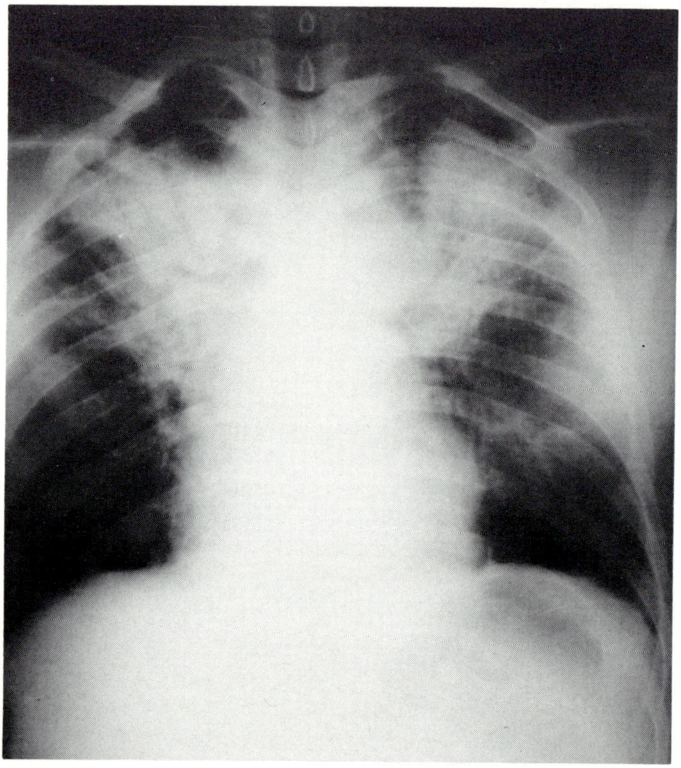

Fig. 16-9. Chest radiograph. Twenty-three year old black male, who worked for approximately two years sandblasting. Large areas of consolidation extending from both hilar regions. Note the "air bronchograms" secondary to filling of the alveoli with proteinaceous material. Rapid downhill course and death from pulmonary insufficiency three years after. Hilar and mediastinal adenopathy are not uncommon in these cases but the perihilar regions are obscured by the surrounding alveolar filling process. (With permission of Paul M. Suratt, M.D., Charlottesville, West Virginia.)

pneumothorax in classical silicosis, there is an especially high incidence in the acute form of the disease. Mediastinal adenopathy may occasionally be a feature in the early stages until finally obscured by the confluent alveolar infiltrate. Although the disease is very similar to alveolar proteinosis, the primary change is in the upper and middle lung zones. (Alveolar proteinosis predominates more often in the lower lung zones.) The temporal sequence is critical; with the presence of lung disease—inexorably progressive on a time scale of months—the possibility of acute silicosis should immediately be considered in patients with an appropriate work history.

When exposure has been relatively severe, but not severe enough to cause acute silicosis, some of the features of both classical, chronic and acute silicosis may be found in the same subject. Under these circumstances the condition is often referred to as subacute silicosis.

CLINICAL FEATURES OF CLASSICAL SILICOSIS

Although silicosis exists in three forms (classical, acute, and subacute), classical silicosis is by far the most common. It is subdivided clinically into simple and complicated, or conglomerate silicosis. Simple silicosis is diagnosed on the basis of a suitable history of exposure, plus the presence of multiple, small, rounded opacities in the chest film. It is further subdivided into categories 1, 2, and 3, according to the profusion of the opacities. Complicated silicosis occurs on a background of simple silicosis and is characterized by the development of a shadow greater than 1 cm. in diameter on the chest x-ray. Although the radiographic features have already been described in detail, it is important to bear in mind that the category of simple silicosis is related to the amount of silica that is retained in the lungs. Unlike coal workers' pneumoconiosis, silicosis may continue to progress after exposure has ceased. (The reasons for this were discussed under the subheading, *Pathogenesis and pathogenic changes*, above). Simple silicosis has no symptoms and absolutely no physical findings. Many simple silicotics will admit to having persistent cough and sputum, but an equal number of those who were exposed and have *no* radiographic changes will admit to the same symptoms.[10] In the latter case the symptoms indicate industrial bronchitis and are a consequence of the continued inhalation and deposition of larger particles in the conducting airways.[11,12]

Although simple silicosis offers few symptoms and causes little impairment, it often progresses to the complicated form of the disease. Conglomerate silicosis, in contrast, leads to severe shortness of breath, cough, and sputum. The severity of the shortness of breath is related to the sizes of the conglomerate masses in the lungs; when the masses become extensive, the affected subject may become completely disabled. Terminally, right ventricular hypertrophy supervenes and overt cor pulmonale later develops.

EFFECTS ON PULMONARY FUNCTION

Simple silicosis has little effect on pulmonary function and is certainly not associated with disabling pulmonary impairment. Nevertheless, categories 2 and 3 occasionally lead to a slight reduction of lung volumes, although the values are seldom outside the predicted range.[13] Although the nodular fibrosis that characterizes this condition spares the alveoli and the interstitial tissues, it affects the lymphoid aggregates that surround the respiratory bronchioles and the intrapulmonary lymph nodes. The fibrosis, being nodular rather than generalized, has little effect on the mechanical properties of the lungs, but does lead to a slight increase in their stiffness, which in turn is associated with a slight decrease in both vital capacity and total lung capacity.[13] Furthermore, static lung compliance tends to be on the low side of the normal range. When obstruction is present it is best explained by cigarette smoking or by the presence of industrial bronchitis. Measurements of the diffusing capacity are normal in simple silicosis,[14] however, perfusion lung scans do occasionally show a slight loss of the vascular bed. This in itself is insufficient to lead to pulmonary hypertension, which is rare in simple silicosis.

The symptoms and degree of pulmonary impairment of stage A complicated silicosis vary only slightly from those seen in the simple form of the disease. In contrast, in stages B and C complicated disease, gross derangements of pulmonary function occur. Lung volumes are decreased and the decrement is clearly related to the size of opacities, with the vital capacity being particularly affected. Coincident and often severe airways obstruction is also present, although the pathophysiological mechanism involved in this phenomenon is difficult to explain. It may resemble the occasional severe airways obstruction that is seen in far advanced tuberculosis, which is best explained by distortion occurring in the airways attributable to traction from the tuberculous fibrotic infiltrates. The diffusing capacity is likewise reduced, and again, the size of the decrement is related to the size of the opacities. A low arterial pO_2 in the presence of a normal arterial pCO_2 is the rule. This is usually the result of ventilation and perfusion mismatching. The lungs tend to be stiffer than normal, while compliance is reduced, as is the maximal elastic recoil pressure at total lung capacity. Pulmonary hypertension that is present at rest, but worsened by exercise, is often the rule in stages B and C conglomerate silicosis, and perfusion lung scans show large avascular areas at the site of the opacities.[15]

PREVENTION OF SILICOSIS

Prevention can only be achieved by lessening the exposure to respirable particles of silica. The problem can be approached by modifying mining equipment so as to reduce the generation of dust particles. The cutting edges of tools, for example, should be sprayed with water, and exhaust ventilation should be adequate. In the case of acute silicosis, even self-contained breathing units are ineffective; many particles bypass the unit and are inhaled. There is little doubt that sandblasting should be banned, as should blasting with other less dangerous substitutes. Regular monitoring of the dust levels in silica-exposed subjects and of their respiratory status should be carried out. The development of radiographic changes is an indication that a given worker should be removed from his dusty environment so that he is no longer exposed to significant concentrations of silica.

RELATIONSHIP BETWEEN SILICOSIS AND TUBERCULOSIS

Virtually all studies that have been carried out over the past 50–60 years have shown that tuberculosis is three to four times more common in men who are exposed to respirable silica.[16] In general, the greater the amount of silica to which the men are exposed, the greater the risk of developing silicosis. Thus, while tuberculosis is most commonly seen in persons with overt radiographic evidence of silicosis, a risk is still present in silica-exposed persons who have negative chest films. It has been shown in silica-exposed animals that tuberculosis may be induced with a smaller number of organisms, and that, once established, it will spread more widely, both hematogenously and by the lymphanes. In addition, it has been shown that the number of tubercle bacilli in the silica-exposed lesions exceed that found in the non-exposed lesions. Silica will not enhance the growth of tubercle bacilli in vitro on media such as the Middlebrook-Dubos; it needs the intervention of a host, and there is good evidence that the host's defenses—in particular the pulmonary macrophage—are compromised by the prior exposure to silica.

Although nationally the incidence of silicotuberculosis may be low, in selected groups of workers the incidence may be quite high. Based on the reports of a high incidence of tuberculosis among patients with silicosis, it is recommended that such persons receive INH preventative therapy if there is reason to believe that they are infected (i.e., a positive skin test reaction), and if the presence of progressive disease has been excluded.[17]

ASSOCIATION BETWEEN PROGRESSIVE SYSTEMIC SCLEROSIS (SCLERODERMA) AND MINERS

It has been suggested that an association between scleroderma and exposure to coal and silica dust exists, and that the incidence of scleroderma is higher among miners than among the general population.[18] The great majority of case reports indicate that exposure to coal and silica dust rather than radiographic evidence of pneumoconiosis seems to be the key factor associated with the presence of scleroderma.

RADIOGRAPHIC MASQUERADERS OF SILICOSIS

Just as it has been found that the unusual features of certain radiographs can be caused by a specific occupational disease and histologically proven, so in contrast it is also known that no occupation allows a worker to remain immune to nonoccupational diseases that can mimick roentgenographically specific fibrogenic dust entities or forms of immunological occupational diseases. VanOrdstrand noted that, traditionally, if an adequate occupational history is obtained in the case of a worker who has been exposed to harmful dusts, the chest x-ray has usually been the main diagnostic tool.[19] In recent years, however, it has been found that in nearly all occupations of this type there may be marked variations in individual susceptibility to pneumoconiosis regardless of the dose relationship. Often, the usual diagnostic studies will not suffice in attempts to differentiate between "masquerading diseases" unrelated to the employment and diseases caused by known hazards of certain types of employment. In some cases, more than the usual work history, routine tests, and chest x-rays will be needed to differentiate occupationally related from nonoccupationally related disease. Frequently, in general clinical work, a detailed dust exposure history is not obtained. In VanOrdstrand's experience, additional tests (particularly lung biopsies) have found equal numbers of previously unsuspected pneumoconioses in workers whose problems had been thought to be nonoccupational, and "masquerading" dust diseases of the lung, which are unrelated to the worker's employment. Unsuspected diagnoses that have been made only after tissue examination include: bronchiolo-alveolar carcinoma, pulmonary alveolar microlithiasis, miliary tuberculosis, lymphangitic metastases, hematogenous metastases, lymphocytic interstitial pneumonitis, sarcoidosis, hemosiderosis secondary to mitral stenosis, retained lipidol, and measles pneumonia.[19] Thus, the differential diagnostic tool of primary importance may frequently be the microscope rather than the radiograph.

REFERENCES

1. Vitums VC, Edwards MJ, Niles RN, et al: Pulmonary fibrosis from amorphous silica dust. Arch Environ Health 32:62–68, 1977
2. Wagner JC, Seal RME: Pathological reactions of the lung to dust, in WKC Morgan and A Seaton (eds), Occupational Lung Diseases. Philadelphia, WB Saunders Company, 1975, pp 39–64
3. IV International Pneumoconiosis Conference: Working Group on Definition of Pneumoconiosis. Bucharest, International Labor Office, September 27–October 2, 1971
4. ILO/UC International Classification of Radiographs of the Pneumoconioses. Med Radiogr Photogr 48:65–110, 1972
5. Lainhart WS, Felson B, Jacobson G, et al: Pneumoconiotic lesions in bituminous coal miners and metal miners. Arch Environ Health 16:207–210, 1968
6. Siemsen JK, Sargent EN, Grebe SF, et al: Pulmonary concentration of Gallium^{67} in pneumoconiosis. Am J Roentgenol 120:815–820, 1974
7. Oechsli WR, Jacobson G, Brodeur AE: Diatomite pneumoconiosis; roentgen characteristics and classification. Am J Roentgenol 85:263–270, 1961
8. Cooper WC, Cralley LJ: Pneumoconiosis in diatomite mining and processing. Washington, DC, United States Department of Health, Education and Welfare Public Health Service, Bureau of States Services, Division of Special Health Services, Occupational Health Program: U.S. Government Printing Office, 1958, pp 1–91
9. Dee P, Suratt P, Winn P: The radiographic findings in acute silicosis. Radiol 126:359–363, 1978

9A. Derom F, Barbier F, Ringoir S, et al: Ten months survival after lung homotransplantation. Man J Thorac Cardiovasc Surg 61:835–837, 1971

10. Irwig LM, Rock P: Lung function and respiratory symptoms in silicotic and nonsilicotic gold miners. Am Rev Respir Dis 117:429–435, 1978
11. Morgan WKC: Industrial bronchitis. Brit J Ind Med. In press.
12. Kibelstis JA, Morgan EJ, Reger R, et al: Prevalence of bronchitis and airway obstruction in American bituminous coal miners. Am Rev Respir Dis 108:886–893, 1973
13. Teculescu DB, Stanescu DC, Pilat L: Pulmonary mechanics in silicosis. Arch Environ Health 14:461–468, 1967
14. Teculescu DB, Stanescu DC: Carbon monoxide transfer factor for the lung in silicosis. Scan J Respir Dis 51:150–159, 1970
15. Lapp NL, Seaton A, Kaplan KC, et al: Pulmonary hemodynamics in symptomatic coal miners. Am Rev Respir Dis 104:418–424, 1971
16. Allison AC, D'Arcy Hart P: Potentiation by silica of the growth of mycobacterium tuberculosis in macrophage cultures. Br J Exp Pathol 49:465–476, 1968
17. Snider DE, Jr: Editorial: The relationship between tuberculosis and silicosis. Am Rev Respir Dis 118:455–460, 1978
18. Rodnan GP, Benedek TG, Medsger TA, Jr, et al: The association of progressive systemic sclerosis (scleroderma) with coal miners' pneumoconiosis and other forms of silicosis. Ann Int Med 66:323–334, 1967
19. VanOrdstrand HS: Pneumoconioses and their masqueraders. J Occupat Med 19:747–753, 1977

Brian T. Butcher
Reynold M. Karr

17
Toluene Diisocyanate-Induced Asthma

Toluene diisocyanate (TDI) belongs to a group of compounds called isocyanates, many of which are used in the manufacture of flexible and rigid foams, fibers, coatings and elastomers. Historically, organic isocyanates were first prepared in 1849 but it was not until the publication of the description of a procedure by Otto Bayer in 1947 that the commercial production and manipulation of these chemicals began to be explored. The estimated world production of isocyanates now exceeds one billion pounds annually, of which over 400 million pounds is TDI (Fig. 17-1). Large numbers of workers are involved in the production and use of isocyanates commercially. In 1973, it was estimated that more than 40,000 persons in the United States alone were involved with TDI. Increasing numbers of individuals are also being exposed in non-commercial settings by using polyurethane paints and varnishes, or by soldering polyurethane-coated electrical wires. In developed countries it is a rare person indeed whose life is not affected by these compounds.

HEALTH EFFECTS

Almost concurrent with the use of isocyanates, reports of untoward effects upon the health of workers began to appear in the medical literature. These adverse reactions were of two main types: toxic and asthmatic.

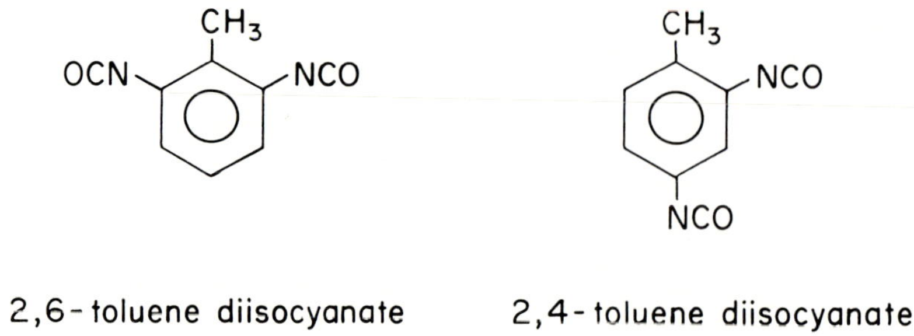

Fig. 17-1. Structure of toluene diisocyanate

Toxic Reactions

Toxic effects are seen at high concentrations (greater than 5 p.p.m.), and affect nearly all individuals. Depending on the vapor pressure of the isocyanate and the method of its use, high levels of isocyanate vapor act as a strong irritant, primarily of the mucous membranes of the upper and middle respiratory tracts and of the cornea and conjunctiva of the eye. These effects are most likely due to reaction of the isocyanate groups with reactive hydrogen atoms present on biochemical structures in tissues, leading to irritation or tissue necrosis. Repeated skin exposure to the isocyanates rarely causes rashes. Such skin eruptions, when they occur, can often be attributed to other chemicals used in the processing of isocyanates, such as aliphatic amines. The high levels of isocyanate capable of causing these adverse effects are usually encountered only as the result of an accident or where safety precautions have not been followed. Acute toxic effects from high levels of exposure are generally reversible, especially if treatment is begun early. However, one report describes continuing neurologic symptoms following exposure of firemen to TDI.[1] While the majority of the toxic reactions are induced by TDI, a few cases are also known to result from exposure to diphenylmethane diisocyanate (MDI) and other isocyanates.[2]

Asthmatic Reactions

Of far greater importance clinically is the asthma induced by TDI. This occurs in approximately five percent of workers exposed to TDI vapor. While TDI is the major cause of sensitivity, there have been occasional reports of asthmatic reactions initiated by MDI or other isocyanates. Such sensitization frequently takes place within the first year of exposure to TDI, and is often associated, anecdotally, with spills or industrial accidents where a worker is exposed to massive doses. The primary symptoms are dyspnea, chest tightness, and wheezing upon or immediately following exposure to TDI, and/or several hours later into the evening or night. Associated toxic symptoms such as headaches, nausea, or vomiting may occur with very intense exposures. Upon removal from areas containing TDI, the respiratory symptoms resolve slowly. Workers developing such sensitivity may react to exposures to concentrations of TDI vapor as low as 0.005 p.p.m. lasting for 15 minutes or less. Since the threshold limit value (TLV) for TDI has been set by the Occupational Safety and Health Administration (OSHA) at 0.02 p.p.m., many workers reacting to lesser levels of TDI are clearly at risk in a work environment containing levels of TDI in the range considered acceptable by government regulation. Once reactivity has been confirmed, sensitive workers should be removed from isocyanate-containing areas.

EARLY STUDIES OF TDI SENSITIVITY

Early studies aimed at determining a mechanism of TDI sensitivity examined environmental TDI levels, the pulmonary function of workers, and immunologic parameters of humoral and cell-mediated immune mechanisms.

Pulmonary testing

Gandevia[3] reported ventilatory changes that occurred in exposed workers. He found reduction in forced expiratory volume (FEV_1) both during the working day and over the week, and demonstrated a cumulative decline in FEV_1 over a two week period. Further, he recognized that overnight recovery was incomplete, and concluded that the fall in FEV_1 was less transient than that seen in byssinosis. He also found that smokers demonstrated a greater fall in FEV_1 than did non-smokers. Environmental testing showed that TDI levels reached as high as 9 p.p.m.

In a report by Peters,[4] who tested workers in the polyurethane foam industry, 34 of 38 workers demonstrated a decline in FEV_1 with a mean fall of 0.22 liters during the day. Although a drop in ventilatory capacity occurred even in workers who were found to have exposures less than the TLV (0.02 p.p.m.), the degree of ventilatory impairment appeared to be related to the level of exposure. In 16 individuals observed over a 2½-year period, there was an overall decline in FEV_1 in excess of that predicted on the basis of aging. Those workers who had shown the greatest drop during individual work days were most likely to develop an excess decline over the 2½-year period. Further, it was shown that reduction of FEV_1 over the study period was greater in TDI-exposed workers than in patients with chronic obstructive pulmonary disease of undetermined etiology.

Although the most widely recognized adverse effect of inhaled TDI is asthma, at least two reports in the literature link TDI exposure to an infiltrative pulmonary reaction. Blake and coworkers[5] reported four cases of developing pulmonary opacities on chest x-rays following isocyanate exposure. More recently, Charles and associates[6] studied four isocyanate workers with apparent restrictive as well as obstructive airway changes whose gas transfer was reduced. One of these subjects additionally demonstrated bilateral pulmonary infiltrates in an alveolar filling pattern. Lung biopsy revealed acute inflammation and fibrosis, most prominent around the respiratory bronchioles in the centrilobular area. Large numbers of eosinophils were found to be infiltrating interalveolar septae and filling alveoli as is seen in allergic bronchopulmonary aspergillosis; skin tests and Ouchterlony double diffusion analyses, however, failed to demonstrate any reactivity to aspergillus antigens. Response to corticosteroids was good, but the disease recurred with corticosteroid withdrawal. These case reports do not unequivocally prove that TDI is the etiologic agent in a unique form of hypersensitivity pneumonitis, but the data do suggest a possible causal role for this agent in the production of infiltrative lung disease.

Environmental Monitoring

Environmental evaluation and control of industrial exposure to TDI has been reviewed by Reilly.[7] The Marcali method has been used to provide periodic point atmospheric sampling for TDI levels, which have been shown to vary according to the manufacturing process used, humidity, ventilation control, and accidental spillage. This approach has demonstrated frequent excursions above the time weighted average (TWA) set by OSHA standards.

Immunological Analyses

Immunological investigations to identify a mechanism of TDI sensitivity have yielded numerous conflicting reports. Some workers reported the presence of homocytotropic and "complement inactivating" antibodies, as well as peripheral lymphocyte transformation that was induced by TDI-protein conjugates. Other workers were not able to duplicate these findings and the immunologic picture has remained confused.

Challenge studies performed by Pepys and his colleagues in England[8] showed that "TDI activator" and varnish could elicit immediate, late and dual pulmonary reactions resembling the immediate, late and dual reactions produced by provocative inhalation challenge with certain fungi, animal protein, and organic dust antigens (e.g., *Aspergillus fumigatus*, house dust, pigeon protein, and *Dermatophagoides sp.*), which have been shown to be IgE mediated.

CURRENT STUDIES OF TDI SENSITIVITY

Recent studies of TDI sensitivity have concentrated on prospective surveys of workers in the manufacturing and foaming industries. These studies have consisted of epidemiological monitoring by questionnaire, pulmonary function testing, measurements of immunoglobulin levels, surveys for the development of TDI-specific antibody, and the monitoring of areas and personnel in TDI plants, to quantitate exposure of workers.

Other studies have been directed at the mechanisms of TDI sensitivity. These include the provocative inhalation challenge of TDI-sensitive workers and the assessment of immunological and pharmacological characteristics of the disease.

Epidemiological Surveys

A prospective survey of workers employed in the manufacture of TDI was begun by us in 1973. The questionnaire used was a National Heart and Lung Institute modification of the British Medical Research Council questionnaire with additional questions relevant to TDI manufacturing. To date, the data show no significant increase in the prevalence of bronchitis, atopic disorders, or upper respiratory symptoms. There is, however, a statistically significant ($P < 0.01$) proportion of workers reporting onset of lower respiratory symptoms following exposure to TDI. Further, a significant number ($P < 0.05$) of these symptomatic workers reporting lower respiratory symptoms were non-smokers.

Pulmonary Function

The results of prospective pulmonary function testing and pre- and post-shift measurements of lung function vary. Saia and his colleagues[9] have shown significant decreases of respiratory function below predicted values for workers exposed to both TDI and MDI. Wegman[10] has reported dose response relationships between exposure to TDI and abnormal lung function. In our own prospective studies of workers engaged in the manufacture of TDI, we have been unable to show a loss of lung function either during the working day or over a period of years.[11]

Immunological Studies

As part of our prospective study of TDI workers, we measured total serum immunoglobulin levels (IgG, IgA, IgM, IgE, IgD) and looked for development of TDI-specific IgE antibodies by the radioallergosorbent test (RAST) using TDI complexed to human serum albumin (TDI-HSA), by intradermal skin testing using TDI-HSA, and by Prausnitz-Kustner (P-K) testing in monkeys. We were unable to confirm the earlier positive results of P-K testing by Scheel and his colleagues.[12] Further, although we observed a small number of positive intradermal skin tests with TDI-HSA, these did not correlate with the presence of TDI-induced respiratory symptoms. The RAST yielded a few borderline positive reactions which also failed to correlate with the presence of disease. Neither total eosinophil counts nor immunoglobulin levels changed following TDI exposure.[13] Recently, a positive RAST, using a toluene monoisocyanate-HSA conjugate, has been demonstrated in the serum of some TDI-sensitive individuals.[14]

Pharmacological Studies

Because of the lack of correlation between immunological findings and clinical manifestations of asthma, we examined the ability of TDI to stimulate in vitro histamine release from peripheral leukocytes, as well as the effect of TDI upon stimulation of lymphocyte cyclic adenosine monophosphate (cAMP) by adrenergic agonists. TDI initiated neither specific nor non-specific histamine release from leukocytes.[15] Further, TDI did not affect histamine stimulation of lymphocyte cAMP. However, when TDI was added to lymphocyte suspensions containing the agonists isoproterenol or prostaglandin E_1, cAMP stimulation was depressed. This depression occurred only with certain concentrations of TDI.[15] Subsequent analysis of the kinetics of this in vitro effect indicated that TDI itself appears to be acting as a partial receptor agonist. In light of this finding, we compared TDI reactors to non-reactors by studying lymphocyte cAMP dose response slopes with TDI and adrenergic receptor agonists. Our findings, to date, show that lymphocytes from TDI reactors have a greatly depressed ability to respond to agonists. This suggests that individuals with reactivity to TDI have a qualitative or quantitative deficiency of cell adrenergic receptors, and is consistent with Sventivanyi's β-adrenergic blockade theory of asthma.

Environmental Monitoring

Monitoring of the plant and workers manufacturing TDI has been carried out in a prospective study over the past five years.[11] Environmental monitoring of TDI levels has shown that there are frequent excursions above the threshold limit value (TLV). Personal monitoring confirmed that TDI workers are intermittently exposed to high levels of isocyanate but the levels measured by personal monitoring did not correlate with area monitoring. This indicates that all workers should be individually monitored for exposure to TDI with personal monitors, while area monitors can be used for detection of leaks or high exposures down-wind from the TDI plant.

DIAGNOSTIC AIDS

Workers suspected of TDI sensitivity may be purposefully allowed to re-enter the work environment. Monitoring of TDI levels and pulmonary function tests may demonstrate a relationship between the presence of TDI vapor and the development of an asthmatic reaction coincident with, or occurring shortly after, the occupational exposure. Since, in addition to TDI, other potential offending agents may be present, the only precise method for diagnosing TDI reactivity is to challenge the "sensitive" worker with TDI in a controlled laboratory environment. Further information can be gained by Mecholyl challenge, as discussed below.

Provocative Inhalation with TDI

Provocative inhalation challenge (PIC) with TDI must be performed under carefully controlled conditions. Methods of producing a TDI environment vary among laboratories, but in all cases, monitoring of TDI concentrations is carefully controlled. The "sensitive" worker is exposed for 15 minutes to concentrations starting at 0.005 p.p.m., with daily increases to 0.01 and 0.02 p.p.m. respectively, or until a reaction occurs. Pulmonary function is monitored prior to, and at frequent intervals during the 24 hours following exposure. PIC may produce three types of reactions: 1) an immediate response characterized by at least a 20 percent drop of FEV_1 occurring within 15 minutes of exposure (Fig. 17-2A); 2) a late reaction commencing at least one hour or as much as six to eight hours post challenge (Fig. 17-2B); and 3) a dual reaction consisting of an immediate, followed by a later response (Fig. 17-2C). In some cases, it has been possible to demonstrate a dose response effect by PIC (Fig. 17-2D).[11]

Mecholyl Challenge

Mecholyl (acetyl-β-methacholine) challenge has been used as an adjunct to PIC with TDI in the identification of TDI-sensitive asthmatic workers. Mecholyl is administered by an appropriate pressure-driven nebulizer at concentrations of 5 mg./ml., 10 mg./ml., or 25 mg./ml.,

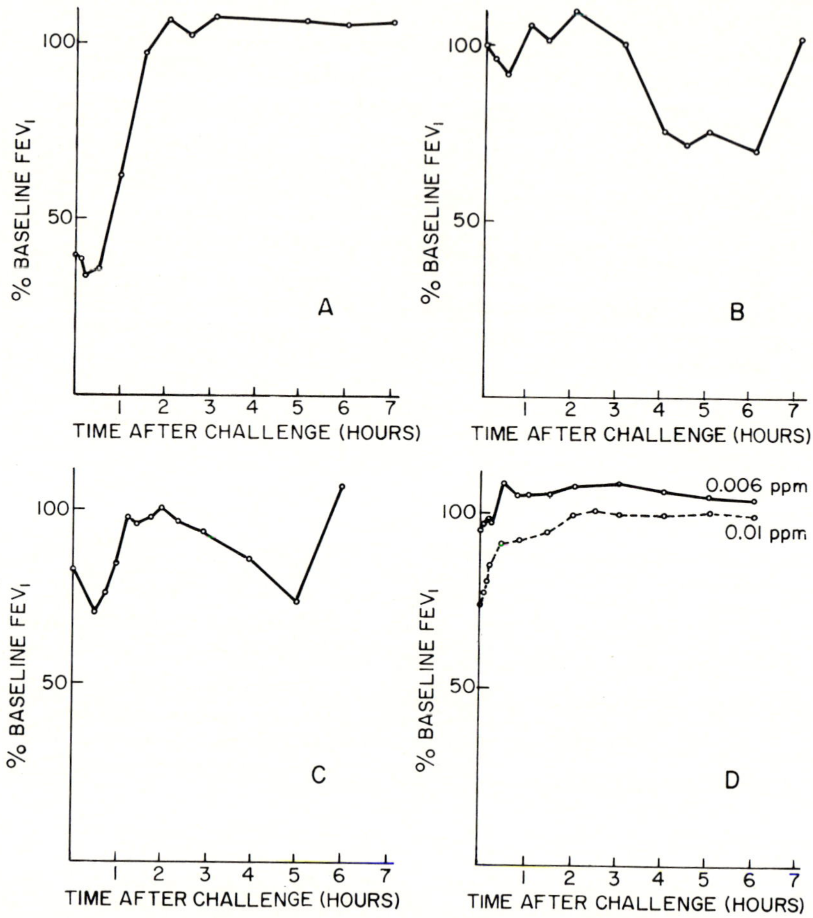

Fig. 17-2. TDI-provocative inhalation challenge results

starting with one breath of the 5 mg./ml. concentration and increasing the number of breaths until five breaths of 25 mg./ml., or a 20 percent drop in FEV_1 is seen. All TDI reactors tested have been shown to respond to Mecholyl challenge, however, an individual with an increased sensitivity to Mecholyl will not necessarily react to TDI.

TREATMENT OF TDI-INDUCED ASTHMA

At present, there is no good treatment for TDI "asthma." Workers proven to have TDI-induced asthma should be removed from environments containing TDI, in which event all asthmatic symptoms will usually

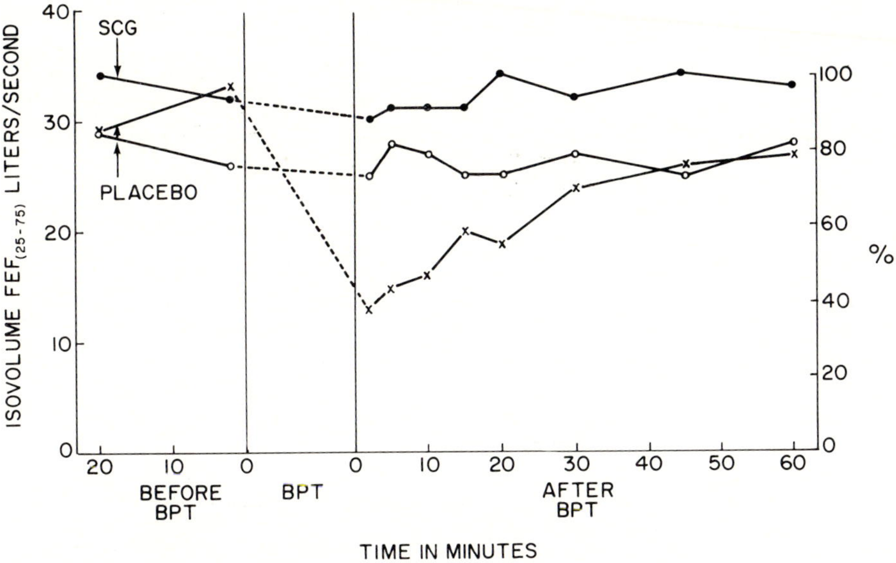

Fig. 17-3. Effect of disodium cromoglycate (SCG) on TDI asthma. ○ — ○ = Saline control; X — X = TDI challenge following placebo; ● — ● = TDI challenge following SCG; BPT = TDI challenge (bronchoprovocation test).

resolve. Should these asthmatic individuals be re-exposed to TDI vapor, they will, again, commonly develop an asthmatic reaction.

Possible prophylactic measures may include inhalation of 40 mg. disodium cromoglycate (DSCG) prior to the work shift, but this has only been shown to be effective in the laboratory environment (Fig. 17-3), at the lowest levels of TDI capable of initiating an asthmatic reaction. The prophylactic use of bronchodilating agents such as theophylline or a β-adrenergic agonist such as isoproterenol or terbutaline may also offer some protection from TDI-induced bronchospasm. The effect of long term, intermittent exposure of normal individuals and of sensitive asthmatic subjects protected with pharmacologic agents is unknown. Therefore, the treatment of choice is to remove the TDI-sensitive worker from any potential exposure to TDI.

SUMMARY

TDI is known to cause asthma-like reactions in approximately five percent of occupationally exposed workers. These asthmatic reactions may be immediate, late or dual responses. With the exception of occasional reports of IgE antibodies detected by toluene monoisocyanate human protein conjugate using the RAST test, there is little evidence for antibody involvement. There is some evidence that TDI may be acting pharmacologically. It has been shown that TDI may be acting as a partial adrenergic receptor agonist. Further, it has been demonstrated that persons reacting to TDI have a decreased ability to respond to adrenergic receptor agonists. TDI reactors also demonstrate increased airway sensitivity to methacholine. These findings indicate that persons who react to TDI are characterized by adrenergic and cholinergic imbalance.

At present there is no adequate treatment for TDI asthma. There is a possibility that prophylactic treatment with disodium cromoglygate and theophylline may be of some use, but the best available approach now is to remove TDI-reactive individuals from environments that may contain TDI vapor. It is hoped that in the near future a pre-employment screening test may be developed to permit identification of high risk individuals, so that they may be excluded from these environments. Possible tests include screening for development of IgE antibodies specific for isocyanates, and pre-employment measurement of lymphocyte cAMP response to adrenergic agonists. Work remains to be done to determine whether workers sensitive to TDI are also sensitive to other organic isocyanates such as MDI and HDI (hexamethyl diisocyanate)—all of which are being used with increased frequency in occupational settings.

REFERENCES

1. LeQuesne PM, Axford AT, McKerrow CB, et al: Neurological complications after a single severe exposure to toluene di-isocyanate. Brit J Indust Med 33:72–78, 1976
2. Munn A: Hazards of isocyanates. Am J Occupat Hygiene 8:163–169, 1965
3. Gaudevia G: Studies of ventilatory capacity and histamine response during exposure to isocyanate vapour in polyurethane foam manufacture. Brit J Indust Med 20:204–209, 1963
4. Peters JM: Cumulative pulmonary effects in workers exposed to tolylene diisocyanate. Proc Roy Soc Med 63:372–375, 1970
5. Blake BL, Mackay JB, Rainey HB, et al: Pulmonary opacities resulting from diisocyanate exposure. J Coll Radiol Aust 9:45–48, 1965
6. Charles J, Bernstein A, Jones B, et al: Hypersensitivity pneumonitis after exposure to isocyanates. Thorax 31:127–136, 1976
7. Reilly DA: A test-paper method for the determination of tolylene di-isocyanate vapour in air. Analyst 93:178–185, 1968
8. Pepys J, Pickering CAC, Breslin ABX, et al: Asthma due to inhaled chemical agents—Tolylene di-isocyanate. Clin Allergy 2:225–236, 1972
9. Saia B, Fabbri L, Mapp C, et al: Epidemiology of chronic non-specific lung disease in a population exposed to isocyanate—I. Analysis of symptoms. Med Lav, 67:278–284, 1976
10. Wegman DH, Pagnotto LD, Fine LJ, et al: A dose-response relationship in TDI workers. J Occupat Med, 16:258–260, 1974

11. Butcher BT, Jones RN, O'Neil CE, et al: Longitudinal study of workers employed in the manufacture of toluene diisocyanate. Am Rev Resp Dis 116:411–421, 1977
12. Scheel LD, Killens R, Josephson A: Immunochemical aspects of toluene diisocyanate (TDI) toxicity. Am Indust Hyg Assoc J 25:179–184, 1964
13. Butcher BT, Salvaggio JE, Weill H, et al: Toluene diisocyanate (TDI) pulmonary disease—Immunologic and inhalation challenge studies. J Allergy Clin Immunol 58:89–100, 1976
14. Karol MH, Ioset HH, Alarie YC: Tolyl-specific IgE antibodies in workers with hypersensitivity to toluene diisocyanate. Am Indust Hyg Assoc J 39:454–458, 1978
15. Davies RJ, Butcher BT, O'Neil CE, et al: The in vitro effect of toluene diisocyanate on lymphocyte cyclic adenosine monophosphate production by isoproterenol, prostaglandin and histamine. A possible mode of action. J Allergy Clin Immunol, 60:223–229, 1977

Dennis J. Stoker
Anthony Leyshon

18

Lumbar Discography: Its Present Status in the Assessment of Disorders of the Intervertebral Disc

Despite medical advances in many fields over the past few decades, low back pain remains a common complaint and a cause of significant morbidity. Radiography is employed routinely in the investigation of the disorder to observe the bony elements of the spine and to exclude specific local lesions of bone. Because standard radiography does not show the soft tissues, information about the intervertebral structures can only be of an indirect nature. As a consequence, the value of radiography in the diagnosis of such common disorders as degenerative disease of the intervertebral disc is in dispute, even though such degeneration, with its associated derangement of the intervertebral joints has long been recognized as a significant cause of low back pain.[1,2]

The main signs relating to disorders of the intervertebral disc, shown on the plain films, comprise reduction in height of the disc space and the formation of osteophytes (spondylosis). Sclerosis of the bony margins of the adjacent vertebral bodies also occurs, probably as a result of abnormal movement at the affected level. The relationship of spondylosis to back pain is neither understood nor generally accepted. The formation of lumbar osteophytes is age-related.[3] As the incidence of rupture of the anulus fibrosus also increases with age,[4] a direct relationship between the two features is possible. Spondylosis is, however, almost as common in the asymptomatic (47 percent) as in the symptomatic (57 percent) patient between the ages of 40 and 70 years, and may not, therefore, be directly related to the causation of back pain.[5]

A variety of radiological contrast examinations are available which help to define the morphological effects of failure of the intervertebral disc mechanism. These include lumbar radiculography, which outlines the nerve roots within their subarachnoid sheaths and ascending lumbar venography, which demonstrates the anatomy of the epidural veins. Disc derangements can thus be identified if they disturb the anatomy of the nerve roots or veins in the region. Discography is the only method of examination which defines the condition of an intervertebral disc by opacifying the nucleus pulposus. Displacement of nerve roots can result from other causes[6]; similar non-specificity limits the value of epidural venography, which can be impossible to interpret in the post-operative patient.[7]

The place of discography in the investigation of disorders of the intervertebral disc is not clearly established. Earlier assessments compared it with less accurate myelography using an oily medium, iophendylate (*Myodil, Pantopaque*). The recent availability of newer methods of investigation such as radiculography[6,8] and epidural venography,[9] both of which are more accurate in the identification of pathological discs, makes it necessary to reassess the position and value of discography. It is, for instance, clear that other lesions may compress nerve roots and mimic a disc protrusion on radiculography[10] and that false positive and even false negative diagnoses[7] may result from venography. McCormick[11] considers that in the diagnosis of intervertebral disc disorders, epidural venography compares poorly with discography and epidurography. (He prefers the latter examination because, in his hands, discography is a painful experience for the patient.)

HISTORICAL

Radiological demonstration of the anatomy of the intervertebral disc was first achieved by Junghanns,[12] who injected red lead into cadaveric specimens. Carl Hirsch of Sweden observed that symptoms from ruptured intervertebral discs could be exacerbated by the injection of normal saline directly into the disc; he reported 16 such cases in 1948.[13] By 1951, his series had extended to 150 cases.[14] At Hirsch's suggestion, Lindblom[15] injected diodrast into 15 discs of 13 patients and described the radiological appearances of normal and ruptured discs, indicating the practical diagnostic value of the technique in sciatica. Any initial fear that disc lesions might be *produced* by this technique was dispelled by Hirsch's observation[16] that puncture or even incision of the anulus during operation resulted in neither an immediate prolapse nor subsequent complications. The intervertebral disc is virtually self-sealing for defects in the anular wall up to 4 mm. in diameter, although changes in physical properties may occur.[17]

Discography was introduced into the United States by Wise and Weiford,[18] who reported their findings in 1950. Numerous reports of small series followed.[19,20,21,22] The center most notably involved in the technique was the Cleveland Clinic; Collis and Gardner published their findings regarding 1,014 cases in 1962[23] and claimed that the method was superior to myelography in the diagnosis of lumbar disc disease. Another large series, of 2,320 cases, was reported by Feinberg.[24] As is often the case after a period of intense enthusiasm, the clinical indications for discography became established and the number of discograms performed diminished. The position of discography at present very much depends on the value placed on it as a diagnostic procedure in disc disease and the relative value of other diagnostic procedures. Despite the promotion of the technique in Sweden and North America, at no time has discography been widely practiced in the United Kingdom or continental Europe. Recently, however, a degree of European interest in discography has been aroused[25,26] and the time seems opportune to assess its value in the diagnosis of intervertebral disc disease.

It has also been contended that with newer contrast media and radiographic equipment, discography has changed. The opportunity will, then, be taken to describe a modern technique.

ANATOMY AND AGING OF THE INTERVERTEBRAL DISC

At birth, the intervertebral disc consists of four distinct parts.[27] On each side an end-plate of hyaline cartilage is attached to the contiguous vertebral body. (Some authors consider the cartilage plate to be part of the centrum, but this is not generally accepted.)[28] Between these are a peripheral fibrocartilaginous ring and a central nucleus pulposus. The nucleus pulposus is sharply demarcated from the fibers of the anulus and has a clear or grayish-translucent appearance; when transected, its surface bulges, reflecting the normal intranuclear pressure. The nucleus pulposus consists of a gel containing vacuolated cells, a collagen framework, and a ground substance consisting mainly of mucopolysaccharide salts and water. In the adult, some fibroblasts and cartilage cells appear. By the third decade, the nucleus is semi-solid and has lost much of its turgidity. The anulus fibrosus is composed of fibrocartilaginous lamellae which are attached to the adjoining vertebrae (Fig. 18-1). The deeper fibers are inserted into the cartilaginous end-plates where a gradual transition from fibrocartilage to hyaline cartilage occurs. The intermediate fibers are inserted into the epiphyseal ring, while the outer fibers skirt the

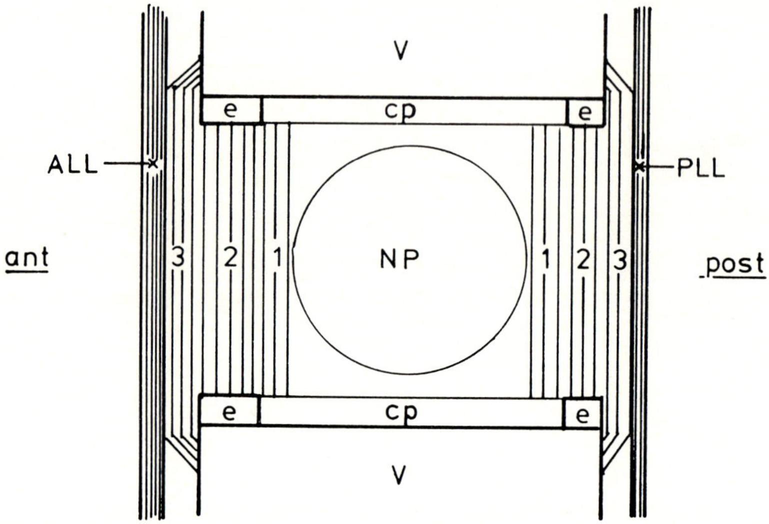

Fig. 18-1. Diagram of intervertebral disc. The attachments of the anulus fibrosus are shown. Its inner fibres (1) attach to the cartilage plates (cp) of the adjoining vertebral bodies (V); the intermediate fibres (2) to the ring epiphysis (e); the outer fibres (3) to the outer aspect of the vertebral bodies. Note that the anterior thickness of the anulus exceeds its posterior thickness. (ALL = anterior longitudinal ligament, PLL = posterior longitudinal ligament, NP = nucleus pulposus).

ring and gain attachment to the adjoining bone of the centrum by means of thickened Sharpey's fibers.[29] Advancing age has an adverse effect on both the nucleus and the anulus.[30] The elastic mechanism of the anulus and the gel properties of the nucleus are progressively lost.[31] Accompanying these changes, fraying and splitting of the innermost anular fibers is observed.[32] The collagenous fibers of the anulus encroach on the nucleus so that, over the years the nucleus changes from a dispersed gel structure to a fibrous dessicated mass of collagen.[33] The tendency towards crystallization and precipitation of collagen from about the fourth decade inhibits the uniform transmission of pressure and may result in abnormally high local stresses on a particular part of the anulus.

DISCOGRAPHIC FINDINGS

Normal. In the adult (Fig. 18-2), the lumbar discogram typically shows two more or less parallel plates of contrast medium communicating posteriorly (Fig. 18-3). Thus, the normal discogram resembles a half-opened clam or oyster shell. This differs from the infant discogram where the entire nucleus pulposus is outlined by the contrast medium.[34] Sung et

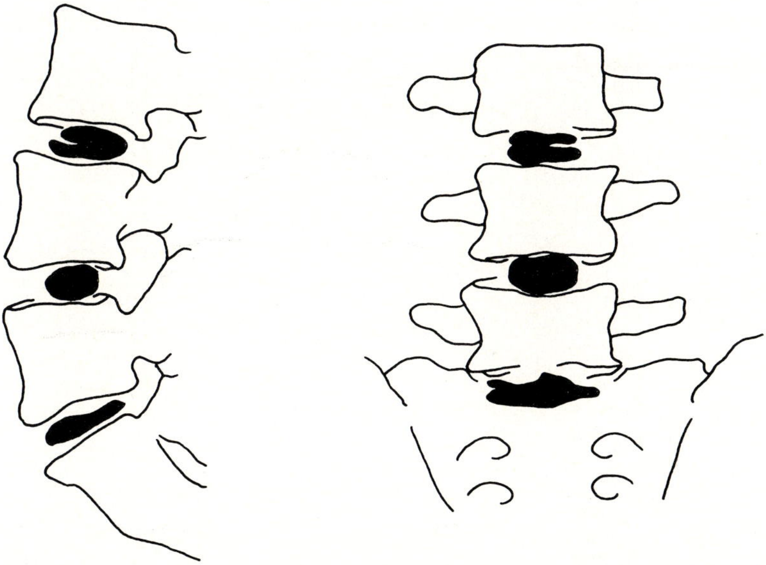

Fig. 18-2. Diagram of normal discographic appearances. From above, descending: L3-4: Normal disc showing bilocular pattern. L4-5: Normal disc showing unilocular pattern ("cotton ball"). L5-S1: Normal disc showing only slight flattening of contour due to anatomical variation at the lumbo-sacral junction.

al.[35] have indicated that the shadow shown in the discogram is not the whole of the nucleus pulposus, and that its periphery does not accept the medium. Occasionally, the condensation that accounts for the anatomical change in adult life invaginates the nucleus posteriorly so that the residual communication is anterior. Rarely, a lateral communication continuous with the posterior one is shown, and even more rarely, a central or collar-stud appearance results. Separate loculi requiring two punctures are also found. The incidence of the various types of communication have been recorded as follows.*

Posterior	19	25	67.5%
Posterior and lateral	6		
Anterior	6		16%
Two separate loculi	5		13.5%
Central	1		

* (Cadaveric discograms in 37 subjects aged 20–49, from Kieffer et al., 1969)[34]

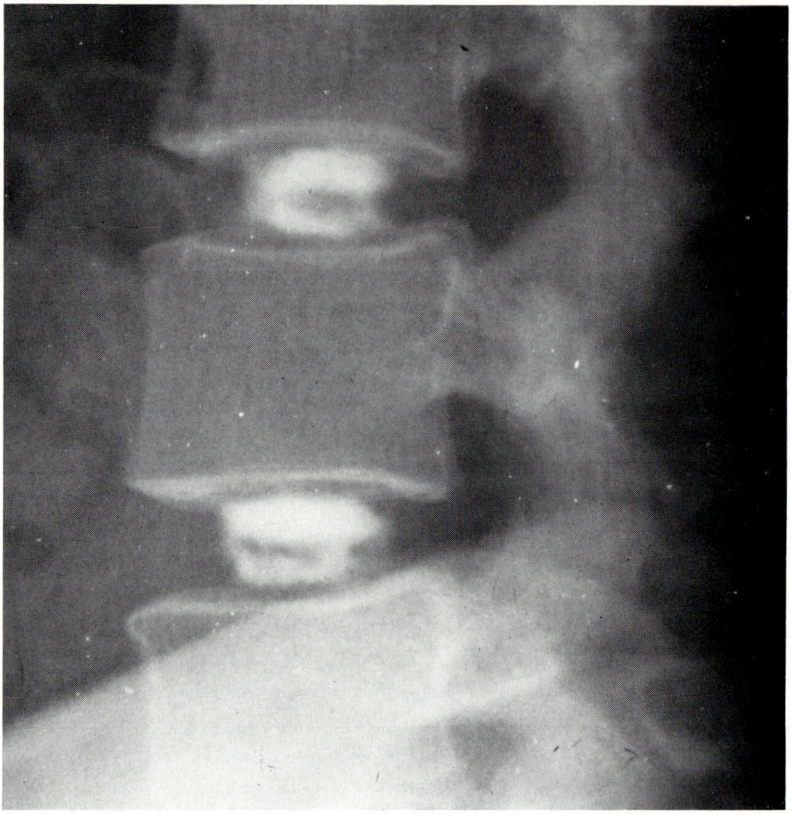

Fig. 18-3. Normal discographic appearance. Discograms at L3-4 and L4-5 show the typical bilocular appearance. The anulus is intact.

Although Butt[36] suggested that in discography, the contrast medium, which lies in the potential space between nucleus and anulus, other does not mix with the substance of the nucleus, but merely coats it, observations do not confirm this view.[34,35]

Abnormal. Anular rupture (Fig. 18-4) is indicated by the passage of contrast medium beyond the normal confines of the nucleus and, with complete rupture, into the extradural space (Figs. 18-5 and 18-6). If a significant amount of disc material has extruded, it may be outlined by the medium. Degenerative change in the disc results in a modification of the round or oval shape of the nucleus; it becomes flatter and broader in outline. Fissures appear within the substance of the nucleus and extend peripherally into the deep surface of the anulus.

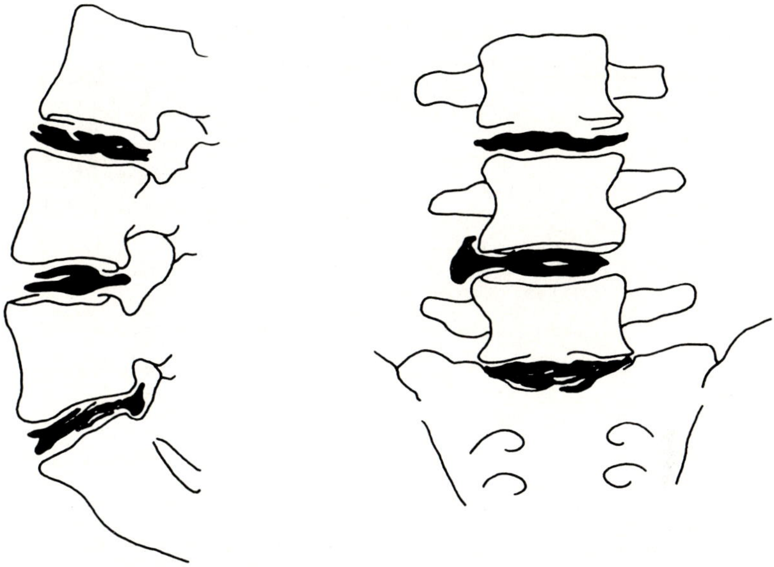

Fig. 18-4. Diagram of abnormal discographic appearances. From above, descending: L3-4: Degenerate disc. L4-5: Non-degenerate disc showing posterolateral protrusion. L5-S1: Degenerate disc with posterior protrusion.

INDICATIONS FOR DISCOGRAPHY

In the many papers following that of Lindblom[15] little agreement has been achieved on the indications for discography. Most authors regard the technique as a substitute for pantopaque myelography and therefore use the same clinical indications. Wiley et al.[37] gave the following indications: (a) patients with low back pain who have no evidence of root irritation and no localizing signs clinically or radiographically; (b) bizarre radiation of back pain, e.g., to the groin; (c) obvious evidence of disc herniation in patients for whom a combination of discotomy with spinal fusion is proposed; and (d) patients who develop recurrent or continuous back pain after laminectomy and discotomy, to determine whether pain originates from that site or another.

Broadly similar indications have been employed by the authors of other large series.[38]

The introduction of water-soluble myelographic media has increased the accuracy of demonstrating entrapment and displacement of nerve roots.[39] Epidural venography has provided another means of demonstrating the space-occupying disc protrusion. Neither of these examinations demonstrates the disc itself. Because water-soluble radiculography does

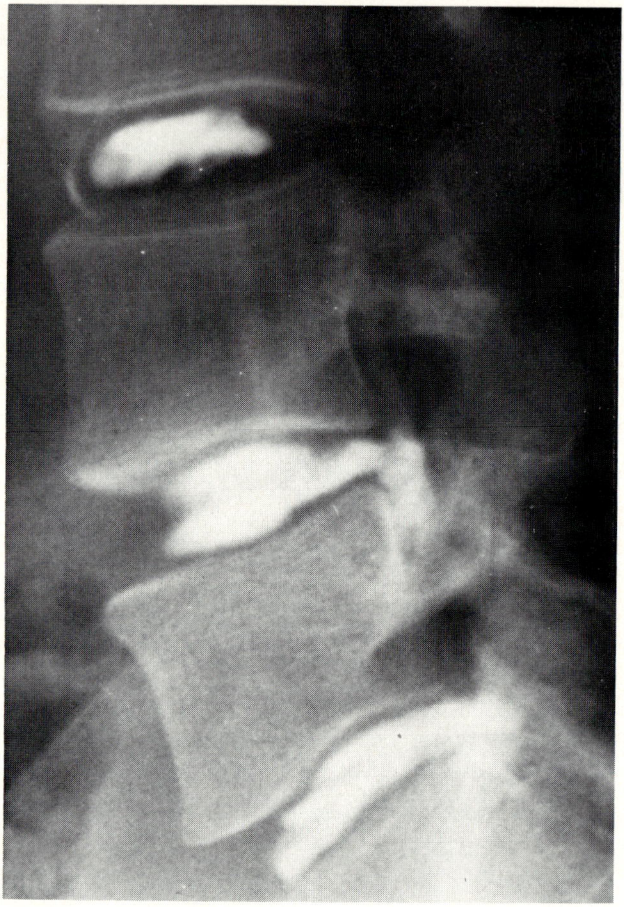

Fig. 18-5. Abnormal discographic appearances. The L3-4 disc is normal. The medium outside the nucleus leaked after the needle was removed. Posterior protrusions are present at L4-5 and L5-S1. The lower disc shows early fissuring of degenerative change.

demonstrate the nerve roots, it should be used as a primary contrast investigation in patients with referred nerve root pain. Discography should not be undertaken before radiculography in such cases, as it may prove to be unnecessary; furthermore, it may result in more severe root involvement.[23] We believe that the advent of accurate radiculography has resulted in an altered emphasis in the indications for discography and a more clearly defined role for the examination. Our indications are: (a) in a patient with suspected disc disease and a normal radiculogram, to

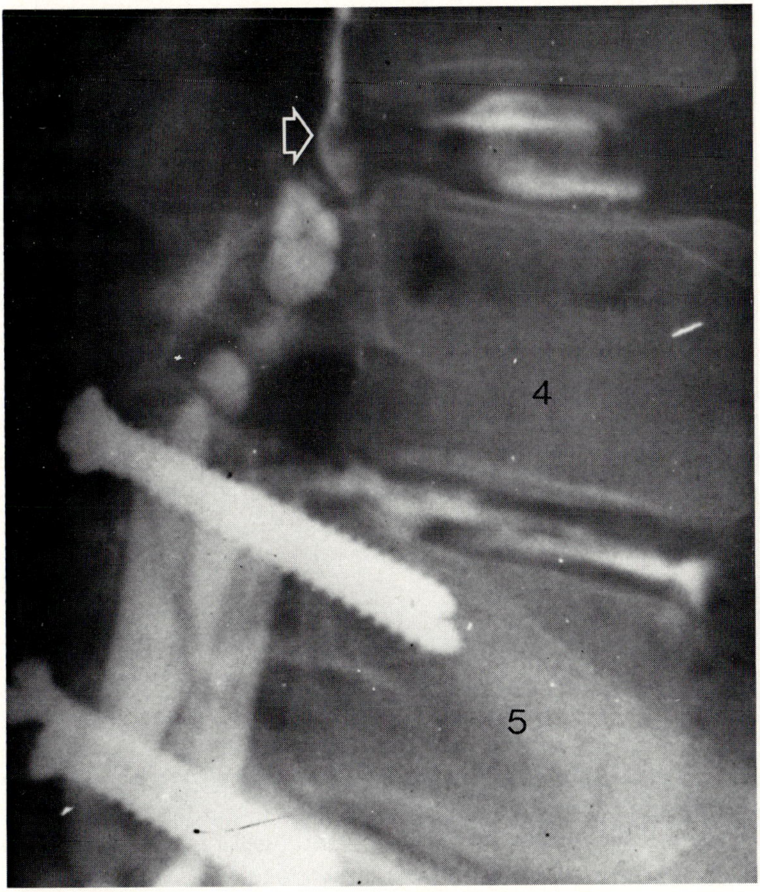

Fig. 18-6. Post-operative discography. The disc at the fused level (L4-5) is degenerate. A posterior anular tear was shown at L3-4, the subdural contrast medium (arrow) appearing during the examination.

confirm or exclude disc disease; (b) to establish, if possible, a symptomatic level where several discs appear to be abnormal on clinical and radiculographic grounds; (c) where arthrodesis is contemplated, to determine the state of the discs above and, if applicable, below the level of proposed fusion (the demonstration of multiple degenerative discs may, indeed, alter the decision to operate; this indication applies to spondylolisthesis as well as primary disc disorders); (d) to confirm normality of the lumbar discs in patients with low back pain and no evidence of root irritation and no localizing sign on routine clinical and radiological examination (this also includes patients where pain of psychogenic origin is suspected); (e) in patients, following spinal fusion, who continue to experience pain in the lumbar region, or who develop further pain after a period of relief (In such cases, the integrity of the discs adjoining the level of fusion are examined.); and (f) prior to chemonucleolysis.[40]

CONTRAINDICATIONS

Because of the seriousness of disc infection, discography is contraindicated in the presence of infection.[36] We especially refer to pyogenic infection of the skin, but defer examination, as well, in cases where the patient is febrile and possible bacteremia cannot be excluded. Discography is contraindicated in the presence of massive disc herniation because of the danger of producing a cauda equina syndrome.[41] Butt[36] cites this as a reason for not using discography as a primary procedure; we would completely discourage discography in this situation. Discography is unnecessary when a patient with lumbar root irritation has radiculographic findings that correlate with the clinical signs. Discography is not indicated in the very young (under 20 years) or the old (over 60 years), except in exceptional circumstances.

TECHNIQUE OF DISCOGRAPHY

The early discograms were performed in the median plane with the patient prone on a special table.[23,42] Using modern fluoroscopic equipment, the examination may be performed by one of three possible approaches: posterior, posterolateral, and lateral. In most reported studies, and in our early cases, the posterior approach was used.

The *posterior* technique involves either the passage of a small needle through a larger spinal needle (in our cases a 26 gauge needle was passed through a 20 or 22 gauge needle at each level) or using a single 22 gauge needle.[37] In both cases only a small puncture (26–22 gauge) breaches the posterior longitudinal ligament and the anulus in the median plane.

The *posterolateral* approach is favored by some workers[43,44,45,46] and offers an alternative should difficulty be experienced with another approach.

Both of these approaches are transdural and result in puncture of the theca with the attendant sequela of leakage of spinal fluid. With the introduction of chemonucleolysis, the requirement that chymopapain be injected only into the nucleus pulposus made a routine extradural approach mandatory. We therefore adopted and modified the technique of Lyman-Smith and Brown[40] for all discograms, whether chemonucleolysis was to follow or not. Such a technique is possible with a combina-

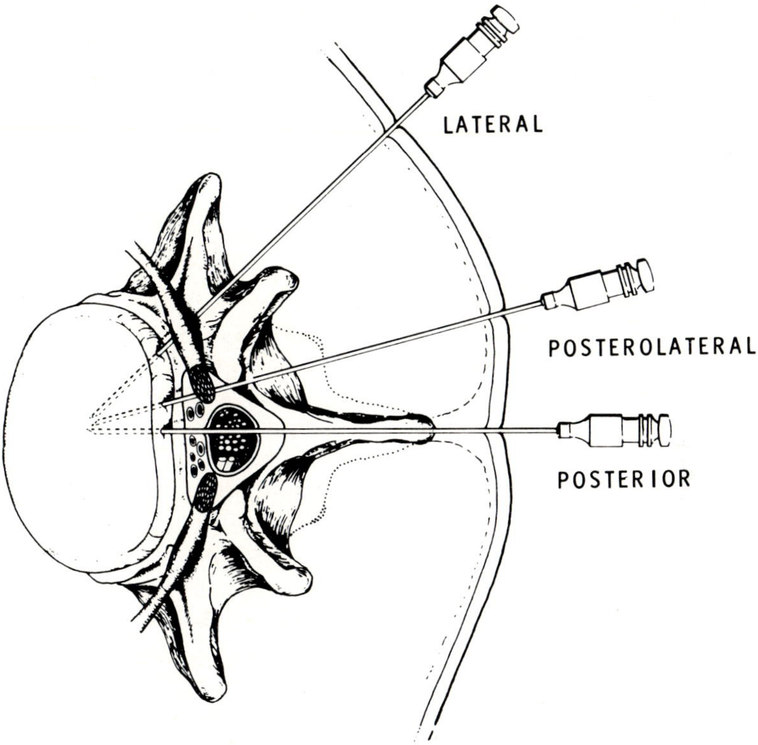

Fig. 18-7. Lumbar discography. Three approaches that may be employed; only the lateral approach is extradural.

tion of vertical fluoroscopy and horizontal beam films to confirm the position of the needles, but is made infinitely quicker and easier by the use of biplane or multiplane fluoroscopy. The availability of such equipment contributed to our conversion to the lateral approach.

The technique described below relates to lumbar discography as a diagnostic radiological procedure. Where it is intended that chemonucleolysis follow discography, only two departures from the technique are employed: a general anesthetic is given, and a larger needle (18 gauge) is used routinely.

The diagnostic examination is performed under sedation and local anesthetic. The use of general anesthesia is extremely rare, and is determined by the patient's temperament or condition. An indwelling intravenous needle is inserted and diazepam ("Valium" Roche) is given in a dose of 10–50 mg., sufficient to produce drowsiness and slurring of the patient's speech.

The patient is placed on his left side on the fluoroscopy table. A firm pad is placed under his left loin; this facilitates access to the L5–S1 disc. The patient is secured by a band or adhesive strapping across the pelvis to reduce unwanted movement (Fig. 18-8).

An aseptic technique is used; the skin is prepared and the radiologist is gowned and masked as for any surgical procedure. With the usual clinical problem, i.e., when a disc disorder is suspected at either the L4–5 or the L5–S1 level, the L4–5 disc is approached first because it is the easier level to puncture and serves as a marker for the later puncture of L5–S1. The skin is infiltrated with 0.5 percent lignocaine at an average distance of 8 cm. from the median plane (range 7–9 cm.), in the transverse plane of the lower margin of the body of L4 (Fig. 18-9). Deeper infiltration with local anesthetic is undertaken through the 6 inch 20 gauge discography needle as it is inserted under fluoroscopic control at an angle which will ensure that the anulus is pierced by the tip of the needle in its posterior third. The needle is carefully positioned so that it rests against the anterior longitudinal ligament at this site and local anesthetic is in-

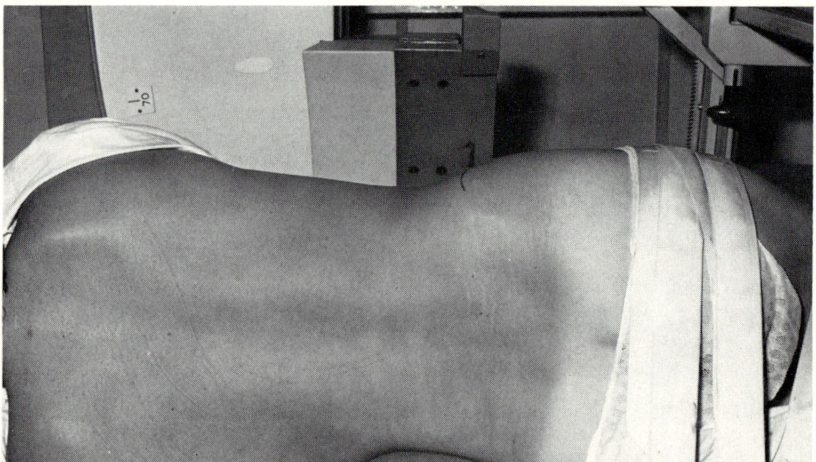

Fig. 18-8. Position for lateral discographic approach. The patient is lying on his left side with a firm pad placed below his right loin. The position is maintained by the use of straps across the hip region. The right iliac crest has been marked for ease of identification.

directly to the nerve root. Pain in such cases may be a form of radiating mesenchymal pain, as described by Inman and Saunders.[51] We have not found injection of meglumine iothalamate solution ("Conray 280") through an accurately placed needle to produce troublesome pain in any but a few patients, and we therefore do not mix local anesthetic with the contrast medium, as does Patrick.[52]

DISADVANTAGES AND COMPLICATIONS

Several authors not practicing discography have commented on the dangers of infecting or permanently damaging an intervertebral disc during discography. Infection is in fact rare; much of the early apprehension about this possible complication stemmed from the report by Pease,[53] who described destruction of the lumbar disc following the inadvertent insertion of a needle through the anulus at lumbar puncture. The relevance of this observation is minimized, however, when it is considered that the series involved the use of large needles and that all the patients were children suspected of purulent meningitis. Of a total of 5,000 discograms collected from the literature,[37] infection was subsequently diagnosed in 30 (0.6 percent); 19 of these came from a group of 88 performed by one researcher. Certainly, proven infection is now very rare, and has never been observed by most authors. Wiley et al.[37] described only one infective discitis following discography at a total of 2,517 levels.

Some concern has been expressed that, even the insertion of a needle into the anulus may cause permanent damage to an intact disc. Little evidence has been produced to support this view, and operative and experimental studies that do exist suggest the opposite. Clinical surveys of large groups of patients following discography do not reveal changes suggesting disc damage on plain x-ray, myelography or surgical exploration.[41] Other authors have expressed the belief that discography does not result in clinical or mechanical damage to a normal disc.[23,54] As with other similar types of examinations, an allergic reaction to the contrast medium may, in rare cases, occur. Such reactions are managed routinely and, indeed, discography has some advantages over certain other contrast examinations. The amount of medium injected, for example, is small, patients are supervised for several hours, and an in-dwelling intravenous needle is employed during the examination. In difficult examinations, especially in obese patients, needles have been known to break.[41] An important complication is exacerbation of root symptoms following discography, rarely progressing, however, to a cauda equina syndrome. Such a complication indicates an immediate need for laminectomy. The danger of this complication makes it imperative that a water-soluble myelogram be performed prior to discography if symptoms and signs of nerve root compression are present.

Discography is absolutely contraindicated in the presence of spinal stenosis. As we have seen, in the early studies much stress was laid on the painful nature of the discographic examination. Cloward[54] comments that discography is painful in comparison with myelography, but that the pain lasts only a matter of minutes. More recently, in a small series employing a transdural approach, McCormick[11] stated that most patients experienced severe pain during the examination. It has been our experience that uncomplicated extradural discography is not a particularly painful procedure, and that most patients prefer it to myelography. The reason for this change in response may be due to the extradural approach, altered premedication and local anesthesia, or the contrast media—now essentially those containing meglumine salts. Certainly, the use of the extradural approach means that headache is not a complication of discography.

MATERIAL

The first 100 patients undergoing discography at the Royal National Orthopaedic Hospital form the subject of this part of the study. They comprise 58 females and 42 males between the ages of 20 and 61 years. Details are provided in Table 18-1. The main clinical diagnosis is shown in Table 18-2. The diagnostic pattern is quite variable, but the patients have been grouped, based on the indications for discography, into those with or without previous spinal surgery (Table 18.3).

The overall failure rate was 6.0 percent. Most of the failures occurred at the lumbosacral level in the early development of the technique. Details of levels attempted are shown in Table 18-4.

Table 18-1
Discography Review: 100 patients,*
Age 20–61 years (Mean age 38.9 years)

20–29 yrs.	16%	10 female : 6 male
30–39 yrs.	37%	25 female : 12 male
40–49 yrs.	32%	16 female : 16 male
50–59 yrs.	14%	7 female : 7 male
60–69 yrs.	1%	1 male

* No previous surgery: 80

Previous surgery: 20 { fusions 12; decompressions 6; discectomy 6 }

Table 18-2
Clinical Diagnosis

Disc degeneration	43
Failed spinal fusion	11
Low back pain ± depression	10
Lumbar instability	8
Prolapsed intervertebral disc (acute)	7
Spondylolysis/listhesis	6
Failed laminectomy	5
Prolapsed intervertebral disc (chronic)	4
Spinal cord claudication	2
"Mechanical backache"	2
"Segmental derangement"	1
Zygapophyseal joint o.a.	1

RESULTS

A positive correlation with the production of pain at discography was obtained in 28 patients (28.0 percent; see Table 18-5). This was most common at the L4–5 level,[17] but also occurred at L5–S1[5] and L2–3 and L3–4 (2 and 4 respectively). The other findings at discography are detailed in Table 18-6.

Table 18-3
Indications for Discography

GROUP 1: No prior spinal surgery, 80 patients		
Assessment prior to posterior spinal fusion	48	60.0 %
As part of the investigatory work up in patients with low back pain	22	27.5 %
To confirm suspected disc normality, e.g., in suspected psychiatric disorder	5	6.25%
To diagnose disc abnormality and determine level prior to chemonucleolysis	3	3.75%
To diagnose disc abnormality and determine level prior to intradiscal injection of hydrocortisone	2	2.5 %
GROUP 2: Prior spinal surgery, 20 patients		
To assess state of adjoining discs following failed posterior spinal fusion	10	50.0 %
To assess the disc state following laminectomy and discectomy prior to possible spinal fusion	8	40.0 %
To diagnose pseudarthrosis following posterior spinal fusion	2	10.0 %

Table 18-4
Disc Levels Attempted*

L2/3	13	0 Failures	0%
L3/4	82	1 Failure	1.2%
L4/5	98	3 Failures	3.1%
L5/S1	74	12 Failures	16.2%

* Total number of discs attempted: 267
Total number of discs injected: 251
Overall failure rate: 6.0%

Table 18-5
Pain Correlation*

L2/3	2
L3/4	4
L4/5	17
L5/S1	5

* 28 of 251 discs (11.2%), or, 28 of 100 patients (28.0%) gave a positive correlation.

Of greatest importance is the effect the investigation has on the clinical management of the individual patient. The implications of the discographic findings for those patients not previously subjected to spinal surgery and for those who had been operated on before are shown in Table 18-7. In 36.2 percent of those without prior surgery, the examination did not alter treatment, but in the remaining 63.8 percent the decision to operate was either abandoned, or the type of operation planned was altered.

Table 18-6

Level	Normal disc	Increased volume	Disc protrusions and anular tears	Disc degenerations
L2/3	10 (13)	3	4	2
	76.9%	23.1%	30.8%	15.4%
L3/4	59 (81)	6	16	11
	72.8%	7.4%	14.7%	13.6%
L4/5	40 (95)	22	41	35
	42.1%	23.2%	43.2%	36.8%
L5/S1	30 (62)	13	19	21
	48.4%	21.0%	30.6%	33.9%

Total No. of normal discs: 139 (55.4%)
Total No. of abnormal discs: 112 (44.6%)

Table 18-7
Decisions Taken After Discography

Decision taken	No prior spinal surgery (80 patients)	Prior spinal surgery (20 patients)
Proceed to surgery planned	29 36.2%	3 15.0%
Prior decision on surgery altered to one of no surgery	17 21.3%	8 40.0%
Need for surgery confirmed but surgical technique altered, e.g., fusion level changed	15 18.8%	5 25.0%
Clinical diagnosis confirmed and decision taken to treat non-surgically, e.g., intradiscal hydrocortisone or chemonucleolysis	9 11.2%	0 0.0%
Disc normality suspected clinically confirmed	7 8.8%	1 5.0%
Surgeon ignored discographic findings	2 2.5%	2 10.0%
Surgery abandoned in favor of other treatment	1 1.2%	2 10.0%

In patients who had had prior surgery, the surgery was abandoned or its type altered in as many as 85.0 percent of the cases.

ILLUSTRATIVE CASE HISTORIES

In order to illustrate the ways in which lumbar discography may be useful in patient evaluation, three case histories that exemplify the particular value of this examination are presented.

Case 1. Mrs. MS, a 42-year-old nurse, presented with a five year history of low back pain without any radiation into the legs. Previous treatment with bed rest, traction and physiotherapy had not relieved her symptoms. Examination of her spine revealed no obvious abnormality and, in particular, the spine was fully mobile and there was no abnormal neurology in the lower limbs. Standard radiographs of the lumbar spine showed possible minimal narrowing of the L4/5 disc space. A radiculogram was normal.

Lumbar discography of L3/4 and L5/S1 levels was normal but, at the L4/5 disc, flattening, degeneration and a posterior protrusion were noted. Injection of contrast medium at this level reproduced the patient's pain exactly.

A discectomy at L4/5 was performed and an isolated posterior screw fusion (Boucher) of L4/5 was performed. The patient was back at work, symptom-free, three months after the operation.

Case 2. Mr. RJ, a 54-year-old truck driver, presented with a ten year history of positional low back pain with some radiation into both thighs. His spine showed excellent movement. There was some local tenderness at L4, but no other positive physical findings were present. Standard radiographs revealed a marked narrowing of the L4/5 disc space with adjacent bony sclerosis and osteophyte formation. The other lumbar disc spaces appeared normal.

On clinical grounds it was felt that he justified a possible fusion at the L4/5 level; further investigations were, therefore, initiated. Radiculography revealed no abnormality. Lumbar discography of all spaces below L2 revealed that all discs were markedly degenerate; injection at each level reproduced the patient's back pain.

In view of the multi-level degeneration, spinal fusion was not performed and he was treated symptomatically with a surgical corset.

Case 3. Mr. DC, a 41-year-old baker, presented in 1974 with a 16-year history of low back pain. In 1963 an L5 laminectomy had been performed and a prolapsed disc excised. Continued symptoms led in 1969 to a posterior spinal fusion at the L5/S1 level which failed to relieve his back pain. Six months prior to admission to this Hospital, an explorative laminectomy at the L4 level had been performed which revealed no pathology. His symptoms were of positional low back pain with some radiation into the left leg to the calf. Examination revealed an exceedingly stiff and painful lumbar spine. There were no abnormal neurological signs in the legs. Standard radiographs revealed a Grade 2 spondylolisthesis at the lumbo-sacral level, and a pseudarthrosis at the fusion site could not be ruled out. The upper lumbar disc spaces appeared normal.

Radiculography was normal, but discography at the L3/4 and L4/5 levels revealed a grossly degenerate disc at the lower level, the upper disc space being normal.

Accordingly, a Wiltse lateral mass fusion from L4 to the sacrum was performed with excellent relief of symptoms at three year follow-up.

CONCLUSION

Lumbar discography should no longer be employed as a primary diagnostic procedure in the investigation of disorders of the intervertebral disc. It has never been used as widely as myelography because of its technical difficulties and problems in interpretation. With the introduction of water-soluble myelographic agents and an increased accuracy in the diagnosis of disc protrusion by this method, the clinical requirement for discography remains a small one. Nevertheless, patients with clinical evidence of a disc disorder and normal or equivocal radiculographic findings do require an additional contrast investigation.[11] Discography remains the only examination that demonstrates the disc itself and not the secondary effects of disc derangement on other tissues. The practice of discography, therefore, is still required in centers treating the complications of disc prolapse and degeneration. In this chapter an attempt has been made to define the current indications for the procedure, to describe the technique, and to assess its value in the clinical management of the patient with backache.

REFERENCES

1. Barr JS, Kubik CS, Molloy MK et al: Evaluation of end results in treatment of ruptured lumbar intervertebral discs with protrusion of nucleus pulposus. Surg Gynec Obstet 125:250–256, 1967
2. Hirsch C: Studies on the pathology of low back pain. J Bone Jt Surg (Br) 41:237–243, 1959
3. Nathan H: Osteophytes of the vertebral column. J Bone Jt Surg (Am) 44:243–268, 1962
4. Farfan HF, Huberdeau RM, Dubow HI: Lumbar intervertebral disc degeneration—the influence of geometrical features on the pattern of disc degeneration—a post-mortem study. J Bone Jt Surg (Am) 54:492–510, 1972
5. Torgerson WR, Dotter WE: Comparative roentgenographic study of the asymptomatic and symptomatic lumbar spine. J Bone Jt Surg (Am) 58:850–853, 1976
6. Hansen EB, Praestholm J, Fahrenkrug A et al: A clinical trial of Amipaque in lumbar myelography. Br J Radiol 49:34–38, 1976
7. Sackett JF, Damm MG, Javid MJ: Unreliability of epidural venography in lumbar disc disease. Surg Neurol 7:35–38, 1977
8. Grainger RG, Gumpert J, Sharpe DM et al: Water-soluble radiculography. A clinical trial of Dimer X—a new contrast medium. Clin Radiol 22:57–62, 1971
9. Gargano EP, Meyer JD, Sheldon JJ: Transfemoral ascending lumbar catheterisation of the epidural veins in lumbar disk disease. Radiology 111:329–336, 1974
10. Macnab I: Negative disc exploration. J Bone Jt Surg (Am) 53:891–903, 1971
11. McCormick CC: Radiology in low back pain and sciatica. An analysis of the relative efficacy of spinal venography, discography and epidurography in patients with a negative or equivocal myelogram. Clin Radiol 29:393–406, 1978
12. Schmorl G, Junghanns H: The human spine in health and disease, 1st American edition. New York & London, Grune & Stratton, 1959
13. Hirsch C: An attempt to diagnose the level of a disc lesion clinically by disc puncture. Acta Orthop Scand 18:132–140, 1948
14. Hirsch C: Studies on the mechanism of low back pain. Acta Orthop Scand 20:261–274, 1951
15. Lindblom K: Diagnostic puncture of intervertebral disks in sciatica. Acta Orthop Scand 17:231–239, 1948
16. Hirsch C: The reaction of intervertebral discs to compression forces. J Bone Jt Surg 37:1188–1196, 1955
17. Markolf KL, Morris JM: The structural components of the intervertebral disc. J Bone Jt Surg (Am) 56:675–687, 1974

18. Wise RE, Weiford EC: X-ray visualization of intervertebral disk; report of a case. Cleve Clin Q 18:127–130, 1951
19. Peterson HO: Discography. Postgrad Med 23:512–517, 1958
20. Walk L: Clinical significance of discography. Acta Radiol (Diagn) (Stockh) 46:36–37, 1956
21. Walker JC: Discography in study and investigation of low back pain. West J Surg 68:240–243, 1956
22. Wise RE, Gardner WJO, Hosier RB: X-ray visualization of the intervertebral disc. N Engl J Med 257:6–10, 1957
23. Collis JS Jr, Gardner WJ: Lumbar discography; an analysis of 1000 cases. J Neurosurg 19:452–459, 1962
24. Feinberg SB: The place of diskography in radiology as based on 2320 cases. Am J Roentgenol 92:1275–1281, 1964
25. Legré J, Dufour M, Debaene A et al: La discographie lombaire; valeur et indications après 300 examens. Neurochirurgie 17:559–578, 1971
26. Patton JT: Proceedings—Discography in assessment of lumbar disc disease. Ann Rheum Dis 34:466–467, 1975
27. Hadley LA: Anatomic–roentgenographic studies of the spine. Springfield, Illinois, Charles C Thomas, 1964
28. Coventry MB: Anatomy of the intervertebral disk. Clin Orthop 67:9–15, 1969
29. McNab I: The traction spur: an indication of segmental instability. J Bone Jt Surg (Am) 53:663–670, 1971
30. Coventry MB, Ghormley RK, Kernohan JW: The intervertebral disc: its microscopic anatomy and pathology. II Changes in the intervertebral disc concomitant with age. J Bone Jt Surg 27:233–247, 1945
31. Naylor A, Happey F, MacRae T: The collagenous changes in the intervertebral disk with age and their effect on its elasticity. An x-ray crystallographic study. Br Med J ii:570–573, 1954
32. Pritzker KPH: Aging and degeneration in the lumbar intervertebral disc. Orthop Clin North Am 8:65–77, 1977
33. Vernon Roberts SB, Pirie CJ: Degenerative changes in the intervertebral discs of the lumbar spine and their sequelae. Rheumatol Rehabil 16:13–21, 1977
34. Kieffer St.A, Stadlan EM, Mohandas A et al: Discographic-anatomical correlation of developmental changes with age in the intervertebral disc. Acta Radiol (Diagn) (Stockh) 9:733–739, 1969
35. Sung HW, Chia Y-M, Kuo H-T et al: Lumbar discography—an experimental and clinical study. Chin Med J (Engl) 83:521–530, 1964
36. Butt WP: Lumbar discography. J Canad Assoc Radiol 14:172–181, 1963
37. Wiley JJ, Macnab I, Wortzman G: Lumbar discography and its clinical application. Canad J Surg 11:280–289, 1968
38. Massare C, Bernageau J: Indications de la discographie. Bilan après 1200 discographies. J Radiol Electrol Med Nucl 53:429–431, 1971
39. Grainger RG: Water-soluble radiculography, in Lodge and Steiner (eds.) Recent Advances in Radiology (No. 5). Edinburgh, Churchill Livingstone, 1975, pp 37–50
40. Smith L, Brown JE: Treatment of lumbar intervertebral disc lesions by direct injection of chymopapain. J Bone Jt Surg (Br) 49:502–519, 1967
41. Collis JS Jr: Lumbar discography. Springfield, Charles C Thomas, 1963
42. Cloward RB, Buzaid LL: Diskography. Am J Roentgenol 68:552–564, 1952
43. Erlacher PR: Direkte Kontrastdarstellung des Nucleus pulposus Zugleich ein Beitrag zur Pathologie der Bandscheibe. Z Orthop 80:40–57, 1950
44. Gleason PG: Technic of discographie. US Armed Forces Med J 3:1831–1837, 1952

45. Keck, C: Discography: technique and interpretation. AMA Arch Surg 80:580–585, 1960
46. Witt AN: Practische Erfahrungen mit der Nukleographie (vorläufig Bericht). Z Orthop 80:57–71, 1950
47. Farfan HF: Mechanical disorders of the low back. Philadelphia, Lea & Febiger, 1973
48. Knutsson F: The instability associated with disc degeneration in the lumbar spine. Acta Radiol (Diagn) (Stockh) 25:593–609, 1944
49. Morgan FP, King T: Primary instability of lumbar vertebrae as a common cause of low back pain. J Bone Jt Surg (Br) 39:6–22, 1957
50. Lettin AWL: Diagnosis and treatment of lumbar instability. J Bone Jt Surg (Br) 49:520–529, 1967
51. Inman WT, Saunders JB de CM: Referred pain from skeletal structures. J Nerv Ment Dis 99:660–667, 1944
52. Patrick BS: Lumbar discography: a five year study. Surg Neurol 1:267–273, 1973
53. Pease CN: Injuries to vertebrae and intervertebral disks following lumbar puncture. Am J Dis Child 49:849–860, 1935
54. Cloward R: Lumbar discography (discussion). J Neurosurg 19:459–460, 1962

Leslie Preger
Landrus Pfeffinger
Jack D. Noyes

19
Lumbar Epidural Venography

The inclusion of the preceding chapters on lumbar discography and this one on epidural venography is predicated on the fact that large numbers of patients are presenting themselves with employment- and industry-related back injuries. Back injuries now number about one-half million per year in the United States. In New York State back injuries without bony involvement are responsible for 16 percent of lost working time, with an average of 46 weeks lost per patient.* It is appropriate to discuss lumbar discography and epidural venography, which may lead to earlier diagnosis of remediable lumbar disc disease and so identify those subsets to whom surgical therapy should be offered and those who should have prescribed a conservative medical program, leading to early return to gainful employment.

Selective epidural venography (EV) has a place in the radiographic assessment of lumbar disc disease. The purposes of this chapter are to describe in some detail a technique that has been found useful, to illustrate normal and abnormal venograms, to summarize much previously published material, to add to this material our own series, and to attempt to indicate the value of EV. The technique is described in greater detail than usual since it represents hard won practical experience.

If the clinical diagnosis of protruded disc (with an intact annulus) or herniated disc (with disruption of annular fibers) was easily and accurately arrived at, then the single radiological examination necessary in the majority of patients would comprise an AP and lateral view of the lumbo-

---

* Russek AS: Biomechanical and physiological basis for ambulatory treatment of low back pain. Orthopaedic Rev 5:21–31, 1976

sacral spine to help exclude an unsuspected metastasis or primary bone disease. Sciatic type pain may have its origin in the thalamus, the exiting foramina, or in or near the vertebral body and its bony appendages, or it may be radicular in origin, due to a variety of diseases within the bony spinal canal; the pain may be due to a lesion of the sciatic plexus or of the sciatic nerve, or it may be a referred pain, not only from disc degeneration but from sources such as sacroiliac joints, hip joints, and the knee. Finally, it may be vascular in origin.[1]

This article is being written at a time when radiculography with metrizamide is replacing myelography with iophendylate in the United States, and discussion of the relative merits of EV and radiculography seems premature on the basis of our data. In the UK, however, an unpublished series[2] indicates an 80 percent correlation between *abnormal* EV and radiculogram and a 100 percent correlation between radiculogram and *normal* EV.

Before the advent of radiculography, EV had an advantage over myelography in that it was more useful in diagnosing disc disease in patients with a high termination of the subarachnoid sac, a lumbosacral epidural space with a wide sagittal, or a subarachnoid sac with a narrow coronal diameter.

Despite the advent of radiculography, EV is not "in vein" because we have found it a most useful out-patient procedure without significant morbidity. Radiculography has a definite morbidity and is not an out-patient procedure.

The confidence that a clinician may have in his ability to diagnose disc herniation is variable, and is the product of many factors, not all of which are medical, in communities where litigation is as common as herniation. Not surprisingly, EV is gratefully accepted by some as a screening investigation, which, if negative, may offer the patient guarded reassurance that the low back pain will probably resolve with a short term, conservative treatment. Other local physicians reserve EV for those who have a high probability of disc herniation based on confirming evidence in the history, examination, and EMG. The remaining physicians will use EV only as a preoperative investigation, to identify segmental level(s) either in combination with radiculography or as an independent examination. It is our impression that, whether the physician falls into the category, "I can't make the diagnosis," or, "I usually can make the diagnosis," or, "I am always right," his decision is not a reflection of diagnostic acumen; it more likely reflects a sensitivity to the difficulties involved in assessing culturally heterogeneous patients, as may be encountered in San Francisco, as well as an awareness of the frequency of professional negligence suits filed by patients with backaches and histories of work-related accidents.

ANATOMY OF LUMBAR EPIDURAL VEINS

Lumbar epidural veins have been described in many recent articles[3–10]; much of the earlier literature of Britain, North America, and Continental Europe contains inaccuracies that are absent from the French literature.

There is an intravertebral and extravertebral venous system, both valveless, which communicate at each lumbar segment via radicular intervertebral veins, and with the IVC via transverse lumbar segmental veins.

Intravertebral Veins

The anterior internal vertebral veins comprise two longitudinal venous channels, the anteromedial and anterolateral internal vertebral veins (AMVV and ALVV) (Figs. 19-1 and 19-2). The AMVV are usually double or triple and may appear plexiform. They lie posterior to the vertebral body, disc, and posterior longitudinal ligament, and medial to the pedicles. At

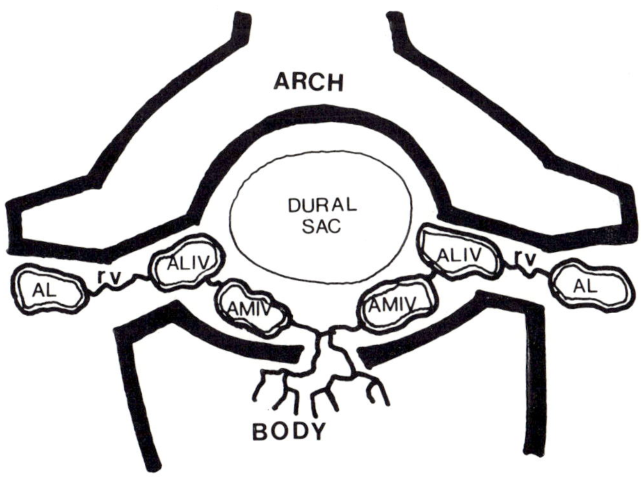

Fig. 19-1. Diagrammatic transverse section of lower lumbar spine to show position of: 1) Paired ascending lumbar veins (AL) anterior to transverse process; 2) paired anteromedial internal vertebral veins (AMIV) posterior to posterior longitudinal ligament and anteromedial to anterolateral internal vertebral vein; 3) paired anterolateral vertebral veins (ALIV) which communicate with ascending lumbar veins via radicular veins (rv) and across midline to other side.

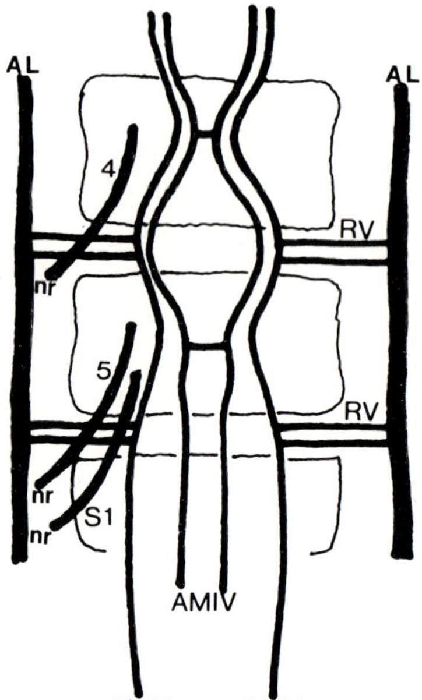

Fig. 19-2. Diagrammatic representation of ascending lumbar vein (AL) and anteromedial and anterolateral internal vertebral veins (AMIV, ALIV). Note convex appearance of AMIV and ALIV at level of discs and separation of AMIV and ALIV at L5-S1 level. Nerve roots (nr) are in close apposition to radicular veins (rv), AMIV, and ALIV.

L5-S1 they take a median course. At the level of each disc the AMVV, except at L5-S1, show a localized lateral excursion.

The anterolateral internal vertebral veins (ALVV) lie immediately lateral and slightly posterior to the AMVV, except at L5-S1, and present a lateral excursion at each disc level, including that of L5-S1, so that at this level they are separated from AMVV.

The radicular veins (also known as intervertebral veins) of the intervertebral foramina are paired so that at each disc level one is superior (the infrapedicular vein of the vertebra above), and one inferior (the suprapedicular vein of the vertebra below) (Fig. 19-3). Either of these veins may be double, or on rare occasions, triple. They communicate with the AMVV and ALVV centrally, and with the ascending lumbar veins laterally.

The AMVV and ALVV of each side communicate across the midline to produce a plexus of varying size at the posterior aspect of the posterior

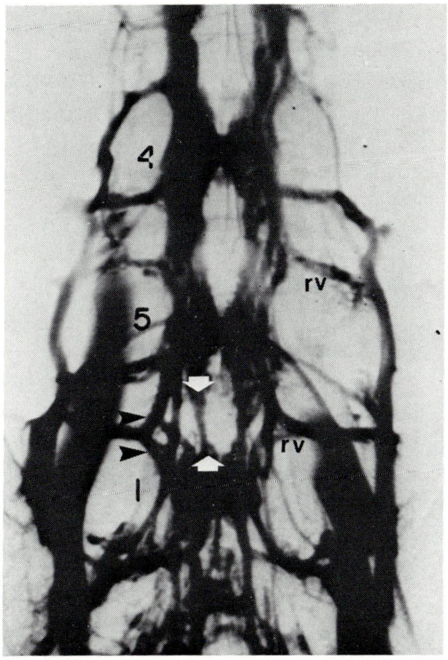

Fig. 19-3. Normal lumbar epidural venogram (LEV). Note diversions of internal vertebral veins at each disc space level; the horizontally disposed radicular veins (rv); the divergence of ALIVV (horizontal black arrows) and AMIVV (vertical white arrows) at L5-S1 level. At L4–5 (R) the AMIV and ALIVV are superimposed; at L4–5 (L) the individual channels are seen separately.

longitudinal ligament at the level of the vertebral bodies (Fig. 19-4). Small emissary veins perforate the posterior longitudinal ligament to communicate with vertebral body diploic veins.

Extravertebral Veins

The ascending lumbar vein (ALV) lies longitudinally on either side of the spine, lateral to the pedicles. It communicates segmentally with the radicular veins. At each level there is an additional communication with the IVC by means of a transverse lumbar vein. This is usually not opacified. Superiorly on the right it communicates with the azygous system; the left ALV communicates with the hemiazygous vein but much of its flow is often diverted by a large anastomotic channel running from

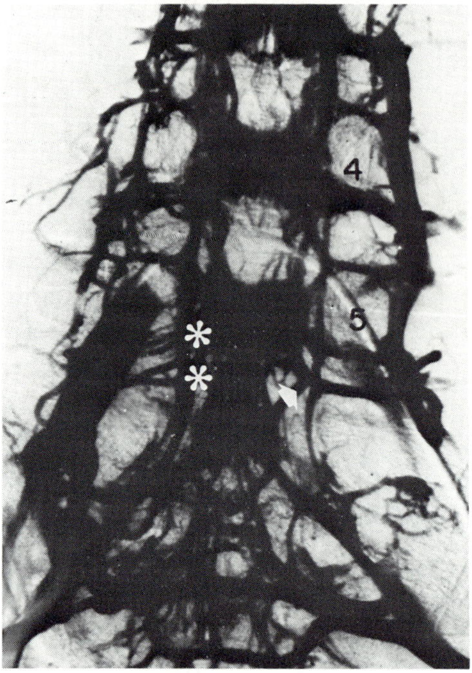

Fig. 19-4. Normal LEV. At L5-S1 (R) the upper star shows triplication of superior radicular vein; the lower star, duplication of inferior radicular vein. The white arrow shows normal lateral divergence of ALIVV at L5-S1.

left to right at about L2–3 level to right ALV. Inferiorly the ALVs arise from the external iliac vein on each side. Occasionally they arise from the iliolumbar vein and rarely from the internal iliac vein.

A posterior external vein lies posterior to the vertebral arch.

Radiological Anatomy

The appearance of the AMVV, ALVV, and RV in frontal projections should be symmetric. The lateral excursions at each disc level suggest a chain of hexagons. The only exception is at L5-S1 where AMVV separate from ALVV and run a more median or paramedian course. The radicular veins need to be differentiated from veins running parallel to them, but projected over the pedicles. These are extravertebral veins and not of significance in the context of epidural venography. There are no internal vertebral veins of any radiographic interest lying posteriorly in the bony spinal canal, despite some conflicting references.[10,11,12] (Meijenhorst[12A]

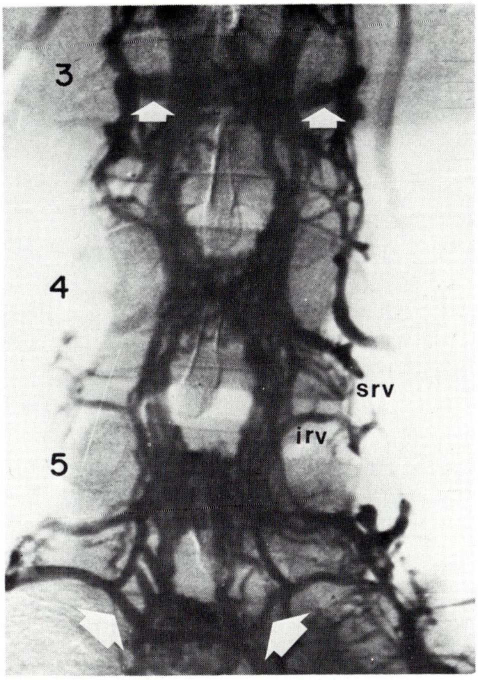

Fig. 19-5. Normal LEV. At L3 body level, a large extravertebral anastomic vein (white arrow) joins (L) and (R) ascending lumbar veins. At L4–5 (L) superior radicular vein (srv) is duplicated, (L) single inferior radicular vein (irv) is bowed slightly, a normal variant. White arrow indicates normal lateral divergence of ALIV at L5-S1.

found a small straight vein in the midline of the vertebral canal in 15 percent of 120 patients, but did not believe it to be of clinical significance.) Veins lying around the posterior spinous processes may be opacified in normal examinations, and are often opacified when they act as collateral channels if the AMV or ALV are obstructed. They appear projected as longitudinal channels near the midline. They need to be differentiated from a medially displaced AMVV, especially at L5-S1. Normal anastomotic channels between left and right ALV may divert opacified blood in such a way that when the left ALV is injected, little contrast material is seen in epidural plexus above the level of the anastomotic channel. These channels are usually at about L2–3, but when they lie more inferiorly, alternate injection sites are usually necessary.

The lateral or presacral veins (PSV) communicate centrally with the ALVV and AMVV where they overlie the sacrum. The segmental PSVs originate from the internal iliac vein. It is wisest to inject one of the more superior PSVs so that contrast is deposited nearer the area of interest, but also because more inferiorly a wide anastomotic channel directing much of the contrast to the opposite internal iliac vein may be present.

The posterior external plexus may be seen as a pair of veins, smaller and less regular than the anterior vertebral veins, that pass medially at the level of the spinous process (unlike anterior internal vertebral veins, which swing medially at the pedicle level) (Fig. 19-12A).

Anomalies such as double IVC are occasionally encountered, making catheterization of PSV difficult; bilateral ALV injection is then needed. The left ALV is easily catheterized; its point of origin from the external iliac vein usually overlies the upper part of the sacroiliac synchondrosis. Occasionally, the true left ALV is small; its function is taken over by an ascending branch of a muscular gluteal branch arising slightly inferior to the ALV. Injection of this vein may cause left buttock pain unless lidocaine is mixed with contrast material. The right ALV arises from the right external iliac vein at a more acute angle than LALV and may be more difficult to catheterize. It may be paired, in which case the larger of the two should be utilized. Rarely, a large vein may arise from the area of confluence of the left and right external iliac veins with IVC. It is of use if no other injection sites are available since it anastomoses with the lateral sacral vein.*

LUMBAR EPIDURAL VENOGRAPHY

Technique

PRIMARY METHOD

The procedure is explained in terms understandable to the patient. We generally state that discs are not seen on ordinary x-rays, but if a disc has "slipped," the adjacent veins will be pushed out of place; by injecting the veins via the groin these veins may be seen on the x-ray and so give indirect evidence of a "slipped disc." After signed permission for the procedure the patient is offered premedication, but this is usually not accepted.

Most catheterizations are done via the left femoral vein. To aid venipuncture the patient may perform a modified Valsalva (with a closed glottis) (Fig. 19-6). A .038 removable core guide wire is inserted and

* Epidural vascular malformations may be identified (Sabil EA, Rowed DW, Gertlbein SD: Epidural vascular malformation demonstrated by epidural venography. Am J Roentgenol 132:987–988, 1979

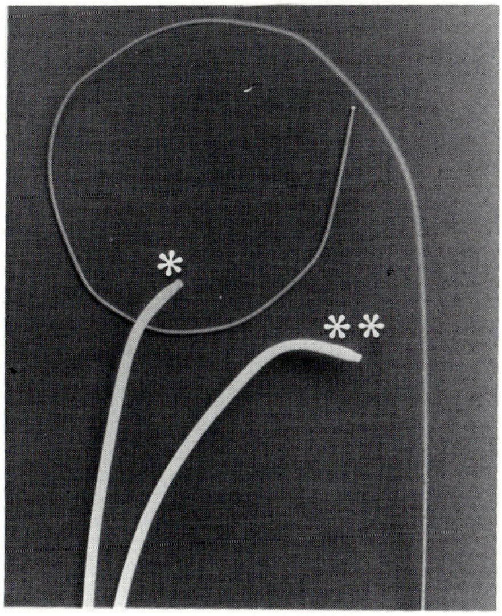

Fig. 19-6. Single curved catheter (single asterisk) used for ascending lumbar vein, and double curved catheter (double asterisk) is used for presacral vein. Typical curve in guide wire to pass from (L) common iliac to (R) internal iliac vein.

frequently will become arrested in the left ascending lumbar vein, which overlies the left sacroiliac joint. It should be withdrawn; if excessive force is used the vein is easily punctured. The wire is positioned over the left sacroiliac joint and a curved six French end hole catheter inserted. An initial attempt is made to pass the catheter from left to right in order to position it in the right internal iliac vein. A test dose of contrast material will show the level of bifurcation. If this initial attempt is unsuccessful the guide wire is withdrawn and curved around two fingers to produce a wide, gentle curve; then the wire and catheter are advanced into the right internal iliac vein. The guide wire is then withdrawn; an acute angle is formed at its tip and reinserted to engage a mid- or upper right presacral vein. The catheter tip may be advanced until resistance is felt; then it is withdrawn about 0.5 cm. to insure that the venous occlusion is not caused. A test dose of contrast with the patient performing a modified Valsalva should give a good filling of the presacral veins across the midline to the left. If only internal iliac vein filling is obtained, further attempts at entering the right presacral vein utilizing different shaped guides and catheters should be attempted, but if these fail injection into the right internal iliac vein is usually successful, provided good abdominal compression is used. If difficulty in entering the right internal iliac vein is encountered a J wire may be used.

In a small proportion of patients a single injection into the right PSV will give complete filling of the epidural plexus and if no abnormality is seen, the procedure is terminated. Usually it is necessary to withdraw the catheter to the left common iliac vein and catheterize left ALV. Initially this is attempted with the same catheter; in about half the patients it is necessary to substitute a catheter with a short distal curve. A second injection is then made.

ALTERNATIVE METHODS

The above method has proven satisfactory in the majority of our patients. If these veins cannot be catheterized, or if, when catheterized, adequate venous opacification is not obtained, the following alternatives may be considered.

One Catheter Technique Using Left Femoral Vein

1. Ipsilateral or contralateral internal iliac vein (IIV) injections: These are frequently successful if the catheter can be positioned inferiorly in IIV and good abdominal compression can be obtained.
2. Ipsilateral or contralateral ALV injections: Catheterization of contralateral ALV usually entails the use of a guided catheter. In either situation there is rarely good filling of the epidural plexus inferior to the body of L5.
3. Ipsilateral left PSV: This usually gives good venous opacification but is technically difficult to perform.

One Catheter Technique Using Right Femoral Vein

1. Ipsilateral or contralateral IIV injections.
2. Ipsilateral or contralateral ALV injections: The right ALV is occasionally double, and each of its branches small. This leads to difficulty in catheterization and poor opacification. In addition, the right ALV arises at a more acute angle from the right external iliac vein than does the left vein, and catheterization is more difficult. Both the left and right ALV may share a common trunk with a gluteal vein. The catheter tip must be distal to this junction to avoid much of the contrast entering the buttock veins; this may be painful.
3. Ipsilateral RPSV: This is technically difficult.

Two Catheter Techniques Using Left and Right Femoral Veins

1. Bilateral ALVs injected simultaneously.
2. Bilateral IIV injection.
3. Combination of IIV, ALV or PSV injections.
4. RALV and RPSV injections.
5. RALV and LPSV injections.
6. LALV and LPSV injections.
7. Bilateral PSV injection.

In each of these instances if veins on both sides of the midline are catheterized, the ALV, PSV or IIV on the side of the catheter may be utilized, or the catheter may be passed across midline to the appropriate contralateral veins.

Two catheter techniques were used by us initially. For most of the later exams consecutive injections of the RPSV and LALV via the left femoral vein have sufficed. The need for bilateral venous puncture is avoided—a consideration in out-patients. Bilateral catheterization is needed if a double IVC that prevents passage of catheters from left to right or an unsuspected left deep venous thrombosis is present, or if technical difficulties occur on one side.

On occasion a supplemental injection of a reduced amount of contrast into a radicular vein may be necessary to confirm that an area of nonopacification is not due to some nonpathologic factor. Abdominal compression is not usually needed when radicular injections are made. A catheter in the radicular vein adjacent to an irritated nerve root may reproduce the patient's pain.[13]

Contrast Material and Filming

Each injection consists of 40 to 50 ml. of 60 percent hypaque meglumine (diatrizoate meglumine USP). If the patient is apprehensive or unable to tolerate strong abdominal compression with a balsa wood block, 5 to 10 mg. of valium (diazepam) is injected slowly through the catheter prior to compression and filming. Injection may be by hand or with an injector at the rate of 8 ml. per second. A scout film is advisable to insure a slight overexposure of the serial films so that satisfactory subtraction films may be made. The first of the serial films is exposed immediately before injection of contrast to provide for subtraction. Films are exposed at the rate of one per second for approximately ten seconds if injection is made into the PSV or ALV. If injection is made into the IIV, filming should continue slightly longer, from 12 to 14 seconds. With good compression, it is probably unnecessary to use modified Valsalva maneuver. A Valsalva maneuver that is too strong may "dam" the opacified blood in the lower lumbar area and prevent visualization above L5. Very firm abdominal compression is the more important factor. If compression is not easily tolerated, this maneuver is needed. The maneuver may be terminated before the last few exposures are made to empty, partially, the epidural plexus at L5-S1 in those cases where overdistension has been produced. AP filming suffices in nearly all patients. There are advocates of the lateral and oblique projections. The radiation dose is increased, and in the case of oblique projections, difficulties in interpretation arise. If lateral projections are used as a supplement, four to five films usually suffice. We originally used contrast reagents with a greater iodine concentration, mixed with 2 ml. of 2 percent lidocaine to alleviate pain. The greater viscosity prevented sufficiently rapid injection.

Subtraction Technique

A one-step subtraction technique usually suffices. Two-step subtraction (double subtraction) may yield a high degree of contrast in well-filled veins, but poorly filled veins, especially thin radicular veins, may become inapparent.

Technical Problems

The bladder should be emptied prior to initiating the procedure. This is very important. Firm compression is impossible with a full bladder, and failures have been encountered in some elderly patients with bladder outlet obstruction.

If there is a history of asthma or of minor reactions to contrast material, 200 mg. of solucortef (hydrocortisone) is injected via the catheter and the contrast injection is delayed five minutes or so. If extravasation of contrast occurs with the test dose, minor pain may be treated with an injection of 3 ml. of two percent lidocaine via catheter at the site of extravasation, followed by 100 mg. of hydrocortisone sodium succinate (solucortef), before the catheter is withdrawn and repositioned at another site. With six French end hole catheter the tip may be in a satisfactory position as judged by test injection but no venous blood may be aspirated. It is tempting to withdraw the catheter to avoid occlusion of the veins. This is not necessary, and usually results in the catheter being withdrawn too far, so that its tip lies in IIV with PSV catheterization.

The internal iliac veins may be occluded or distorted in those who have had prior pelvic surgical operations, especially panhysterectomy.

The femoral vein may lie in an unusually lateral position in those who have had a herniorrhaphy, and may be partly in front of or behind the femoral artery. Before compression is released, patients are warned that they may experience a transient feeling of dizziness as contrast reaches the head.

PATIENTS WITH HIGHER RISKS

Abdominal Aortic Aneurysm. Inspect any prior films or the scout film, or, if your style is to do so, lay a hand on the belly. An aneurysm is a strong contraindication to abdominal compression.

Prior Severe Reaction to Contrast Material. This is a strong contraindication.

Prior Ingestion of Oral Contraceptives. It is wise to wait a month after discontinuing these medicines to lessen the change of post-venography iliofemoral thrombosis.

Prior Iliofemoral Thrombosis or Thrombophlebitis. This is a strong contraindication. Even when such history is inapparent, an occasional patient will be found to have narrowing or occlusion of one of the major deep veins shown by the test injection. The procedure should then be aborted, or, if it is felt necessary to continue, a different injection route should be used and the patient heparinized at the completion of the examination.

Prior Laminectomy or Fusion. ALVs are usually thrombosed after fusion. Only discs above the level of laminectomy may be examined by EV.

COMPLICATIONS

No major complications have ensued. In one patient with acute low back pain, abdominal compression could not be tolerated. The exam was aborted and repeated successfully under general anesthetic. This experience led us to utilize 5 to 10 mg. Diazepam IV through the catheter just before compression is tightened in those patients who are in considerable pain. Local bleeding at the femoral vein puncture site was troublesome in one patient who, unknown to us, had a bleeding diathesis that was compounded by the use of aspirin for low back pain. I have seen films of a patient who had a selective radicular vein injection with rupture so that contrast passed into the extradural space. After a few hours of backache (patient) and headache (radiologist), both had an uneventful recovery.

POSTVENOGRAPHY INSTRUCTIONS

Firm digital pressure to the venipuncture site is applied for ten minutes. All patients are instructed to press on this area for the rest of the day while coughing, micturating, or defecating. Our patients are asked to go to the hospital cafeteria and have tea. If they feel well, they may leave 30 minutes later. If patients returning to the ward are up and about, they are encouraged to ambulate; if they are in traction, this is deferred for a few hours; a patient has to ambulate as much as possible to avoid venous stasis.

INTERPRETATION

The abnormal venographic signs are summarized in Table 19-1 (*see also* Figs. 19-7 through 19-12. Extravertebral veins must first be identified and differentiated from internal intravertebral and radicular veins. The

Table 19-1
Venous Abnormalities Due to Extradural Impressions

1. The internal vertebral veins may show:
   Displacement
   Obstruction or Narrowing
   Bypass enlargement
2. The radicular vein may show:
   Displacement
   Obstruction
3. Abnormal extravertebral collaterals may be present

extravertebral veins that may cause confusion are pedicular veins, posterior veins, and anastomotic veins.

Pedicular Veins. These veins lie horizontally and are projected onto the pedicle; they are posterior extravertebral veins.

Posterior Veins. These appear to lie in the midline. They are adjacent to the spinous processes and are also in a posterior extravertebral position. A small proportion may be within the vertebral canal. They must be differentiated from AIVV that have been displaced centrally by a lateral disc. They usually do not appear to be symmetrical, multiple, or reduplicated as is usual with AIVV. They may be large if they are routes of collateral flow from an obstructed internal vertebral vein.

Anastomotic Veins. A not unusual finding is a large vein that runs upwards and to the right, going from the LALV to the RALV. This vein is extravertebral throughout its course. Where it overlies the spine in the AP projection it must not be confused with internal vein. It may result in areas of nonopacification of IVV, if only ALV is injected, since it directs the flow of opacified blood into the opposite ALV rather than the IVV.

Abnormalities of Internal Vertebral Vein Opacification

TECHNICAL

The films are examined to insure that areas of non- or incomplete filling are not the result of flow defects. These may occur if catheter placement is such that filling of the PSV is inadequate, as may occur if only ALV injections are used, or if large normal anastomotic channels are

A
B
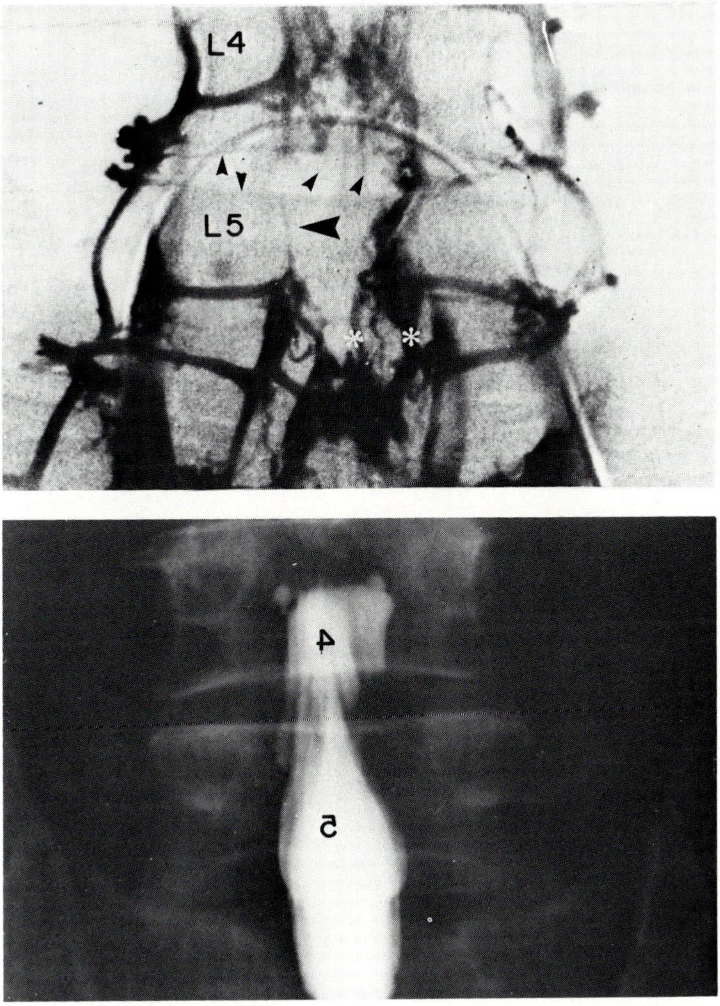

Fig. 19-7 A, B. Patient #14. 45 year male. History: Low back pain 2 yrs.; (R) sciatica 1 month. Exam: Sensation normal; decrease in strength (R) Ext. Hall. Long. and Tib. Ant.; Absent right ankle reflex. LEV: At L4–5; (L) and (R) AMIVV occluded (oblique arrows); (R) ALIVV narrowed (horizontal arrow); (R) superior and inferior radicular veins thinner than (L). At L5-S1: Abnormal shape of (L) AMIVV and ALIV (asterisks) compared with (R). Myelog: At L4–5: (R) extradural defect; At L5-S1: No definite abnormality. Operation: At L4–5: (R) disc protrusion; At L5-S1: (L) disc protrusion.

LEV demonstrated asymptomatic disc protrusion at L5-S1 (L), in addition to symptomatic disc at L4–5 (R).

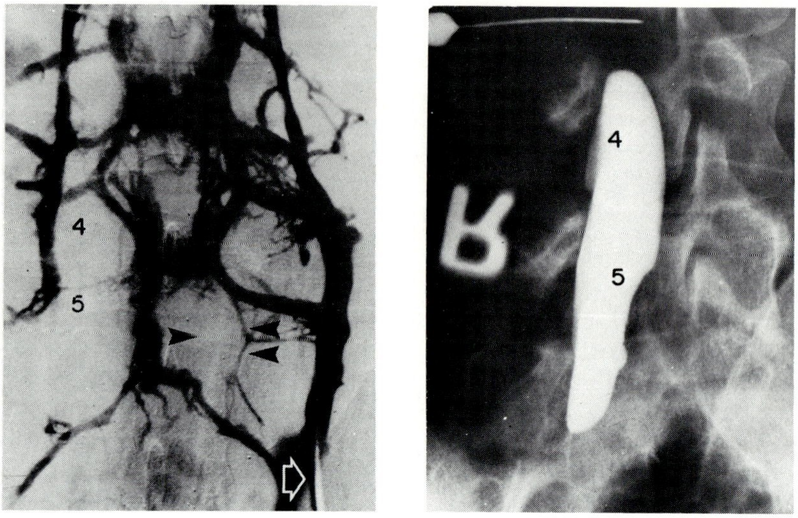

A B

Fig. 19-8 A, B. Patient #25. 29 year male. History: Low back pain, (L) sciatica. Exam: Sensation normal; decrease in strength (L) Ext. Hall. Long. and Tib. Ant.; Deep tendon reflexes normal. LEV: At L5-S1: (L) AMIV completely obstructed (single black arrow); (L) ALIV displaced laterally (double black arrow). Myelog: At L5-S1: (L) extradural defect. Operation: At L5-S1: (L) extruded disc.

The LEV was via (L) ascending lumbar vein injection (white arrow). The (R) ALIV at L5-S1 is not opacified with this injection, but was opacified with a (R) presacral vein injection.

present. Other potential causes include venous spasm if the catheter is too large for the vein to be injected and the release of vasoactive substances by adjacent disc herniation, which causes venous spasm at the next higher disc space.[2] This may be lessened by injection of 10 mg. of lidocaine before a repeat injection is made, or the choice of a different injection route. Each serial film must be scrutinized together with, on occasion, several subtraction films taken at different time intervals and with different degrees of contrast to insure that a vein with reduced or no opacification remains so throughout the series. The IVV and radicular veins are valveless, but turbulence, Valsalva maneuver, compression, or catheter artifacts may produce vagaries in the direction of the *initial* flow of contrast. Similarly, external veins may obscure internal veins at one phase, but not at another, of the series.

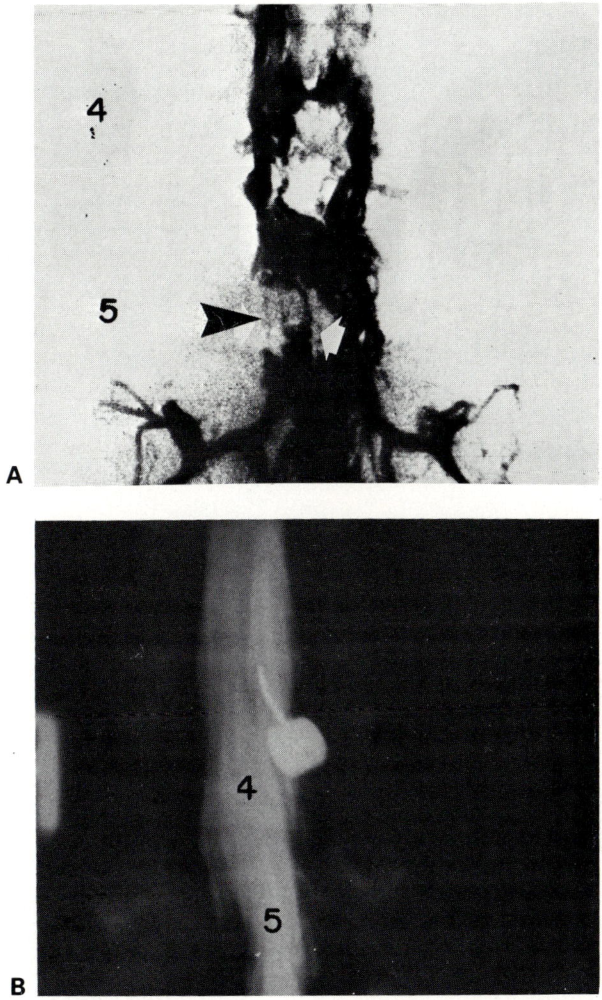

Fig. 19-9 A, B. Patient #4. 57 year male. History: Low back pain 15 years, (R) sciatica 2 months. Exam: Decrease in sensation L5 dermatome (R); decrease in strength (R) Ext. Hall. Long. and Tib. Ant; Absent (L) and (R) ankle reflex. LEV: At L4–5: (L) AMIVV attenuated compared with (R); At L5-S1: (R) AMIV displaced inwards (oblique arrow), (R) ALIV obstructed (horizontal arrow). Myel: At L4–5: Minor root sleeve abnormality; At L5-S1: (R) extradural defect. Operation: At L4–5: (L) and (R) disc protrusion; At L5-S1: (R) disc extrusion.

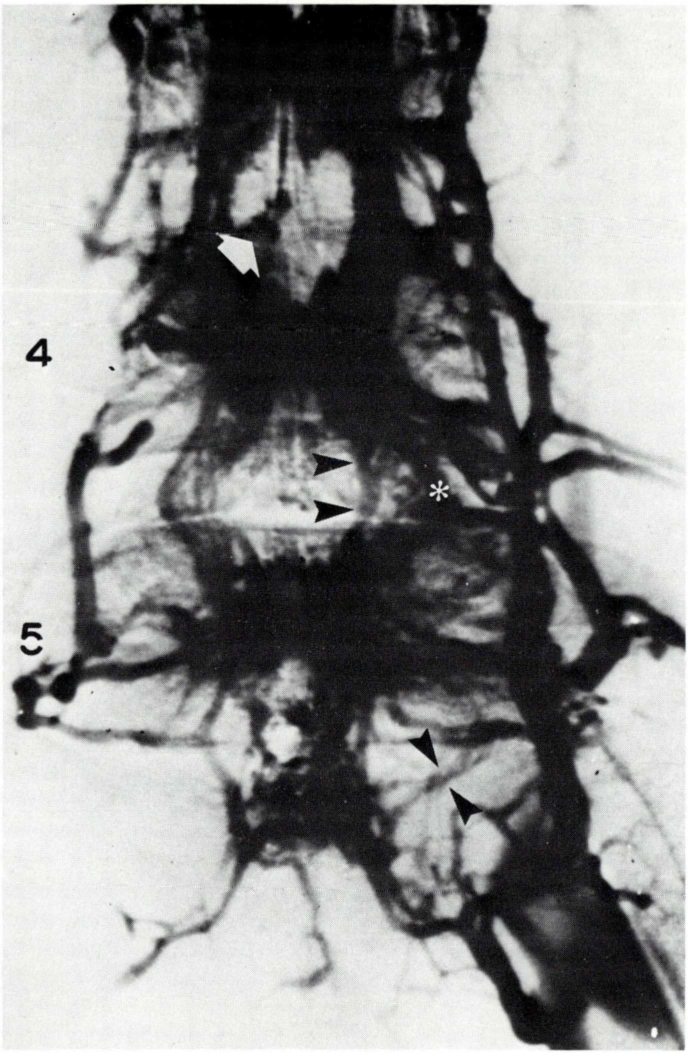

Fig. 19-10. Patient #26. 47 year female. History: Low back pain and (L) sciatica 1 month. Exam: Sensation and strength normal; decrease in (L) ankle reflex. LEV: At L4–5 (L) a short segment is obstructed, and there is excessive separation of AMIV (double horizontal arrows), and ALIV (star) compared with closely applied AM and ALIV on (R). Myel: Extradural defect at L4–5 and L5-S1 (not illustrated). Operation: At L4–5: (L) disc protrusion; At L5-S1: Disc was normal; the ALIV at L5-S1, (L) appears displaced laterally (oblique arrow) despite a normal disc.

Note irregular shaped posterior extravertebral vein passing toward spinous process (white arrow).

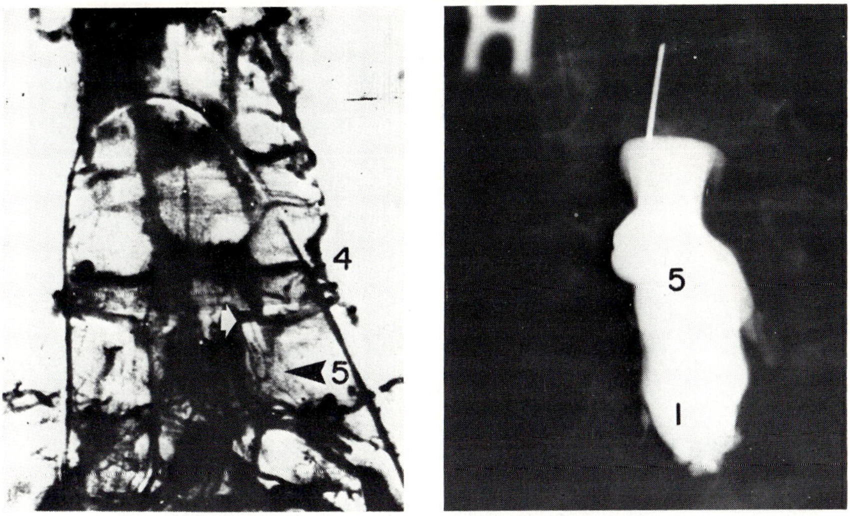

A B

Fig. 19-11 A, B. Patient #11. 44 year female. History: Low back pain and (L) sciatica 1 month. Exam: Hyperesthesia (L) lateral calf; decrease in strength (L) Tib. and Ant. and Ext. Hall. Long.; Reflexes—unsustained clonus at ankle. LEV: At L4–5: (L) AMIV is obstructed; (L) ALIV is distorted into an ⌐ shape (white arrow); At L5: (L) ALIV is irregular in shape (black arrow). Myel: At L4–5: (L) extradural defect; Operation: At L4: (L) disc protrusion compressing L5 (L) root.

PATHOLOGICAL

The longitudinal internal vertebral veins, comprising the anteromedial and anterolateral channels, are so positioned that they are affected early on by disc herniation. They may be displaced, narrowed or completely obstructed. Lack of symmetry at each level should be looked for.

POSTEROLATERAL DISC HERNIATION

This may produce a unilateral deformity of the anteromedial or of both the anteromedial and anterolateral IVV, depending on the severity of herniation. Above the lumbosacral articulation it is usual for the AMVV and ALVV of one side to be involved together, since these veins are in close opposition; the severity of involvement of these two longitudinal channels may differ according to the amount and location of disc herniation. At L5-S1 these two channels diverge so that the degree of involvement may vary more than at other locations; the AMVV, for example, may be completely occluded while the ALVV may be merely displaced. If the involvement is slight, the radicular veins may appear normal. Radicu-

Table 19-2
Scoring of Venograms and Myelograms

True Positive	Positive study	Abnormal disc
True Negative	Negative study	Normal disc
False Positive	Positive study	Normal disc
False Negative	Negative study	Abnormal disc

level and 24 patients at the L5 level. It should be mentioned that there is little opportunity to visualize epidural vein occlusion intraoperatively, therefore, standard terminology regarding herniation, i.e., bulging, protrusion and extrusion was used to express and identify pathology.

RESULTS

The results of the myelograms and venograms for each level were compared statistically in terms of sensitivity and specificity. Sensitivity for this particular study is defined as the number of true positive tests divided by the total number of abnormal discs found at surgery; whereas specificity is the number of true negative tests divided by the total number of normal discs found at surgery. Thus, sensitivity indicates percentage of patients who have an abnormal disc and in whom the venogram was abnormal. Specificity indicates percentage of normal persons in whom the venogram was normal. Both sensitivity and specificity should approach one if the test is accurate. The results of these two parameters at each disc considered are noted in Table 19-3.

At the L3 level, the numbers indicate the myelogram to be more sensitive and more specific. This reflects the difficulties that at times may be encountered in filling the epidural veins at higher disc levels.

At the L4 level, the numbers indicate little difference in terms of sensitivity, but there is considerable difference in specificity, with venography at 0.66 and myelography at 0.52.

To consider the L5 level is of particular interest, since, as predicted in other articles,[3,4] the venogram is more accurate than the myelogram (the specificity being 0.77 and 0.57 respectively). This reflects the traditional

Table 19-3
Sensitivity and Specificity Values

	Sensitivity		Specificity	
Disc Level	Venogram	Myelogram	Venogram	Myelogram
L3	0.62	0.93	0.50	0.75
L4	0.82	0.86	0.66	0.52
L5	0.84	0.73	0.77	0.57

difficulty with myelography in localizing herniated discs at the L5-S1 interspace using oil-based contrast media. In general it appears that:

1. The venogram and myelogram consistently display a higher index of sensitivity than specificity.
2. In terms of specificity, both the venogram and myelogram values fall precipitously.
3. Venography is more accurate at the L5 disc level.

Finally, it should be noted that, although the raw scores indicate differences, when statistical analysis is applied, there is no significant difference between the sensitivity and specificity values of myelography and venography, and the probabilities are greater than 0.10. A larger series will be needed to determine if there is any true statistical difference between venography and myelography. No article to date (that we have reviewed) has subjected data to such statistical analysis. The reading of venograms and myelograms by the radiologists *without* any clinical information is critical in determining the accuracy of each test. This particular point has not been made clear in articles reviewed.

DISCUSSION

The clinician is confronted daily with "the low back pain patient" who may or may not also present with sciatica and/or neurological deficit. The clinical evaluation of the patient is of utmost consideration in the overall course of treatment. It should be mentioned that 90 percent of patients with clearly defined motor or reflex deficits, and 97 percent of patients with a positive contralateral straight leg raising test will have a herniated intervertebral disc.[34] Therefore, negative myelograms and venograms should not defer surgery if the history, physical examination and hospital course indicate that it should be performed.

It is generally agreed that when surgery is indicated or clarification of a questionable diagnosis of herniated disc is needed, clinical tests for the purpose of localization and documentation are often obtained. The use of lumbar myelography, radiculography and electromyography is well established for these purposes. The risks, artifactual results, and limitations of these procedures—particularly those of myelography and radiculography—have been well established elsewhere and consequently underscore the importance of the clinical evaluation of the patient.[31-35]

Certainly any clinical test that can more accurately localize a lesion with minimal risk to the patient is a welcome addition to present methods. The experiences of others are summarized in Table 19-4. At French Hospital, San Francisco, California, since 1975, lumbar venography has been used for preoperative evaluation in addition to lumbar myelography and EMG studies on a comparative study basis. Most of the venograms

Table 19-4
Surgical Confirmation of EV Findings

Reference		Number of Cases	Percentage with Abnormal EV	Comments
Roland, 1978	No Herniation	10	60	% Accuracy L3–4 100
Ref. 6	Herniation	101	93	L4–5 96
				L5–S1 88
Giustra, 1978				
Ref. 17, 18	(a) No Herniation	2	100	
	Herniation	25	100	
	(b) Herniation	40	100	8 patients with normal or equivocal EV had herniated disc at surgery
MacNab, 1976 Ref. 26	Herniation	50	98	
Sackett, 1977 Ref. 27	Herniation	69	87	23% of venograms were non-diagnostic or suboptimal, or on patients who had been operated on previously. Does not indicate numbers of previously operated patients making up the 13% error rate.
Kistler, 1976	Herniation	20	98	
Ref. 28	No Herniation	2	50	
O'Dell, 1977 Ref. 11	Herniation	19	86	
Clarke, 1977 Ref. 29	Herniation	29	66	Series included 4 patients with extra-dural disease other than herniated disc.

Beavis, 1978 Ref. 2	Herniation	38	74	In 10 out of 38 patients the protruding disc material was one level lower than indicated on venogram (see discussion p. 370)
Garagano, 1974 Ref. 12	Herniation	30	93	
Handel, 1977 Ref. 14	Herniation	37	97	Specificity 25% of 12 patients with normal EV, only 3 had normal surgical findings.
Gershater, 1976 Ref. 15	Herniation	130	99	Includes other causes of extradural and intradural disease.
Miller, 1976 Ref. 16	Herniation	27	92	No false positive venograms
McCormick, 1978 Ref. 30	Herniation No herniation	20 2	76	Of 25 exams, 3 were inconclusive, 2 false positive and 1 false negative. All these patients had negative or equivocal iophendylate myelograms
Gershater, 1979 Ref. 37	Herniation No herniation	552 337	99	Of cases with surgical proof, error rate 1.5% (false positive 0.3%, false negative 0.4%)

were performed on out-patients for screening purposes. Over 300 venograms have been performed at French Hospital.

The preliminary analysis of the data in our limited retrospective study has encouraged us to continue its use. Further, the limited morbidity and ability to perform on an out-patient basis, with resultant lower cost to the patient, have been an added attraction of venography.

SUMMARY

Lumbar venography is a relatively new technique which can be performed on an out-patient basis and with low morbidity to the patient. Preliminary analysis of the data in our limited series seems to indicate that venography may correlate with the operative findings as well as or better than lumbar myelography using iophendylate.

At the time of writing (1978) we do not have sufficient data to compare metrizamide radiculography with EV. Our tentative opinion is that despite the greater accuracy of radiculography over myelography and partly because of its greater morbidity, EV remains a valuable initial choice and is the procedure generally used at our institution. Those with an unequivocally abnormal EV and appropriate clinical findings may subsequently undergo radiculography, or occasionally proceed directly to surgery. Those with an equivocal EV or one at variance with clinical findings will be ordered to undergo radiculography, while those with a normal EV will have prescribed conservative therapy and reassessed later.

ACKNOWLEDGMENTS

We greatfully acknowledge the cooperation of the following members of the Department of Orthopedics, French Hospital, San Francisco: Doctors Hartwig, Civello, von Rogov, Wong, Gordon, Ferretti, and White. Their transition from dogged scepticism via uncontrolled enthusiasm to ungrudging acceptance proves that not all has been "in vein".

REFERENCES

1. MacNab I: Backache. Baltimore, Williams & Wilkins, 1978, p 206
2. Beavis J: Lumbar venography. Lecture at Royal Postgraduate Med School, London, May, 1978
3. Theron J, Houteville JP, Adam H, et al: La phlebographie lombaire. Rev Rhum Mal Osteoartic 44:165–171, 1977
4. Theron J, Houteville JP, Ammerich H, et al: Lumbar phlebography by catheterization

of the lateral sacral and ascending lumbar vein with abdominal compression. Neuroradiol 11:175–182, 1976
5. Meijenhorst GCH: Methods of transfemoral lumbar epidural venography in the diagnosis of lumbar disc herniation. Radiologia Clin 46:439–457, 1977
6. Roland J, Larde D, Masson J-P, et al: Les veines lombaires epidurales. J Radiol Electrol 58:35–38, 1977
7. Roland J, Treil J, Larde D, et al: Lumbar phlebography in the diagnosis of disc herniation. J Neurosurg 49:544–550, 1978
8. Renard M, Masson J-P, Larde D: Les veines epidurales lombaire. Bull Assoc Anat (Nancy) 60:801–803, 1976
9. Renard M, Masson J-P, Larde D: Les veines du canal sacre. Bull Assoc Anat (Nancy) 60:801–803, 1976
10. Mosnier H: Study of anastomoses between left renal vein and internal vertebral plexus. Bull Assoc Anat (Nancy) 61:237–241, 1977
11. O'Dell CW, Coel MN, Ignelzi RJ: Ascending lumbar venography in lumbar disc disease. J Bone & Joint Surg 59-A:159–163, 1977
12. Gargagno FP, Meyer JD, Sheldon JJ: Transfemoral ascending lumbar catheterization of the epidural veins in lumbar disc disease. Radiol 111:337–339, 1974
12A. Meijenhorst GCH: Epidural double-catheter venography in the diagnosis of lumbar disc herniation; unknown vein in the vertebral canal. Roentgenol 129:581–587, 1978
13. Wilmink JT, Penning L, Beks JWF: Techniques in transfemoral lumbar epidural venography. Neuroradiol 15:273–286, 1978
13A. Gargagno FP, Bakst S, Donovan Post MJ: Extradural venography. Orth Rev VI:59–61
14. Handel S, Miller M: Lumbar epidural venography. Orth Rev VI:65–68, 1977
15. Gershater R, Holgate RC: Lumbar epidural venography in the diagnosis of disc herniation. Am J Roentgenol 126:992–1002, 1976
16. Miller MH, Handel SF, Coan JD: Transfemoral lumbar epidural venography. Am J Roentgenol 126:1003–1009, 1976
17. Giustra PE, Wiekenden JW, Furman RS: Multiple contrast injections in epidural venography. Am J Roentgenol 131:448–488, 1978
18. Giustra PE, Wiekenden JW, Furman RS: Epidural venography. J Maine Med Assoc 69:16–19, 1978
19. Mace BEW: Vertebral venography in disc disorders. Proc Roy Soc Med 69:433–437
20. Rettig A, Jackson DW, Wiltse L, et al: The epidural venogram as a diagnostic procedure in the young athlete with symptoms of lumbar disc disease. Am J Sports Med 5:158–164, 1977
21. Le Page JR: Transfemoral ascending lumbar catheterization of the epidural veins. Radiol 111:337–339, 1974
22. Smith P: Lumbar epidural venography. Radiography XLII:125–129, 1976
23. Bucheler E, Janson R: Combined catheter venography of the lumbar venous system and inferior vena cava. Brit J Radiol 45:655–661, 1973
24. Helander CG, Lindblom A: Sacrolumbar venography. Act Radiol 44:410–416, 1955
25. Drasin GF, Cooke MA, Schum JM, et al: Epidural venography. J Kentucky Med Assoc 76:217–219, 1978
26. MacNab I, St Louis EL, Grabias SL, et al: Selective ascending lumbosacral venography in the assessment of lumbar disc herniation. J Bone & Joint Surg 58-A:1096–1098, 1976
27. Sackett JF, Damm MG, Manucher JJ: Unreliability of epidural venography in lumbar disc disease. Surg Neurol 7:35–38, 1977
28. Kistler MW, Pribram HW: Epidural venography in the diagnosis of lumbar disc disease. Surg Neurol 5:287–291, 1976

29. Clarke AK, Beavis J, Irving JD, et al: Ascending lumbar venography in the diagnosis of lumbar disc disease. Rheumatol Rehabil 16:83–87, 1977
30. McCormick CC: Radiology in low back pain and sciatica. An analysis of the relative efficacy of spinal venography, discography and epidurography in patients with a negative or equivocal myelogram. Clin Rad 29:393–406, 1978
31. LaJoie WJ: Nerve root compression. Correlation of electromyographic, myelographic and surgical findings. Arch Phys Med Rehab 53:390–392, 1972
32. Lane ME, et al: Variance in correlation of electromyography, myelography and surgical findings in back disorders. Bull Hosp Joint Disease 36:30–33, 1975
33. MacLean IC, Curtiss PH Jr: The value of electromyography in lumbar disc lesions. Ohio State Med J 71:769–770, 1975
34. Rothman RH, Cambell RE, Menkowitz E: Myelographic patterns in lumbar disc degeneration. Clinical Ortho and Related Research 99:18–28, 1974
35. Eldevik OP, Nakken KO, Haughton VM: The effect of dehydration on the side effects of metrizamide myelography. Radiol 129:715–716, 1978
36. Gershater R, St Louis EL: Lumbar epidural venography. Am J Roentgenol 126:1003–1009, 1979
37. Gershater R, St Louis EL: Lumbar epidural venography. Radiol 131:409–421, 1979

Appendix

Clinical Information

Name Age Sex	Clinical	Lumbar Venogram	Lumbar Myelogram	EMG	Operative Findings
1. M., M. 69 yrs. old female	*(L)LE pain and parathesia × 22 yrs. *P.E.:* Sensation intact strength: normal DTR: absent (L)AJ.	Abn: L_3 RCL L_4 RL L_5 LC	Abn: L_3 RCL L_4 RCL L_5	Denervation L_5 (R) nerve root distribution	L_3 stenosis Scarring and adhesion of L_5 nerve root on (L) L_5 disc extruded on (L)
2. J., E. 57 yrs. old female	LBP × 1 yr. (R)LE pain × 1 mo. *P.E.:* Sensation intact Decrease in strength (R) EHL DTR: absent (R)AJ	Abn: L_4 RCL L_5 RCL	Abn: L_4 RCL	Re-innervation L_5-S_1 distribution on (R) Mild active denervation in S_1 distribution (R)	L_4 disc extruded on (R) L_5 stenotic root foramina bilaterally
3. C., M. 40 yrs. old male	LBP × 5 yr. (R)LE pain × 1 mo. *P.E.:* Sensation intact	Abn: L_4 CR L_5 CR	Abn: L_4 RCL L_5 CR	Denervation in $L_{4\text{-}5}$ root distribution particularly L_5 on the (L).	HNP $L_{4\text{-}5}$ with extruded fragment on the (L) and (R) No abnormality at L_5-S_1 interspace.

Appendix (con't) p. 2

Name Age Sex	Clinical	Lumbar Venogram	Lumbar Myelogram	EMG	Operative Findings
	Decrease in strength (R) EHL and TA DTR: Normal				
4. D., J. 57 yrs. old male	LBP × 15 yrs. (R)LE pain × 2 mo. *P.E.*: Decrease in sensation L_5 Decrease in strength (R) EHL and TA. DTR: absent (L)AJ (R)AJ	Abn: L_4 C L_5 CR	Abn: L_4 RCL L_5 CR	Denervation and re-innervation of S_1 root distribution (R) Minor abn. L_4 and L_5 on (R)	L_4 disc extruded on (R). L_5-S_1 disc protrusion bilat
5. A., L. 34 yrs. old male	LBP × 11 mo. Bilateral LE pain × 3 mo. *P.E.*: Slight sensation L_5 Strength normal DTR: absent (L)AJ (R)AJ	Abn: L_4 L L_5 LC	Abn: L_4 RCL L_5 CL	Normal	L_4 disc protrusion bilat. L_5 disc extruded on (L)

6. T, S.S. 37 yrs. old male	LBP × 3 yrs. (R)LE pain *P.E.:* Decrease in strength EHL(R) and sensation: R-ankle, lat. aspect DTR's intact	Abn: L_4 RLC L_5 RLC	Abn: L_4 RC L_5 RC	Denervation of R-EHL compatible with a (R) L_5 root lesion	L_4 disc protrusion on (R) L_5 disc protrusion on (R) Tight L_5 root foramen exit
7. D., D. 35 yrs. old female	LBP × 1½ yrs. (R)LE pain × 1 mo. *P.E.:* Decrease in strength (R) EHL Decrease in sensation L_4, L_5, S_1 (R) DTR: absent (R) Achilles reflex	Abn: L_5 RLC	Abn: L_4 C L_5 RCL	Denervation of (R) EHL L_5 root level	L_4-L_5 interspace no path L_5 extruded on (R)
8. B., G. 62 yrs. old male	LBP and (R)LE pain × 1½ mo. *P.E.:* Hyperesthesia of (R) foot Decrease in strength (R) EHL, TA, Quads DTR: Absent (R) Achilles tendon and RKJ	Abn: $L_{3\text{-}4\text{-}5}$ RLC	Abn: $L_{3\text{-}4\text{-}5}$ RCL	Mildly abnormal Re-innervation potentials in $L_{4\text{-}5}$ distribution on (L) No active signs of denervation	L_4 disc protrusion on (L) L_5 disc protrusion on (R) L_3 stenosis L_5 Stenotic foramen on (L) S_1 stenotic foramen on (R)

Appendix (con't) p. 3

Name Age Sex	Clinical	Lumbar Venogram	Lumbar Myelogram	EMG	Operative Findings
9. J., M. 33 yrs. old female	LBP × 6 yrs. (R)LE pain × 1 mo. *P.E.:* Sensation: intact Decrease in strength (R) EHL DTR: R-AJ decreased	Abn: L_4 RC L_5 R	Abn: L_4 LR L_5 R	Normal	L_5 disc protrusion on (R) L_4 disc protrusion on (R) L_5 stenotic foramen on (R)
10. M., W. 48 yrs. old male	LBP and (L)LE pain × 3 yrs. *P.E.:* Sensation intact Decrease in strength (L) EHL DTR: normal	Abn: L_4 C	Abn: L_4 RCL L_5 RCL	Normal	L_4 disc protrusion on (L) L_5 disc no pathology
11. M., E. 44 yrs. old female	LBP and (L)LE pain × 1 mo. *P.E.:* Hyperesthesia (L)lat calf. Decrease in strength (L)TA, EHL	Abn: L_4 CL	Abn: L_4 RCL	Slight neuropathy. EMG abn. in the (L) L_5 root distribution	L_4 protrusion on (L) compressing L_5 root

	DTR: unsustained clonus				
12. M., D. 41 yrs. old male	LBP and (R)LE pain × 5 mo. *P.E.:* Sensation normal Decrease in strength (R)EHL DTR: absent (R)AJ	Abn: L_4 RC L_5 R	Abn: L_4 R L_5 R	L_5 root denervation (R)	$L_{4\text{-}5}$ protrusion on (R) L_5 protrusion on (R) adherent to S_1 nerve root
13. M., L. 38 yrs. old male	LBP and (L)LE pain × 1½ mo. *P.E.:* Sensation normal Strength normal DTR: absent (L)AJ	Abn: L_4 CL L_5 CL	Abn: L_4 C L_5 L	S_1 root denervation (L)	L_4 protrusion on (L) L_5 extrusion on (L)
14. C., D. 45 yrs. old male	LBP × 2 yrs. (R)LE pain × 1 mo. *P.E.:* Sensation normal Decrease in strength (R)EHL, TA, EDL DTR: absent (R)AJ	Abn: L_4 RC	L_3 C Abn: L_4 RCL	L_5, S_1 denervation on (R)	L_3 protrusion on (R) L_4 extrusion on (R) L_4 extrusion on (L)

Appendix (con't) p. 4

Name Age Sex	Clinical	Lumbar Venogram	Lumbar Myelogram	EMG	Operative Findings
15. B., R. 48 yrs. old male	LBP × 8 yrs. (L)LE pain × 5 mo. *P.E.:* Sensation normal Decrease in strength (L)EHL DTR: absent (L)AJ	Abn: L_4 LC L_5 CL	Abn: L_4 RCL L_5 RCL	L_5 denervation on (L) S_1 denervation on (L)	L_4 protrusion on (L) L_5 protrusion on (L)
16. H., S. 52 yrs. old female	LBP and (L)LE pain × 1 mo. *P.E.:* sensation (L) lat. calf. decreased Decrease in strength (L)TA and (L) EHL. DTR: Decrease in (L)EHL	Abn: L_3 CL L_4 RCL L_5 RCL	Abn: L_3 LCR L_4 RCL L_5 C	Normal	$L_{3\text{-}4}$ disc protrusion on (L) $L_{4\text{-}5}$ disc extruded on (L) No visualization of disc on (R)'
17. K., L. 51 yrs. old male	LBP × 7 mo. (L)LE pain × 2 mo. *P.E.:* Sensation normal Strength normal DTR: absent (L)AJ	Abn: L_4 LCR L_5 RCL	Abn: L_4 RCL L_5 RCL	Denervation in the L_5 and S_1 root distribution, mainly S_1	L_4 disc extrusion bilat. L_5 disc extrusion bilat.

18. M., C. 41 yrs. old male	LBP and (L) hip pain × 1 mo. *P.E.:* Sensation normal Decrease in strength (L)EHL and (L) EDL DTR: normal	Abn: L_4 CL	Abn: L_4 C	Normal	L_4 disc extrusion on (L)
19. S., W. 40 yrs. old male	LBP and (L)LE pain × 6 mo. *P.E.:* Sensation normal Decrease in strength (L)EHL DTR: absent (L)AJ	Abn: L_4 C L_5 LR	Abn: L_4 C L_5 RCL	Re-innervation of S_1 distribution on (L) No sign of denervation	L_4 disc extrusion on (L) L_5 disc no pathology
20. W., M.B. 44 yrs. old male	LBP and (L)LE pain × 1 mo. *P.E.:* Decrease in sensation over S_1 Decrease in strength (L)EHL, (L)peronei DTR: absent (L)AJ	Abn: L_4 CL L_5 C	Abn: L_3 RCL L_4 RCL	Suggestive of L_5 radiculopathy on (L)	L_4 disc extrusion on (L)

Appendix (con't) p. 5

Name Age Sex	Clinical	Lumbar Venogram	Lumbar Myelogram	EMG	Operative Findings
21. C., W. 48 yrs. old male	LBP and (L)LE pain × 2 mo. *P.E.:* sensation: decrease in lateral calf strength: decrease in (L) EHL DTR: decrease in (L) KJ	Abn: L_3 CL L_4 CL L_5 CL	Abn: L_3 C L_4 RCL L_5 RCL	Denervation and reinnervation L_4, L_5, S_1 roots on (L)	Lumbar stenosis L_3, L_4 disc levels L_4 disc protrusion on (L)
22. A., M. 40 yrs. old female	LBP × 2 yrs., (L)LE pain × 1 mo. *P.E.:* sensation: normal strength: normal DTR: decrease in (L) AJ	Abn: L_4 C L_5 C	Abn: L_4 RCL L_5 C	Normal	L_4 disc central protrusion
23. R., D. 42 yrs. old male	LBP × 10 yrs and bilateral leg pain × 3 mo *P.E.:* sensation: normal strength: decrease in (L) and (R) TA DTR: normal	Abn: L_4 R L_5 R	Abn: L_4 R	Denervation and reinnervation L_5 roots on (L) and (R)	L_4 disc extruded (L) and (R)

24. B., G. 53 yrs. old male	LBP and (L)LE pain × 1 mo. *P.E.:* sensation: decrease in lateral calf (L) strength: decrease in (L) EHL and EDL DTR: normal	Abn: L_4 RL L_5 L	Abn: L_4 L L_5 L	Denervation L_5 root on (L)	L_4 disc extruded on (L) into L_5 root foramen
25. H., D. 28 yrs. old male	LBP and (L)LE pain × 1 yr *P.E.:* sensation: normal strength: decrease in (L) EHL and (L)TA DTR: normal	Abn: L_4 R L_5 L	Abn: L_4 R	History of polio with residual electrical findings	L_5 disc extruded on (L)
26. F., B. 47 yrs. old female	LBP and (L)LE pain × 1 mo. *P.E.:* sensation: normal strength: normal DTR: Decrease in (L) AJ	Abn: L_4 L L_5 L	Abn: L_4 RCL L_5 C	Denervation of L_5 and S_1 root on (L)	L_4 disc protrusion on (L)
27. K., J. 63 yrs. old male	LBP × 10 yrs and (R)LE × 2 mo. *P.E.:* sensation: normal strength: normal DTR: normal	Abn: L_4 CR L_5 RCL	Abn: L_4 RCL L_5 RCL	Normal	Lumbar stenosis L_4 disc level L_5 disc bulging centrally

Appendix (con't) p. 6

Name Age Sex	Clinical	Lumbar Venogram	Lumbar Myelogram	EMG	Operative Findings
28. R., R. 52 yrs. old male	LBP × 10 yrs. (L) hip pain × 2 mo. *P.E.:* Sensation normal Decrease in strength (L)TA, EHL DTR: Decrease in (L)AJ	Abn: L_4 LR	Abn: L_4 LR	None	L_4 disc extrusion on (R) and (L) L_5 root compression on (R) and (L)
29. E., F. 47 yrs. old female	LBP and (R)LE pain × 3 mo. *P.E.:* Sensation: normal Strength: decrease in (R)EHL DTR: absent (R)AJ	Abn: L_4 C L_5 C	Abn: L_4 L L_5 CR	None	L_4 disc protrusion on (R) Osteophyte of (R) L_3 and L_4 root foramena Calcified anulus of $L_{3\text{-}4}$
30. L., T. 57 yrs. old female	LBP and (R)LE pain × 6 mo. *P.E.:* Sensation normal Strength normal. DTR: absent (R)AJ	L_4 C Abn: L_5 R	L_5 R Abn: L_4 L	None	L_5 disc protrusion on (R) with compression of nerve

31. W., R. 68 yrs. old male	LBP and (R)LE pain × 2 mo. *P.E.:* Sensation normal Decrease in strength (R)EHL DTR: 1+(R)AJ	Abn: L_3 RL L_4 RL	Abn: L_3 RCL L_4 C L_5 R	None	L_3 disc protrusion on (R) L_4 disc protrusion on (R)

* LEGEND
LBP = low back pain
(L)LE = left lower extremity
(R)LE = right lower extremity
P.E. = physical examination
DTR = deep tendon reflex
EHL = extensor hallucis longus
EDL = extensor digitorum longus
TA = tibialis anterior

Index

a b c d e f g 0 h 1 i 8 2 j

THE SQUIBB INSTITUTE FOR MEDICAL RESEARCH
LIBRARY
APR 11 1980
PRINCETON, N. J.